GASTROINTESTINAL CANCERS

Endoscopic Imaging and Treatment

System requirements:

Operating System – Windows XP or above
Web Browser – Internet Explorer 8 or above, Google Chrome, Mozilla Firefox, and Safari
Essential Plugins – Java & Flash player

- Facing problems in viewing content – it may be your system does not have java enabled
- If Videos don't show up – it may be the system requires Flash player or need to manage flash setting. To learn more about flash setting click on the link in the troubleshoot section
- You can test java and flash by using the links from the troubleshoot section of the CD/DVD.

Accompanying CD/DVD ROM is playable only in Computer and not in DVD player.

CD/DVD has Autorun function – it may take few seconds to load on your computer. If it does not work for you then follow the steps below to access the contents manually:

- Click on my computer
- Select the CD/DVD drive and click open/explore – this will show list of files in the CD/DVD
- Find and double click file – "launch.html".

DVD Contents

DVD-1

1. **Esophageal Squamous Cell Carcinoma: Early Diagnosis**
   Lee Guan Lim, Khek Yu Ho
   - Early esophageal SCC delineated by NBI and Lugol's iodine
   - Esophageal SCC with intrapapillary capillary loop under magnified WLE and magnified NBI observation
2. **Endoscopic Resection and Dissection of Early Squamous Cell Carcinoma of Esophagus**
   Hironori Yamamoto, Naohisa Yahagi
   - Endoscopic submucosal dissection of esophageal SCC
3. **Barrett's Esophagus and Esophageal Adenocarcinoma: Wide Field Imaging Techniques**
   Jayan Mannath, Krish Ragunath
   - Barrett's esophagus: Acetic acid enhanced endoscopy
   - Barrett's esophagus: Indigo carmine endoscopy
   - Barrett's esophagus: NBI magnification endoscopy
   - Barrett's esophagus: Trimodal imaging
4. **Barrett's Esophagus and Esophageal Adenocarcinoma: Endomicroscopy and Spectroscopy**
   Michael B Wallace, Ralf Kiesslich
   - Endoscopic examination of BE using acetic acid chromo-endoscopy with magnification
   - Endoscopic examination of BE with HGD using white light and NBI
   - Endoscopic examination of BE with LGD using white light, NBI, pCLE and endoscopic resection of the area using a multi-band ligation mucosectomy complicated by bleeding, treated by endoclip placement
   - Nodular BE with HGD examined with white light, NBI, and pCLE then resected using multi-band ligation mucosectomy complicated by bleeding, treated by endoclip placement
   - Multiple methods of mucosal imaging of high-grade dysplasia including NBI, AFI, and FICE (a-c)
5. **Endoscopic Eradication Therapies for Barrett's Neoplasia**
   Oliver Pech, Gary W Falk
   - 5fach ER BFK
   - HALO 360
   - Meister Blutungnach ER
6. **Detection of Premalignant and Malignant Gastric Lesions**
   Philip WY Chiu, Joseph JY Sung
   - Endoscopic examination of gastric intestinal metaplasia and early gastric cancer with WLE and NBI
   - NBI magnifying OGD and indigo carmine chromoendoscopy for type 0-IIc + IIb early gastric cancer
7. **Endoscopic Management of Early Gastric Cancer**
   Brigitte Schumacher, Horst Neuhaus
   - ESD of early gastric cancer, located in the antrum by use of IT knife
   - ESD of early gastric cancer (type IIa + IIc) using R-scope
   - ESD of early gastric cancer located in the cardia using Hybrid-knife.

DVD-2

8. **Imaging for Small Bowel Neoplasms: Capsule Endoscopy and Deep Enteroscopy**
   Lauren B Gerson
   - Hemangioma (a, b)
   - Lymphoma
   - GIST
9. **Solid and Cystic Lesions of Pancreas: Role of Endosonography**
   Mohammed A Qadeer, Girish Mishra
   - Side-branch IPMN with FNA
   - Pancreatic mass with liver metastasis with FNA of each
   - Mucinous cystadenocarcinoma with FNA
10. **Endoscopic Therapy for Ampullary and Pancreatic Neoplasms**
    Alessandro Repici, Cesare Hassan, Daniel de Paula Pessoa Ferreira
    - Endoscopic papillectomy for adenomas of the major duodenal papilla
    - Metallic biliary stent
11. **Biliary Tumors: Early Detection and Endotherapy**
    Guido Costamagna, Ivo Boškoski, Paola Cesaro, Pietro Familiari
    - Cholangioscopy (Spyglass) guided biopsies of malignant biliary stricture
    - CLE of normal bile duct epithelium
    - CLE of malignant bile duct epithelium
12. **Endoscopic Imaging of Colorectal Polyps and Cancer**
    Anna M Buchner, Douglas K Rex
    - High resolution endoscopy combined with pCLE in assessment of benign colon polyp
    - High resolution endoscopy combined with pCLE of adenomatous colon polyps
13. **Endoscopic Resection of Advanced Mucosal Neoplasia and Early Cancer in the Colon**
    Michael Bourke
    - Endoscopic resection (piecemeal) of granular LST in transverse colon (a, b)
    - Endoscopic resection (piecemeal) of sessile polyp in transverse colon
    - Endoscopic resection (piecemeal) of granular LST in cecum
    - Endoscopic resection (piecemeal) of granular LST in rectum (a, b)
    - Endoscopic resection (piecemeal) of granular LST in ascending colon
    - Endoscopic resection (piecemeal) of sessile polyp in descending colon.

GASTROINTESTINAL CANCERS
Endoscopic Imaging and Treatment

Editors

Prateek Sharma MD
Professor of Medicine
Director, GI Fellowship Training Program and
Clinical Research
University of Kansas School of Medicine
Kansas City, USA

D Nageshwar Reddy MD DM DSc FAMS FRCP
Chairman and Chief of Gastroenterology and
Therapeutic Endoscopy
Asian Institute of Gastroenterology
Hyderabad, Andhra Pradesh, India

Foreword

Guido NJ Tytgat MD PhD FRCP
Professor Emeritus in Gastroenterology
University of Amsterdam
Academic Medical Center, Amsterdam
The Netherlands

JAYPEE BROTHERS MEDICAL PUBLISHERS (P) LTD

New Delhi • Panama City • London • Dhaka • Kathmandu

Jaypee Brothers Medical Publishers (P) Ltd.

Headquarters
Jaypee Brothers Medical Publishers (P) Ltd.
4838/24, Ansari Road, Daryaganj
New Delhi 110 002, India
Phone: +91-11-43574357
Fax: +91-11-43574314
Email: jaypee@jaypeebrothers.com

Overseas Offices
J.P. Medical Ltd.
83 Victoria Street London
SW1H 0HW (UK)
Phone: +44-2031708910
Fax: +02-03-0086180
Email: info@jpmedpub.com

Jaypee-Highlights Medical Publishers Inc.
City of Knowledge, Bld. 237, Clayton
Panama City, Panama
Phone: +507-317-0160
Fax: +507-301-0499
Email: cservice@jphmedical.com

Jaypee Brothers Medical Publishers (P) Ltd
17/1-B Babar Road, Block-B, Shaymali
Mohammadpur, Dhaka-1207
Bangladesh
Mobile: +08801912003485
Email: jaypeedhaka@gmail.com

Jaypee Brothers Medical Publishers (P) Ltd
Shorakhute, Kathmandu
Nepal
Phone: +00977-9841528578
Email: jaypee.nepal@gmail.com

Website: www.jaypeebrothers.com
Website: www.jaypeedigital.com

Inquiries for bulk sales may be solicited at: jaypee@jaypeebrothers.com

Gastrointestinal Cancers: Endoscopic Imaging and Treatment/Editors Prateek Sharma, D Nageshwar Reddy

First Edition: **2013**

ISBN 978-93-5025-893-4

Printed at Ajanta Offset & Packagings Ltd., New Delhi

To

My parents – my teachers
My brother Sandeep – my best friend
My wife Priyanka – my guide, and
My son Paranjay – my life, for
their constant support and love

—Prateek Sharma

Contents

Contributors

EDITORS

Prateek Sharma MD
Professor of Medicine
Director, GI Fellowship Training Program and Clinical Research
University of Kansas School of Medicine
Kansas City, USA

D Nageshwar Reddy MD DM DSc FAMS FRCP
Chairman and Chief of Gastroenterology and Therapeutic Endoscopy
Asian Institute of Gastroenterology
Hyderabad, Andhra Pradesh
India

CONTRIBUTING AUTHORS

Ivo Boškoski MD
Digestive Endoscopy Unit
Agostino Gemelli University Hospital
Università Cattolica del Sacro Cuore
Largo Gemelli
Rome, Italy

Michael Bourke MBBS FRACP
Director of Gastrointestinal Endoscopy
Westmead Hospital
Sydney, Australia

Anna M Buchner MD PhD
Assistant Professor of Medicine
Division of Gastroenterology
Hospital of the University of Pennsylvania
Philadelphia, USA

Paola Cesaro MD
Digestive Endoscopy Unit
Agostino Gemelli University Hospital
Università Cattolica del Sacro Cuore
Largo Gemelli
Rome, Italy

Philip WY Chiu MBChB(CUHK) MD(CUHK) FRCSEd(Gen) FCSHK FHKAM(Surgery)
Professor of Surgery
Member, Management Committee
Institute of Digestive Disease
The Chinese University of Hong Kong
Hong Kong, China

Guido Costamagna MD FACG
Professor of Medicine and Head
Digestive Endoscopy Unit
Agostino Gemelli University Hospital
Università Cattolica del Sacro Cuore
Largo Gemelli, Rome, Italy

Gary W Falk MD MS
Professor of Medicine, Division of Gastroenterology
Hospital of the University of Pennsylvania
Philadelphia, USA

Pietro Familiari MD
Digestive Endoscopy Unit
Agostino Gemelli University Hospital
Università Cattolica del Sacro Cuore
Largo Gemelli, Rome, Italy

Daniel de Paula Pessoa Ferreira MD
Digestive Endoscopy Unit
IRCCS Istituto Clinico Humanitas
Milano, Italy

Lauren B Gerson MD MSc
Associate Professor of Medicine
Division of Gastroenterology
Stanford University School of Medicine
Stanford, USA

Cesare Hassan MD PhD
Digestive Endoscopy Unit
IRCCS Istituto Clinico Humanitas
Milano, Italy

Khek Yu Ho MD FRACP FAMS FRCP (Glasgow)
Professor and Head
Department of Medicine
Yong Loo Lin School of Medicine
National University of Singapore
Head, Department of Gastroenterology and Hepatology
Chief and Senior Consultant
Department of Medicine
Clinical Director, Endoscopy Centre
Director, NUH Referral Laboratories Pte Ltd
Singapore

Ralf Kiesslich MD PhD
Professor of Medicine
Head of Endoscopic Unit
Med. Clinic, University of Mainz
Germany

Lee Guan Lim MBBS MRCP
Consultant, Director of Clinical Services, and Assistant Professor
Department of Gastroenterology and Hepatology
National University Hospital
Singapore

Jayan Mannath MD MRCP
Nottingham Digestive Diseases Centre and NIHR Biomedical Research Unit
Nottingham University Hospitals NHS Trust
Nottingham, NG7 2UH, UK

Girish Mishra MD MS
Associate Professor of Internal Medicine
Director of Endoscopic Ultrasound Services
Section of Gastroenterology
Wake Forest University Baptist Medical Center
Winston-Salem, USA

Horst Neuhaus MD
Professor of Medicine
Department of Internal Medicine
Evangelisches Krankenhaus Düsseldorf
Kirchfeldstrasse 40
Düsseldorf, Germany

Oliver Pech MD PhD
Department of Gastroenterology
HSK Wiesbaden
Ludwig-Erhard-Str. 100
65199 Wiesbaden, Germany

Mohammed A Qadeer MD MPH
Assistant Professor of Internal Medicine
Section of Gastroenterology
Wake Forest University Baptist Medical Center
Winston-Salem, USA

Krish Ragunath MD DNB MPhil FRCP
Associate Professor and Reader in GI Endoscopy
Nottingham Digestive Diseases Centre and NIHR Biomedical Research Unit
Queens Medical Centre Campus
Nottingham University Hospitals NHS Trust
Nottingham, NG7 2UH, UK

Alessandro Repici MD
Digestive Endoscopy Unit
IRCCS Istituto Clinico Humanitas
Milano, Italy

Douglas K Rex MD FACP FACG
Professor of Medicine
Indiana University School of Medicine
Chancellor's Professor
Indiana University Purdue University Indianapolis
Director of Endoscopy
Indiana University Hospital
Indianapolis, USA

Brigitte Schumacher MD
Department of Internal Medicine
Evangelisches Krankenhaus Düsseldorf
Kirchfeldstrasse 40
Düsseldorf, Germany

Joseph JY Sung MBBS MD PhD FRCP FRCPE FRACP FACG FHKCP FHKAM
Professor of Medicine
Associate Dean (General Affairs)
Chairman, Department of Medicine and Therapeutics
Director, Center for Emerging Infectious Diseases
Faculty of Medicine
The Chinese University of Hong Kong
Prince of Wales Hospital
Shatin, New Territories
Hong Kong, China

Michael B Wallace MD MPH
Professor of Medicine
Mayo Clinic, Jacksonville, FL, USA

Naohisa Yahagi MD PhD
Professor of Medicine
Tumor Center, Keio University, School of Medicine
35 Shinanomachi, Shinjuku-ku
Tokyo, Japan

Hironori Yamamoto MD PhD
Chairman and Chief
Department of Endoscopic Research and International Education
Jichi Medical University
Tochigi, Japan

Foreword

Gastrointestinal, hepatic, and pancreatic cancers are responsible for the largest cancer load worldwide and, consequently, for a high mortality. The prevalence of digestive cancers is expected to increase for many more years, which is mainly related to the rapidly rising population longevity. Currently, the overall quality of digestive cancer cure and care is mediocre to poor. Worldwide improvement and harmonization of the quality of digestive oncology teaching and training seems essential to ameliorate the situation. This can be done through the creation of a superspecialized oncogastroenterologist. Such oncogastroenterologists would be responsible for many diverse tasks, such as initiating and supervising population screening, detection and ablation of early malignancy, accurate staging of advanced cancer (mainly via endosonography), monitoring neoadjuvant and adjuvant chemotherapy, expert performance of all palliative modalities, including nutritional support dealing with complications, supervision of psychosocial support, etc. Furthermore, the oncogastroenterologist should be the central orchestrator of a multidisciplinary digestive cancer team, surrounded by an expert oncogastrointestinal surgeon, radiotherapist, diagnostic and therapeutic radiologist, medical oncologist, dedicated nursing staff, etc. Such a multidisciplinary team would guarantee maximal concentration of expertise, optimized continuity of patient care, improved data collection with respect to disease prevalence and outcome, etc.

Bringing all the diagnostic and therapeutic digestive cancer-related novelties together in a single lavishly illustrated textbook is timely and fulfills a major gap in our current gastrointestinal and endoscopic teaching material. It is particularly in the field of digestive neoplasia, which is on its way to become the most important workload of the gastroenterologist that substantial progress has been and is being made. Expertise in resecting and ablating neoplastic lesions is rapidly spreading over the world. This parallels the rising fraction of digestive malignancies that is being discovered in an early, still curable phase of development. This fraction is expected to further enlarge, as novel technology is being developed (e.g., microRNA) for early detection of patients at risk or with early malignancy through screening and surveillance. Optimal teaching of all novel developments especially in therapeutic endoscopy cannot be realized during the standard gastroenterology training program. An additional year would seem mandatory to 'superspecialize' in all aspects of advanced top-quality diagnostic and therapeutic endoscopy.

The editors, Prateek Sharma and D Nageshwar Reddy, pioneers in modern gastroenterology, are to be congratulated for bringing together worldwide top-class contributors, all highly experienced in their various areas of interest. This collective wisdom, condensed in this superb textbook-atlas represents a landmark in the digestive endoscopy dedicated library. International organizations dedicated to digestive oncology, such as International Digestive Cancer Alliance (IDCA) should endorse this endeavor and propagate this book through its various regional chapters to contribute to their teaching goals and to guarantee global exposure to this state-of-the-art production. One may only hope and wish that the superb content of this book will be met with great enthusiasm by the gastrointestinal fraternity and is helpful in further raising the level of expertise in academic and clinical practice.

Guido NJ Tytgat MD PhD FRCP
Professor Emeritus in Gastroenterology
University of Amsterdam
Academic Medical Center, Amsterdam
The Netherlands

Preface

Gastrointestinal cancers continue to be a major challenge and a health concern not just in western countries but globally. Increasing attention has been focused on the diagnosis and detection of early neoplastic lesions in the GI tract; improving our understanding of the possible etiologies, leading to a rise in cancer incidence and minimally invasive therapies, including endoscopic therapy. With the increasing incidence of esophageal, hepatobiliary, and other GI cancers, it is time to take stock of the information base, and the recent rapid expansion of scientific discoveries has included insights into the epidemiology, pathophysiology, and importantly endoscopic approaches to patients with these lesions.

The uses of endoscopic techniques, such as high-definition endoscopy, chromoendoscopy with or without magnification, as well as endoscopic optical techniques, such as narrow band imaging and confocal microscopy, allow us to obtain "realtime" biopsies of the GI tract. Accurate risk stratification of patients, i.e., identifying those at the highest risk for cancer would reduce the number of patients requiring surveillance and limited healthcare resources could then be focused to this group. Both risk stratification as well as our methods for diagnosing dysplasia and cancer could be enhanced leading to significant improvements in screening and surveillance programs. Finally, endoscopic techniques, including endoscopic mucosal resection and submucosal dissection, play a major role in the treatment of neoplastic lesions of the GI tract.

We have assembled a highly distinguished group of physicians who have presented their state-of-the-art views on the topics of clinical importance in this field, and each of these reviews and chapters included in this book has been written to provide comprehensive discussion on the relevant issues. These articles have attempted to focus on new and evolving concepts with regards to GI cancers. Experts in the field of gastrointestinal oncology discuss the etiology, epidemiology, endoscopic diagnosis, use of endoscopic techniques, and the role of endoscopic interventions for all major GI cancers. All the contributing authors have provided an in-depth review of their topics with extremely useful clinical information. This should provide clinicians a better and informed knowledge about the various approaches for the endoscopic diagnosis and treatment of patients with premalignant and malignant diseases of the GI tract.

We wish to thank all the contributing authors for providing uniformly outstanding and detailed reviews. We hope that this book will provide new insights to our understanding and treatment of patients with GI cancers. Our work was greatly facilitated by the expert assistance of Dr Gokul B, Dr Srinivas G, and Dr Neil Gupta, without whose efforts this book would not have been possible. We are indebted to the critical role played by them. We also wish to express our gratitude to the editorial and production team members of M/s Jaypee Brothers Medical Publishers for their integrated and conscious efforts in bringing out this book.

Prateek Sharma

D Nageshwar Reddy

1 Esophageal Squamous Cell Carcinoma: Early Diagnosis

Lee Guan Lim, Khek Yu Ho

ABSTRACT

Esophageal cancer is an important cause of cancer mortality. Detection of esophageal squamous cell carcinoma (SCC) at the premalignant or early malignant stage is of great clinical importance. Nonendoscopic modalities, such as serum markers and esophageal balloon cytology are currently not good enough for widespread use in the early diagnosis of esophageal SCC. White light endoscopy (WLE) performs suboptimally for the diagnosis of early SCC. Chromoendoscopy using Lugol's iodine as the staining agent has high sensitivity for detecting early esophageal SCC, and the performance characteristics are enhanced by using the pink color sign. Narrow band imaging (NBI) with or without magnification is useful for the detection and diagnosis of early esophageal SCC. The performance characteristics of autofluorescence imaging (AFI) for the diagnosis of early esophageal SCC are generally poor. The role of other endoscopic imaging modalities in the diagnosis of early esophageal SCC needs to be further evaluated.

INTRODUCTION

Esophageal cancer is the 8th most common cancer worldwide, accounting for 4% of all cancers in 2008, and is the 6th most common cause of death from cancer.[1] These figures encompass both adenocarcinoma and squamous cell carcinoma (SCC) types. The highest rates of esophageal SCC are in north and central China, northeastern Iran, and the countries inbetween the two.[2] Although the incidence of esophageal SCC is reported to be declining,[3,4] esophageal SCC is associated with significant mortality.[5] In a 13.5-year follow-up study of 682 endoscoped subjects from Linxian, China, which has one of the highest rates of esophageal SCC in the world, squamous dysplasia and carcinoma *in situ* were the only histological lesions associated with a significantly increased risk of developing esophageal SCC.[6] Patients with esophageal carcinoma *in situ* had a significantly better survival rate than those with invasive esophageal SCC.[7] Surgery for esophageal SCC at earlier stages can improve the prognosis in patients with esophageal SCC.[8,9] Therefore, detection of esophageal SCC at the premalignant or early malignant stage is of great clinical importance.

Esophageal cancer rarely presents symptomatically at an early stage, as the expansible nature of the esophagus allows circumferential involvement or significant penetration into the lumen to occur before symptoms appear. This makes diagnosis of early esophageal SCC difficult. Various techniques for the diagnosis of early esophageal SCC have been described in this chapter.

NONENDOSCOPIC MODALITIES

A population-based screening study, which used ELISA tests to measure the serum concentrations of matrix metalloprotease-9, tissue inhibitor of matrix metalloprotease-1, copper/zinc superoxide dismutase, anti-p53 autoantibodies, and soluble serum interleukin-2 receptor, showed that only serum matrix metalloprotease-9 concentration was significantly different by esophageal squamous dysplasia status, but the maximum sensitivity and specificity were low.[10] Serum autoantibodies against matrix metalloproteinase-7 demonstrated sensitivity and specificity for detection of esophageal SCC of 78 and 81%, respectively.[11] In another study, serum antibody levels to esophageal carcinoma SEREX antigen (ECSA) -1, -2, and -3 were significantly higher in patients with esophageal

SCC than in healthy donors.[12] Although there are some promising serum markers, currently, none is good enough for routine clinical use.

Esophageal balloon cytology has been studied for the diagnosis of esophageal SCC, but the sensitivity for cytological diagnosis of biopsy proven cancers was low at 14–36%.[13] In attempts to improve these screening characteristics, gene methylation in esophageal balloon cytology specimens was studied, but the sensitivity of methylation of each individual gene and of combinations of these genes to detect biopsy proven high-grade squamous dysplasia was poor.[14] The performance characteristics of esophageal balloon cytology are currently not good enough for widespread use in the diagnosis of esophageal SCC.

ENDOSCOPIC MODALITIES

Endoscopy is the main diagnostic modality for esophageal SCC. The ability to diagnose early esophageal SCC is enhanced with techniques, such as chromoendoscopy, virtual chromoendoscopy, and endomicroscopy.

White Light Endoscopy

White light endoscopy (WLE) performs suboptimally for the diagnosis of early SCC. In a study by Dawsey et al., 63 patients in Linxian, China, with balloon cytological evidence of esophageal squamous dysplasia or early cancer had WLE, and biopsy specimens taken every 4 cm, and additional specimens were taken from all visually abnormal areas. Twenty-five of 31, at least moderately dysplastic specimens, including all 9 specimens of invasive cancer, came from visually abnormal sites, such as friability, focal red area, erosion, nodule, or plaque. Importantly, more than a quarter (27%) of the sites containing high-grade dysplasia could not be identified visually by WLE.[15]

Chromoendoscopy

Chromoendoscopy using Lugol's iodine as the staining agent was first described in the 1970s.[16,17] Esophageal epithelial capacity for staining with Lugol's solution appears to be associated with the glycogen content of the squamous epithelium and is based on the color reaction between iodine and glycogen within the tissue with the reaction intensity increasing with greater glycogen content. As a significant amount of glycogen is found in mature squamous cells, iodine reacts with the glycogen in normal squamous mucosa to produce brown stain. Normal esophageal epithelium is stained brown or dark-brown with 5% Lugol's solution, and shows a "silk-crape" like surface appearance when observed close-up. Lesions unstained by Lugol's iodine are likely to be invasive SCCs, carcinomas *in situ*, or severe dysplasia.[18-20]

The role of chromoendoscopy in the diagnosis of esophageal SCC in high-risk populations with atypical cytology has been explored by various investigators. Freitag et al. evaluated 96 asymptomatic subjects in southern Brazil, who were found to have atypia after exfoliative cytology and were at risk for esophageal SCC. Biopsies were obtained in Lugol's stained and unstained areas in the esophageal mucosa. Stained areas in these 96 subjects showed 1 high- and 1 low-grade dysplasia. Unstained areas were present in 64 instances yielding 4 high- and 4 low-grade dysplasias. In this study, Lugol's unstained areas diagnosed dysplasia with a sensitivity of 80% and a specificity of 63%.[21] Dawsey et al. reported that in 225 adults in Linxian with balloon cytology showing dysplasia or carcinoma, WLE yielded a sensitivity of visible lesions identifying high-grade dysplasia or cancer of 62%, and a specificity of 79%. With Lugol's iodine chromoendoscopy, the sensitivity of unstained lesions for identifying high-grade dysplasia or cancer was 96%, and the specificity was 63%. Preneoplastic and neoplastic lesions were larger or more clearly defined with Lugol's iodine chromoendoscopy. A total of 38% of dysplastic lesions were identified only after the staining.[22]

Lugol's iodine chromoendoscopy has also been evaluated in alcoholics and smokers. In a study conducted by Meyer et al., it was found that 12 out of 158 patients who were chronic alcoholics and/or smokers had cancerous lesions detected before iodine staining. Lugol's iodine staining improved the diagnostic accuracy moderately, yielding 17 cancers in 13 patients.[23] Yokoyama et al. studied a cohort of 629 male alcoholics with Lugol's iodine chromoendoscopy, which identified distinctly demarcated iodine unstained lesions in 162 patients, out of which 36 such unstained lesions in 21 patients turned out to be SCCs of the superficial type, yielding an unexpectedly high rate of 3.3%.[24] Fagundes et al. studied 190 males older than 35 years of age attending an outpatient unit for alcoholics who consumed more than 80 g of alcohol, more than 10 cigarettes, and more than 500 mL 'maté' (a hot infusion of herbs) per day over 10 years. There was a high prevalence of dysplastic lesions of 6.9% in these individuals, and occult dysplasia was significantly more frequent in iodine unstained (26%) than stained areas (4%).[25]

Dubuc et al. reported the largest prospective endoscopic screening study for esophageal SCC in high-risk patients. A total of 1,095 patients were included from 62 endoscopy centers. Overall, cancer, high-grade dysplasia, or low-grade dysplasia was found in 6% of the patients. Lugol chromoendoscopy significantly increased the number of detected lesions to 67 from the 35 lesions detected before iodine staining. There was no death related to the endoscopic procedure. The overall morbidity was 0.7%, which included reversible bradycardia in 1 patient, severe cough in 3 patients, significant agitation and esophageal spasm in 2 patients, and suspected diagnosis of iodine allergy in 1 patient.[26]

Despite its high sensitivity for detecting esophageal cancer, iodine chromoendoscopy has a low specificity. More recently, the pink color sign for iodine chromoendoscopy had been described. Shimizu et al. studied 79 patients who were found to have demarcated iodine unstained areas. After a target lesion was found following Lugol's iodine spray, the lesion was observed for about 3 minutes and its discoloration was evaluated. The lesion was regarded as being positive for pink color, if a light pink part appeared in the iodine unstained area. If no light pink part was observed in the lesion within 3 minutes, the lesion was regarded as being negative for pink color. Thirty-four of the 39 lesions diagnosed as pink color positive were histologically proven to be high-grade intraepithelial squamous neoplasia or SCC, whereas only 3 of the 82 lesions diagnosed as pink color negative were histologically confirmed to be high-grade intraepithelial squamous neoplasia ($p < 0.0001$). The sensitivity was 91.9% and specificity was 94% when using the pink color sign as a diagnostic index for high-grade intraepithelial squamous neoplasia and SCC.[27] Ishihara et al. verified the performance characteristics of the pink color sign for the diagnosis of esophageal squamous neoplasms with the quantitative analysis of 45 iodine unstained lesions images. Among these, 19 out of 22 pink color negative lesions were diagnosed as low-grade intraepithelial neoplasias or nonneoplastic lesions, and 22 out of 23 pink color positive lesions were diagnosed as high-grade intraepithelial neoplasias or invasive cancers. The area under the receiver operating characteristic curve was 0.94, indicating excellent validity of the test, with an optimal cut-off, yielding a sensitivity of 88% and specificity of 95%.[28]

Peng et al. described double vital staining with Lugol's iodine and methylene blue (MB) for diagnosing superficial esophageal lesions. Suspicious esophageal lesions identified with conventional endoscope were sprayed with 3% Lugol's iodine and 0.5% MB in order and were inspected after each staining. The sensitivity and specificity of Lugol's lightly stained and unstained areas for identifying esophageal squamous neoplasia were 100 and 35%, respectively. The sensitivity and specificity of double vital staining, hyperstained, and lightly stained areas for identifying esophageal squamous neoplasia were 100 and 98%, respectively.[29]

Narrow Band Imaging

Narrow band imaging (NBI) utilizes the illumination of 400–430 nm and 525–555 nm narrow bandwidth lights instead of red/green/blue broadband light. Penetration depth of the illuminated light corresponds with its wavelength. Short wavelength accentuates contrasted epithelial surface structure because light reflects and scatters at the superficial layer of the mucosa. In addition, blue/green light is well absorbed by hemoglobin, making NBI ideal for examining vascular architecture in the superficial mucosa.[30]

The microscopic intrapapillary capillary loop (IPCL) pattern can be clearly visualized with NBI, because of the effect of capillary enhancement. Yoshida et al. assessed the magnifying NBI esophageal images of 41 patients using numerical analysis, which showed that both the ratio and the contrast value between the IPCL and background mucosa were statistically different. Based on an evaluation of actual images, the accuracy for NBI images was higher than that for regular images for both experienced endoscopists and novices.[31] This was further studied by Ishihara et al. who reviewed magnifying NBI video images of 56 esophageal Lugol's unstained lesions (26 high-grade squamous neoplasias, 15 low-grade neoplasias, and 15 nonneoplasias) for brownish dots (dilated IPCL), tortuous IPCL, elongated IPCL, caliber change in IPCL, variety in IPCL shapes, demarcation line, brownish epithelium, and protrusion or depression. Brownish epithelium and brownish dots were the only factors confirmed to be associated significantly with diagnosis of mucosal high-grade neoplasia on multivariate analysis. Intraobserver agreement was substantial for brownish epithelium and brownish dots. The sensitivity was 85% and specificity was 79%, when the diagnosis of mucosal high-grade neoplasia was based on brownish epithelium and brownish dots.[32]

Ishihara et al. assessed the role of experience in the NBI diagnosis of esophageal squamous neoplasia. NBI for esophageal neoplasia followed by iodine chromoendoscopy was performed in patients with a history of esophageal neoplasia or head and neck cancer. Biopsy specimens were obtained from iodine unstained lesions and the histological results of squamous high-grade neoplasias served as the reference standard. Endoscopic examination was performed by experienced endoscopists in 170 patients and by less experienced endoscopists in 180 patients. A total of 42 new mucosal high-grade neoplastic lesions (25 in the experienced endoscopist group and 17 in the less experienced endoscopist group) were detected. The sensitivity was significantly higher in the experienced endoscopist group (100%; 25/25) compared with the less experienced endoscopist group (53%; 9/17) ($p < 0.001$) as per lesion-based analysis. The sensitivity of NBI in the less experienced endoscopist group improved from 43% in the former half of patients to 60% in the latter half of patients. The sensitivity of NBI was significantly higher in the experienced endoscopist group (100%) than in the less experienced endoscopist group (69%). Therefore, experience appeared to be essential for NBI diagnosis of squamous neoplasia.[33]

NBI has been shown to be superior to WLE for the diagnosis of esophageal squamous neoplasia. Lee et al. enrolled 69 patients with documented head and neck cancers, who underwent WLE followed by NBI and finally magnifying NBI. The sensitivity and accuracy of detection were 62.9 and 64.4% for WLE, 100 and 86.7% for NBI alone, and 100 and 95.6% for magnifying NBI, respectively. The sensitivity and accuracy of NBI alone was significantly superior to that of WLE, but the gain in accuracy was not statistically significant, when magnifying NBI was compared with nonmagnifying NBI.[34] In a multicenter prospective randomized controlled trial, Muto et al. randomly assigned 320 patients with esophageal SCC to WLE followed by magnifying NBI (162 patients) or magnifying NBI followed by WLE (158 patients) in a back-to-back fashion. Magnifying NBI detected significantly more superficial cancer than did WLE in both the head and neck region and the esophagus (100 vs. 8%, $p < 0.001$; 97 vs. 55%, $p < 0.001$, respectively). The sensitivity of magnifying NBI for diagnosis of superficial cancer was 100 and 97% in the head and neck region and the esophagus, respectively. The accuracy of magnifying NBI for diagnosis of superficial cancer was 87 and 89% in these regions, respectively. The sensitivity and accuracy were significantly higher using magnifying NBI than WLE in both regions ($p < 0.001$ and $p = 0.02$ for the head and neck region; $p < 0.001$ for both sensitivity and accuracy for the esophagus, respectively). Although magnifying NBI required a statistically significantly longer examination time than WLE, the investigators were of the opinion that the actual time difference between NBI and WLE of 20–42 seconds was clinically acceptable.[35]

NBI appears to perform better than iodine chromoendoscopy for diagnosing early esophageal squamous cell neoplasia. Takenaka et al. studied 142 patients with head and neck SCC who were examined by magnifying NBI endoscopy followed by iodine chromoendoscopy. Magnifying NBI had significantly better specificity (95 vs. 85%; $p < 0.001$) and accuracy (95 vs. 86%; $p < 0.01$, but similar sensitivity 91 vs. 100%; $p = 1$) compared to iodine chromoendoscopy for the diagnosis of esophageal high-grade intraepithelial neoplasia and SCC.[36] Kuraoka et al. evaluated 49 patients with NBI endoscopy followed by iodine chromoendoscopy. The sensitivity and specificity of NBI positive areas for cancer were 100 and 59%, respectively, and the corresponding values for iodine chromoendoscopy were 100 and 4%, respectively.[37]

A recent consensus stated that NBI is useful for detection of superficial esophageal SCC and that magnifying NBI can distinguish esophageal neoplasia from nonneoplasia.[38] Figure 1-1 shows an esophageal SCC, which was not evident on WLE but became easily detectable on NBI and after staining with Lugol's iodine.

Autofluorescence Imaging

Autofluorescence refers to the emission of a longer wavelength of light from tissue when it is excited by short wavelength light. Differences in the composition of autofluorescent light and the emission spectra resulting from the differences in the proportion of lysosomes and mitochondria between normal, hyperplastic, and adenomatous tissue can be used to clinically differentiate between neoplastic and nonneoplastic tissue.[39]

The performance characteristics of autofluorescence imaging (AFI) for the diagnosis of early esophageal SCC are generally poor. Ishihara et al. studied 364 patients with known history of esophageal neoplasia or head and neck cancer with AFI endoscopy followed by iodine chromoendoscopy, from whom 43 new mucosal high-grade neoplasias were detected. The sensitivities of AFI in the experienced and less experienced endoscopist groups were 71 and 50% (95% CI 32–68%), respectively. The specificity of AFI in the experienced and the less experienced endoscopist groups was 24 and 30%, respectively. The sensitivity of AFI in lesions ≤10 mm was only 31%. The sensitivity and specificity of AFI for the detection of new squamous mucosal high-grade neoplasias, especially the smaller lesions, was too poor for clinical utilization.[40]

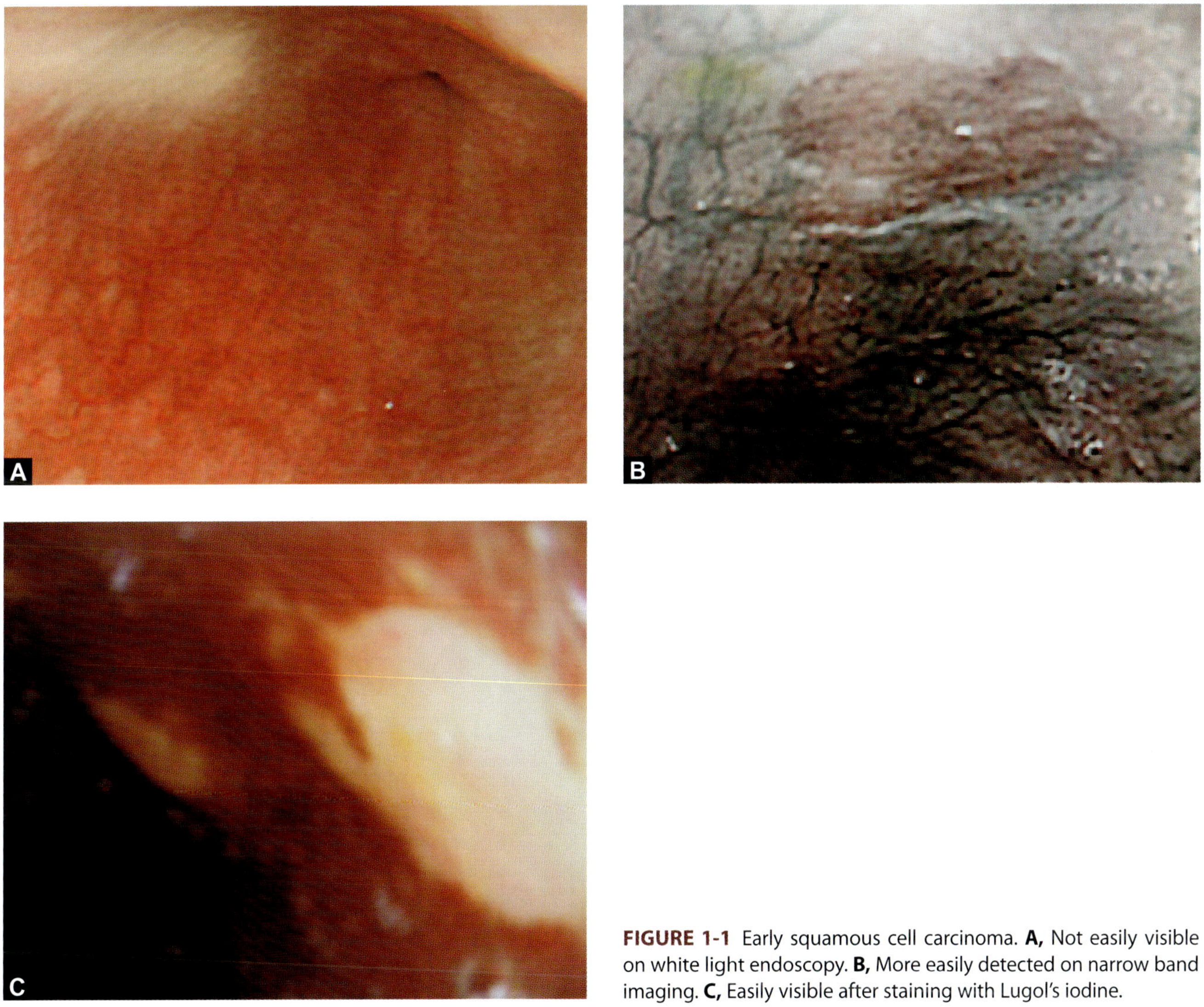

FIGURE 1-1 Early squamous cell carcinoma. **A,** Not easily visible on white light endoscopy. **B,** More easily detected on narrow band imaging. **C,** Easily visible after staining with Lugol's iodine.

A study by Yoshida et al. aimed to assess the ease of detection of esophageal SCC using various modalities of WLE, NBI, AFI, and iodine chromoendoscopy. Twenty sets of endoscopic images of esophageal SCC were prepared, each of which contained still images from WLE, NBI, AFI, and Lugol chromoendoscopy. These images were shown to 25 endoscopists, who then scored the ease of detection of esophageal SCC for each endoscopic modality. According to the scores, the lesions were more easily visualized on NBI and iodine chromoendoscopy compared to AFI and WLE.[41]

Confocal Laser Endomicroscopy

Confocal laser endomicroscopy (CLE) is an innovative technology, which focuses a low-powered laser onto a single point in a defined microscopic field of view, and the laser light reflected from the tissue is refocused onto the detection system by the same lens. The term "confocal" refers to the illumination and detection systems being in the same focal plane. CLE allows the generation of high-resolution microscopic images of living tissue, as far as 200 μm beneath the surface epithelium, enabling *in vivo* evaluation of any pathologic changes therein, realtime during endoscopy.[42] There are currently two CLE systems available in the market: an endoscopy-mounted CLE (eCLE) and a probe-based CLE (pCLE).

Liu et al. performed eCLE for 27 patients with histologically confirmed esophageal SCC and 30 controls. CLE images were evaluated for features, which differentiate esophageal SCC from normal squamous tissue. On CLE, abnormal cells or increased diameter of IPCLs had a high sensitivity of 94.1% for predicting esophageal SCC. The combinations of abnormal cells and increased diameter of IPCLs, abnormal cells, and tortuous IPCLs both had a specificity of 100% in diagnosing esophageal SCC. As CLE can distinguish squamous cell neoplasia from normal epithelium, it can potentially help in early detection of esophageal SCC.[43] Although the diagnosis of late stage malignancy can be easily made on CLE images by even endoscopists with minimal confocal experience, the accurate diagnosis of premalignant or early neoplastic changes on CLE images require sufficient experience in CLE.[44] In addition, CLE is available in only a small proportion of the medical facilities worldwide. Therefore, the widespread use of CLE is unlikely to happen in the near future, and the role of CLE in the diagnosis of esophageal SCC will need to be further studied.

Endocytoscopy

Kumagai et al. described a prototype endocytoscopy system with magnification of up to 1125×, which was used in tandem with MB staining to examine 12 patients with pretreatment esophageal SCC. On examination, cancer cells demonstrated extreme heterogeneity, with the nuclei having different size, shape, and staining.[45] Inoue et al. reported an overall accuracy of endocytoscopy in differentiating between nonmalignant and malignant esophageal pathology of 82%.[46] Fujishiro et al. acquired evaluable pairs of an endocytoscopic image and a histological picture at 12 cancerous and 14 normal areas from 27 esophageal SCC. The mean numbers of the total nuclei per image of 129 at the normal area was significantly lower than that of 550 at the cancerous area.[47] Kumagai et al. performed *ex vivo* examination of 57 iodine-unstained areas in the resected esophageal SCC specimens from 28 patients, followed by an *in vivo* investigation of 71 lesions of esophageal SCC. The sensitivity and specificity of endocytoscopy for malignant lesions was 95 and 84%, respectively.[48]

OTHER MODALITIES

The sensitivity and specificity of esophageal capsule endoscopy in 68 patients with known history of head and neck neoplasia were 61 and 86%, respectively, when iodine chromoendoscopy guided biopsy was used as the reference standard. Therefore, esophageal capsule endoscopy had inadequate sensitivity to be used in first-line screening for SCC among high-risk patients.[49] Fluorescein enhanced AFI has been reported to have good sensitivity and specificity for differentiating between neoplastic and nonneoplastic lesions, and might have a potential role in the diagnosis of esophageal SCC in the future.[50]

CONCLUSION

Lugol chromoendoscopy and NBI with and without magnification have good performance characteristics for the diagnosis of early esophageal SCC. The role of other diagnostic modalities is less clear.

REFERENCES

1. Ferlay J, Shin HR, Bray F, Forman D, Mathers C, Parkin DM. GLOBOCAN 2008 v1.2, Cancer Incidence and Mortality Worldwide: IARC CancerBase No. 10 [Internet]. Lyon, France: International Agency for Research on Cancer; 2010. Available from: http://globocan.iarc.fr. Accessed on 13.8.2010.
2. Lambert R, Hainaut P. Esophageal cancer: cases and causes (part I). *Endoscopy*. 2007;39:550-5.
3. Fernandes ML, Seow A, Chan YH, Ho KY. Opposing trends in incidence of esophageal squamous cell carcinoma and adenocarcinoma in a multi-ethnic Asian country. *Am J Gastroenterol*. 2006;101:1430-6.
4. Cook MB, Chow WH, Devesa SS. Oesophageal cancer incidence in the United States by race, sex, and histologic type, 1977-2005. *Br J Cancer*. 2009;10:855-9.
5. Gertler R, Stein HJ, Langer R, Nettelmann M, Schuster T, Hoefler H, et al. Long-term outcome of 2920 patients with cancers of the esophagus and esophagogastric junction: evaluation of the New Union Internationale Contre le Cancer/American Joint Cancer Committee staging system. *Ann Surg*. 2011;253:689-98.
6. Wang GQ, Abnet CC, Shen Q, Lewin KJ, Sun XD, Roth MJ, et al. Histological precursors of oesophageal squamous cell carcinoma: results from a 13 year prospective follow up study in a high risk population. *Gut*. 2005;54:187-92.
7. Song PI, Liang H, Fan JH, Wei WQ, Wang GQ, Qiao YL. Long-term survival after esophagectomy for early esophageal squamous cell carcinoma in Linxian, China. *J Surg Oncol*. 2011;104:176-80.
8. Zhu ZJ, Hu Y, Zhao YF, Chen XZ, Chen LQ, Chen YT. Early recurrence and death after esophagectomy in patients with esophageal squamous cell carcinoma. *Ann Thorac Surg*. 2011;91:1502-8.
9. Yuequan J, Shifeng C, Bing Z. Prognostic factors and family history for survival of esophageal squamous cell carcinoma patients after surgery. *Ann Thorac Surg*. 2010;90:908-13.
10. Chen W, Abnet CC, Wei WQ, Roth MJ, Lu N, Taylor PR, et al. Serum markers as predictors of esophageal squamous dysplasia and early cancer. *Anticancer Res*. 2004;24:3245-9.
11. Zhou JH, Zhang B, Kernstine KH, Zhong L. Autoantibodies against MMP-7 as a novel diagnostic biomarker

in esophageal squamous cell carcinoma. *World J Gastroenterol.* 2011;17:1373-8.

12. Kagaya A, Shimada H, Shiratori T, Kuboshima M, Nakashima-Fujita K, Yasuraoka M, et al. Identification of a novel SEREX antigen family, ECSA, in esophageal squamous cell carcinoma. *Proteome Sci.* 2011;9:31.
13. Dawsey SM, Shen Q, Nieberg RK, Liu SF, English SA, Cao J, et al. Studies of esophageal balloon cytology in Linxian, China. *Cancer Epidemiol Biomarkers Prev.* 1997;6:121-30.
14. Adams L, Roth MJ, Abnet CC, Dawsey SP, Qiao YL, Wang GQ, et al. Promoter methylation in cytology specimens as an early detection marker for esophageal squamous dysplasia and early esophageal squamous cell carcinoma. *Cancer Prev Res (Phila).* 2008;1:357-61.
15. Dawsey SM, Wang GQ, Weinstein WM, Lewin KL, Liu FS, Wiggett S, et al. Squamous dysplasia and early esophageal cancer in the Linxian region of China: distinctive endoscopic lesions. *Gastroenterology.* 1993;105:1333-40.
16. Toriie S, Kohli Y, Akasaka Y, Kawai K. New trial for endoscopical observation of esophagus by dye scattering method. *Endoscopy.* 1975;7:75-9.
17. Toriie S, Akasaka Y, Yamaguchi K, Nishino H, Kohli Y, Kawai K, et al. New trial for endoscopical observation of esophagus by dye spraying method. *G E N.* 1976;30:159-65.
18. Mori M, Adachi Y, Matsushima T, Matsuda H, Kuwano H, Sugimachi K. Lugol staining pattern and histology of esophageal lesions. *Am J Gastroenterol.* 1993;88:701-5.
19. Sugimachi K, Kitamura K, Baba K, Ikebe M, Kuwano H. Endoscopic diagnosis of early carcinoma of the esophagus using Lugol's solution. *Gastrointest Endosc.* 1992;38:657-61.
20. Misumi A, Harada K, Murakami A, Arima K, Kondo H, Akagi M, et al. Role of Lugol dye endoscopy in the diagnosis of early esophageal cancer. *Endoscopy.* 1990;22:12-6.
21. Freitag CP, Barros SG, Kruel CD, Putten AC, Dietz J, Gruber AC, et al. Esophageal dysplasias are detected by endoscopy with Lugol in patients at risk for squamous cell carcinoma in southern Brazil. *Dis Esophagus.* 1999;12:191-5.
22. Dawsey SM, Fleischer DE, Wang GQ, Zhou B, Kidwell JA, Lu N, et al. Mucosal iodine staining improves endoscopic visualization of squamous dysplasia and squamous cell carcinoma of the esophagus in Linxian, China. *Cancer.* 1998;83:220-31.
23. Meyer V, Burtin P, Bour B, Blanchi A, Cales P, Oberti F, et al. Endoscopic detection of early esophageal cancer in a high-risk population: does Lugol staining improve videoendoscopy? *Gastrointest Endosc.* 1997;45:480-4.
24. Yokoyama A, Ohmori T, Makuuchi H, Maruyama K, Okuyama K, Takahashi H, et al. Successful screening for early esophageal cancer in alcoholics using endoscopy and mucosa iodine staining. *Cancer.* 1995;76:928-34.
25. Fagundes RB, de Barros SG, Pütten AC, Mello ES, Wagner M, Bassi LA, et al. Occult dysplasia is disclosed by Lugol chromoendoscopy in alcoholics at high risk for squamous cell carcinoma of the esophagus. *Endoscopy.* 1999;31:281-5.
26. Dubuc J, Legoux JL, Winnock M, Seyrig JA, Barbier JP, Barrioz T, et al. Endoscopic screening for esophageal squamous-cell carcinoma in high-risk patients: a prospective study conducted in 62 French endoscopy centers. *Endoscopy.* 2006;38:690-5.
27. Shimizu Y, Omori T, Yokoyama A, Yoshida T, Hirota J, Ono Y, et al. Endoscopic diagnosis of early squamous neoplasia of the esophagus with iodine staining: high-grade intra-epithelial neoplasia turns pink within a few minutes. *J Gastroenterol Hepatol.* 2008;23:546-50.
28. Ishihara R, Yamada T, Iishi H, Kato M, Yamamoto S, Yamamoto S, et al. Quantitative analysis of the color change after iodine staining for diagnosing esophageal high-grade intraepithelial neoplasia and invasive cancer. *Gastrointest Endosc.* 2009;69:213-8.
29. Peng G, Long Q, Wu Y, Zhao J, Chen L, Li X. Evaluation of double vital staining with lugol's iodine and methylene blue in diagnosing superficial esophageal lesions. *Scand J Gastroenterol.* 2011;46:406-13.
30. Gono K, Obi T, Yamaguchi M, Ohyama N, Machida H, Sano Y, et al. Appearance of enhanced tissue features in narrow-band endoscopic imaging. *J Biomed Opt.* 2004; 9:568-77.
31. Yoshida T, Inoue H, Usui S, Satodate H, Fukami N, Kudo SE. Narrow-band imaging system with magnifying endoscopy for superficial esophageal lesions. *Gastrointest Endosc.* 2004;59:288-95.
32. Ishihara R, Inoue T, Uedo N, Yamamoto S, Kawada N, Tsujii Y, et al. Significance of each narrow-band imaging finding in diagnosing squamous mucosal high-grade neoplasia of the esophagus. *J Gastroenterol Hepatol.* 2010; 25:1410-5.
33. Ishihara R, Takeuchi Y, Chatani R, Kidu T, Inoue T, Hanaoka N, et al. Prospective evaluation of narrow-band imaging endoscopy for screening of esophageal squamous mucosal high-grade neoplasia in experienced and less experienced endoscopists. *Dis Esophagus.* 2010; 23:480-6.
34. Lee CT, Chang CY, Lee YC, Tai CM, Wang WL, Tseng PH, et al. Narrow-band imaging with magnifying endoscopy for the screening of esophageal cancer in patients with primary head and neck cancers. *Endoscopy.* 2010;42: 613-9.
35. Muto M, Minashi K, Yano T, Saito Y, Oda I, Nonaka S, et al. Early detection of superficial squamous cell carcinoma in the head and neck region and esophagus by narrow band imaging: a multicenter randomized controlled trial. *J Clin Oncol.* 2010;28:1566-72.
36. Takenaka R, Kawahara Y, Okada H, Hori K, Inoue M, Kawano S, et al. Narrow-band imaging provides reliable screening for esophageal malignancy in patients with head and neck cancers. *Am J Gastroenterol.* 2009;104:2942-8.
37. Kuraoka K, Hoshino E, Tsuchida T, Fujisaki J, Takahashi H, Fujita R. Early esophageal cancer can be detected by screening endoscopy assisted with narrow-band imaging (NBI). *Hepatogastroenterology.* 2009;56:63-6.
38. Uedo N, Fujishiro M, Goda K, Hirasawa D, Kawahara Y, Lee JH, et al. Role of narrow band imaging for diagnosis

of early-stage esophagogastric cancer: current consensus of experienced endoscopists in Asia-Pacific region. *Dig Endosc.* 2011;23:58-71.

39. DaCosta RS, Andersson H, Cirocco M, Marcon NE, Wilson BC. Autofluorescence characterisation of isolated whole crypts and primary cultured human epithelial cells from normal, hyperplastic, and adenomatous colonic mucosa. *J Clin Pathol.* 2005;58:766-74.
40. Ishihara R, Inoue T, Hanaoka N, Takeuchi Y, Tsujii Y, Kanzaki H, et al. Autofluorescence imaging endoscopy for screening of esophageal squamous mucosal high-grade neoplasia: a phase II study. *J Gastroenterol Hepatol.* 2012;27:86-90.
41. Yoshida Y, Goda K, Tajiri H, Urashima M, Yoshimura N, Kato T. Assessment of novel endoscopic techniques for visualizing superficial esophageal squamous cell carcinoma: autofluorescence and narrow-band imaging. *Dis Esophagus.* 2009;22:439-46.
42. Kiesslich R, Goetz M, Neurath MF. Confocal laser endomicroscopy for gastrointestinal diseases. *Gastrointest Endosc Clin N Am.* 2008;18:451-66.
43. Liu H, Li YQ, Yu T, Zhao YA, Zhang JP, Zuo XL, et al. Confocal laser endomicroscopy for superficial esophageal squamous cell carcinoma. *Endoscopy.* 2009;41:99-106.
44. Lim LG, Yeoh KG, Salto-Tellez M, Khor CJ, Teh M, Chan YH, et al. Experienced versus inexperienced confocal endoscopists in the diagnosis of gastric adenocarcinoma and intestinal metaplasia on confocal images. *Gastrointest Endosc.* 2011;73:1141-7.
45. Kumagai Y, Monma K, Kawada K. Magnifying chromoendoscopy of the esophagus: in-vivo pathological diagnosis using an endocytoscopy system. *Endoscopy.* 2004;36:590-4.
46. Inoue H, Sasajima K, Kaga M, Sugaya S, Sato Y, Wada Y, et al. Endoscopic in vivo evaluation of tissue atypia in the esophagus using a newly designed integrated endocytoscope: a pilot trial. *Endoscopy.* 2006;38:891-5.
47. Fujishiro M, Takubo K, Sato Y, Kaise M, Niwa Y, Kato M, et al. Potential and present limitation of endocytoscopy in the diagnosis of esophageal squamous-cell carcinoma: a multicenter ex vivo pilot study. *Gastrointest Endosc.* 2007; 66:551-5.
48. Kumagai Y, Kawada K, Yamazaki S, Iida M, Momma K, Odajima H, et al. Endocytoscopic observation for esophageal squamous cell carcinoma: can biopsy histology be omitted? *Dis Esophagus.* 2009;22:505-12.
49. Heresbach D, Leray E, d'Halluin PN, Cholet F, Lapalus MG, Gaudric M, et al. Diagnostic accuracy of esophageal capsule endoscopy versus conventional upper digestive endoscopy for suspected esophageal squamous cell carcinoma. *Endoscopy.* 2010;42:93-7.
50. Lim LG, Bajbouj M, von Delius S, Meining A. Fluorescein-enhanced autofluorescence imaging for accurate differentiation of neoplastic from non-neoplastic colorectal polyps: a feasibility study. *Endoscopy.* 2011;43:419-24.

2 Endoscopic Resection and Dissection of Early Squamous Cell Carcinoma of Esophagus

Hironori Yamamoto, Naohisa Yahagi

ABSTRACT

Squamous cell carcinoma (SCC) is still the most common type of esophageal cancer in the developing world. The development of newer endoscopic modalities has made early diagnosis of esophageal cancer a reality. Endoscopic management for early SCC of esophagus includes endoscopic mucosal resection (EMR) and endoscopic submucosal dissection (ESD). Endoscopic treatment is now a very feasible alternative to surgical resection of early esophageal cancer. These strategies have been shown to be safe and effective with the availability of long-term data. In this chapter, we will discuss the role of endoscopic resection (ER) techniques for esophageal SCC, especially focusing on ESD.

INTRODUCTION

Recent advancements in the technologies in the field of endoscopy have made it possible to make a diagnosis of gastrointestinal (GI) cancers at an early stage. As long as a cancer is detected at a very early stage, local treatment, such as endoscopic resection (ER) and endoscopic dissection can provide a cure for the disease.[1]

In the esophagus, squamous cell carcinoma (SCC) develops in elderly persons with a history of considerable amount of smoking and alcohol consumption. Screening endoscopy for asymptomatic patients who are considered to have high risk of developing esophageal SCC would increase the chance of detection of SCC in the early stages. New imaging technologies, such as narrow band imaging (NBI)[2] and flexible spectral imaging color enhancement (FICE)[3] could increase the detection rate of early SCC by enhancing the color contrast between the lesion and the surrounding normal mucosa.

After the detection of esophageal SCC at an early stage, detailed evaluation of the lesion is necessary in order to select appropriate treatment for the patients. ER is indicated for superficial SCC with an estimated risk of lymph node metastasis lower than the risk of fatal complications of surgery. The risk of lymph node metastasis strongly correlates to the depth of invasion. Magnifying endoscopy with NBI or FICE is useful for detailed diagnosis using the intraepithelial papillary capillary loop (IPCL) pattern.[4] Endoscopic ultrasonography is also useful for the diagnosis of the depth of invasion and Lugol chromoendoscopy is useful to determine the extent of SCC. The detail of endoscopic diagnosis of esophageal SCC is described in Chapter 1: Esophageal Squamous Cell Carcinoma: Early Diagnosis.

Although pretreatment endoscopic diagnosis has become dependable, histopathologic diagnosis of resected specimen is still the most reliable diagnosis to determine the risk of lymph node metastasis. Histopathologic type, depth of invasion, and presence or absence of vessel involvement are important factors to estimate the risk. En bloc resection is essential for accurate histopathologic diagnosis of the lesion. Therefore, endoscopic submucosal dissection (ESD), which provides a reliable en bloc resection of the entire lesion, is considered a superior method to determine the curability of the treatment and the necessity of additional surgical resection.

ENDOSCOPIC RESECTION OF SQUAMOUS CELL CARCINOMA OF THE ESOPHAGUS

Endoscopic mucosal resection (EMR) using lifting of the lesion with submucosal injection and snaring of

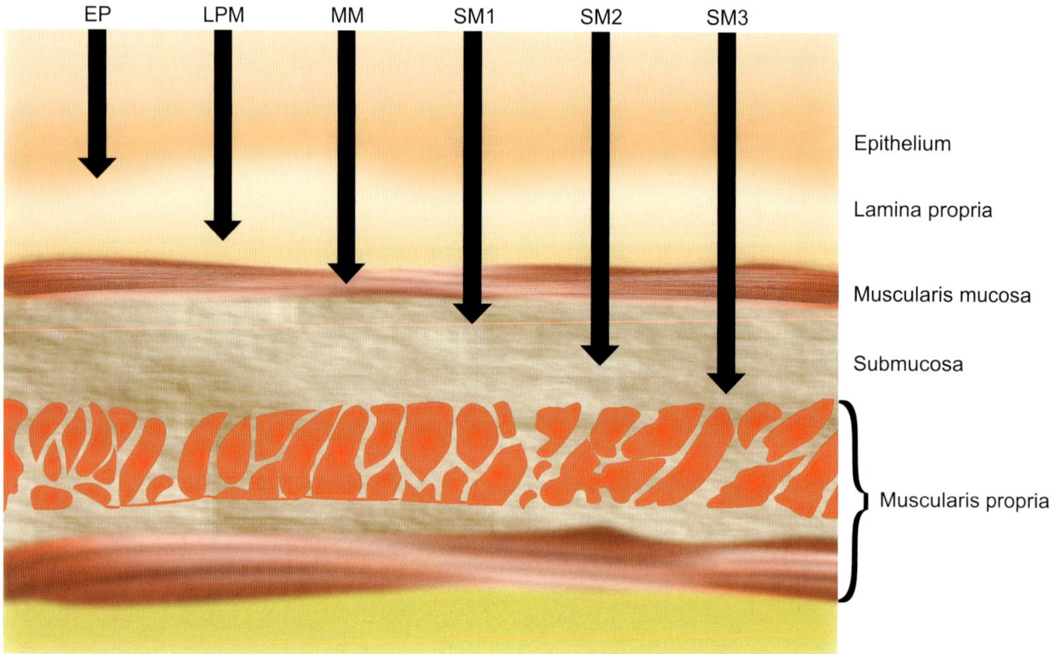

EP, intraepithelial carcinoma; LPM, lesions restricted within the proper mucosal layar; MM, lesions invading or adjacent to but not beyond the muscularis mucosa; SM1, lesions invading the submucosal layer to a depth of 1/3rd; SM2-3, lesions invading the submucosal layer to a depth of more than 1/3rd.

FIGURE 2-1 Squamous cell carcinoma of the esophagus and its depth of invasion.

the lesion has been used for endoscopic resection of SCC in the esophagus. Conventional esophageal EMR procedures include the endoscopic esophageal mucosal resection (EEMR) tube method described by Makuuchi et al.,[5] endoscopic mucosal resection using a cap (EMRC) method described by Inoue et al.,[6] and the EMR with an oblique aspiration mucosectomy device (EAM) method described by Tanabe et al.[7] In all of these procedures, a flat lesion is deformed into a polyp-like shape to be snared using aspiration or a grasper as an extension of a polypectomy. All are simple, but the rate of en bloc resection was as low as 23–57%, because the resected area per resection was limited to 15.1–23.9 mm.[7,8] Therefore, the local recurrence rate was reported to be as high as 7.8–20%.[9,10] In addition, more fractionated resections tended to lead to a higher local recurrence rate. ESD was developed to overcome these shortcomings of EMR. ESD can provide precise and large en bloc resections for superficial esophageal SCC.

Indications

ESD is indicated for cancer with no or minimal risk of lymph node metastasis. When the lesions are classified according to the depth of invasion as intraepithelial carcinoma (EP), restricted within the proper mucosal layer (LPM), adjacent to or invading, but not beyond the muscularis mucosa (MM), and invading the submucosal layer to a depth of 1/3rd (SM1), or more than 1/3rd (SM2 and 3) of the layer thickness (Figure 2-1), then the incidence of lymph node metastasis was reported to be 0%, 0–5.6%, 8–18%, 11–53%, and 30–54%, respectively (Table 2-1).[11,12] Therefore, according to the 2007 Japan Esophageal Society guidelines for the treatment of esophageal cancer, the absolute indication for ER is

TABLE 2-1 Incidence of Lymph Node Metastasis According to the Depth of Invasion of Esophageal SCC

Depth of invation	*Incidence of lymph node metastasis*
EP	0%
LPM	0–5.6%
MM	8–18%
SM1	11–53%
SM2-3	30–54%

EP, intraepithelial carcinoma; LPM, lesions restricted within the proper mucosal layar; MM, lesions invading or adjacent to but not beyond the muscularis mucosa; SM1, lesions invading the submucosal layer to a depth of 1/3rd; SM2-3, lesions invading the submucosal layer to a depth of more than 1/3rd.

TABLE 2-2 Indications for Endoscopic Resection of Esophageal SCC

Absolute indications	*Relative indications*
1. Depth of invasion: EP-LPM	1. Depth of invasion: MM-SM1
2. Extension: 2/3rd or less of the circumference	2. Extension: 3/4th or more mucosal defect after ER

Source: Guidelines for the treatment of esophageal cancer. The Japan Esophageal Society; 2007.

defined as EP-LPM esophageal cancer as well as 2/3rd or less extension of the circumference, while the relative indication is defined as MM-SM1 esophageal cancer with as well as 3/4th or more mucosal defect after ER (Table 2-2).[13]

Techniques

In order to perform ESD in the esophagus successfully, anatomical characteristics of the esophagus should be considered. In the esophagus, endoscopic approach to the lesion becomes tangential in most cases, which are suitable for ESD techniques. However, control of endoscope is limited by the narrow lumen of the esophagus. Therefore, rotation of endoscope shaft should be used rather than the angle of the endoscope tip to control the movement of devices inserted through the accessory channel. Submucosal tissue of the esophageal wall is soft and easy to dissect, as long as fibrosis is absent. However, control of bleeding is sometimes difficult because of abundant blood vessels. Moreover, esophageal wall can be easily perforated, as it is thin and lacks serosa outside the muscle layer. Esophageal perforation could lead to catastrophic complications, such as pneumomediastinum, pneumothorax, and cardiac tamponade, which can cause respiratory and cardiac arrest.

Considering the above mentioned characteristics of the esophagus, ESD techniques, which allow direct visualization of the tissue at dissection, should be selected. Transparent hood attached to the tip of the endoscope is useful for visualization of the tissue and stabilization of the control of dissecting devices.

Endoscopic Submucosal Dissection Procedure

Marking

Coagulation dots placed with the tip of ESD knives are used for marking and indicating the incision line around the lesion. Lateral margins of SCC lesions should be determined by NBI or FICE with magnification recognizing the IPCL pattern in the lesion (Figure 2-2). Lugol staining is also useful to determine the margins of the lesion, as the SCC lesion can be easily recognized as an unstained area (Figure 2-3). Marking dots should be placed at about 3–5 mm outside the margins using a soft coagulation mode. It is important to place the marking dots accurately before starting the ESD procedure, as the margins of the lesion could become difficult to determine after starting the injection, incision, and dissection.

Injection

In order to obtain safety margin from the muscle layer for mucosal incision and submucosal dissection, mucosal elevation should be created by injecting a solution into the submucosal layer. The injection solutions currently used for ESD include normal saline, glycerol solution, and sodium hyaluronate solution. An injection solution that has a long duration of action is preferable, as it makes ESD safe and easy to perform. Glycerol solution has a somewhat longer duration of action than normal saline, however, sodium hyaluronate solution is most suitable for esophageal ESD because it has the longest duration in maintaining the thickening of the submucosal layer.[14,15]

A small amount of adrenaline (epinephrine; 0.01 mg/mL) can be added to the injection solution to prevent bleeding during dissection. A small amount of indigo carmine (0.02–0.04 mg/mL) can also be used to generate slight submucosal staining, which is useful to distinguish between the submucosal layer and the muscularis propria.

Knives

Several kinds of ESD knives have been developed. While selecting an ESD knife, the operator should understand its specific use and features. In the esophagus, the operator should select a knife, which is suitable for direct visualization of the tissue at dissection, as described above.

Such knives include the Needle knife, Flush knife, Dual knife, Flex knife, and Hook knife. All these knives are a type of electrocautery knife, which are used for incision and coagulation with the application of current. It is therefore important to place the knife on the tissue to be incised and to point the knife in a safe direction (i.e., away from or parallel to the muscle layer), before the current is applied.

Recently released new ESD knife, Safe knife has a unique feature to make the ESD procedure easy and

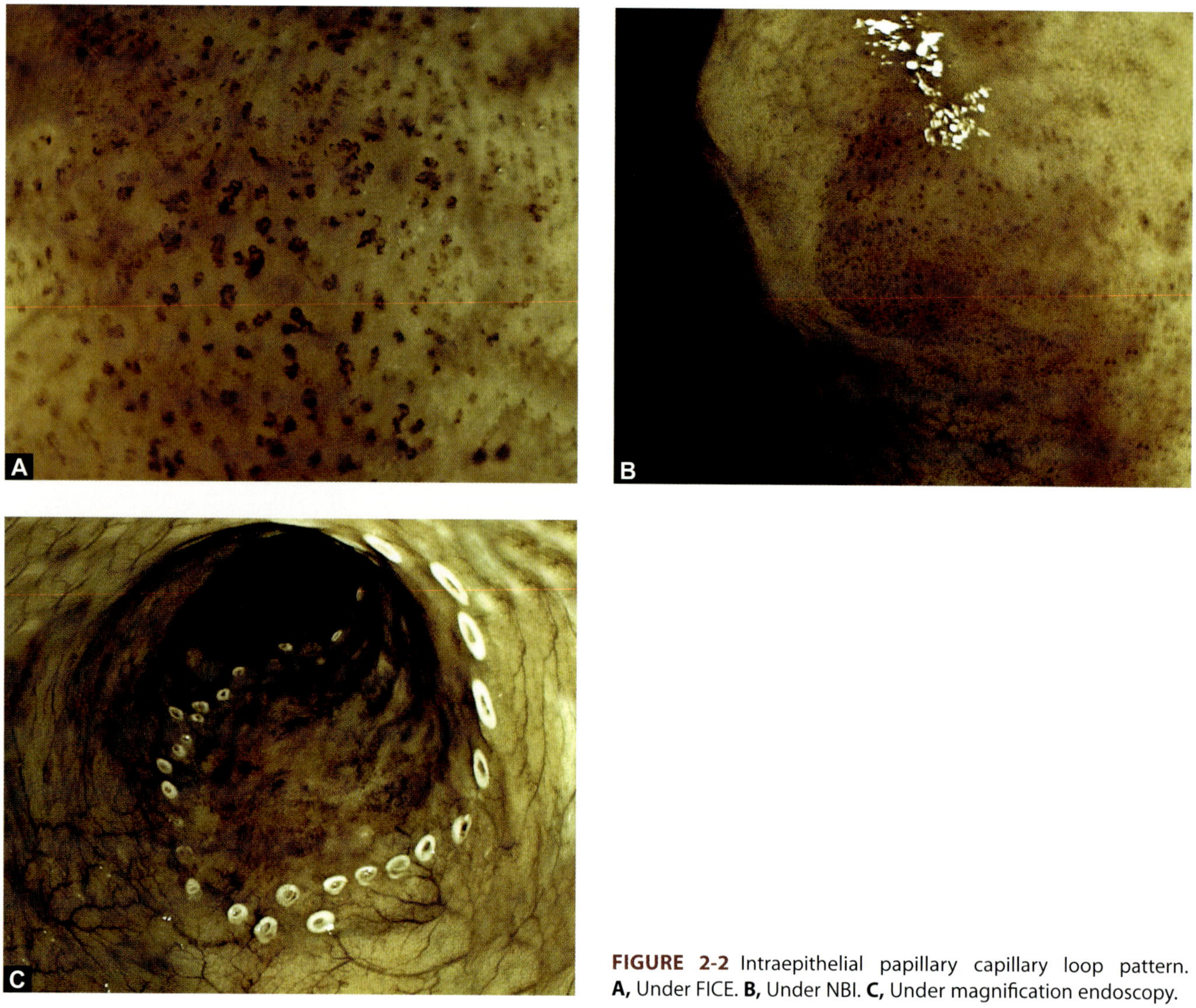

FIGURE 2-2 Intraepithelial papillary capillary loop pattern. **A,** Under FICE. **B,** Under NBI. **C,** Under magnification endoscopy.

safe. There are two kinds of Safe knives (Figure 2-4). One is for the vertical approach (Safe knife V) and the other is for the horizontal approach (Safe knife H). In esophageal ESD, Safe knife H (horizontal type) is suitable for submucosal dissection because the approaching angle becomes horizontal in most of the cases. Electrodes of Safe knife H are arranged at the depressions between protrusions of the insulated tip at both the front and rear edges (Figure 2-5). When the tip of the knife is inserted into the submucosal layer by horizontal approach, soft submucosal tissue can be inserted into the depressions to touch the electrodes. However, muscle layer does not easily touch the electrodes, because it is not as elastic as submucosal tissue. Therefore, submucosal tissue can be selectively cut by applying electric current to the knife. This knife, therefore, makes the esophageal ESD an easy and safe procedure.

Hood

A transparent hood is attached to the distal end of the endoscope, which helps ensure safe and well-controlled use of an ESD knife. The operator can open the incised wound with the tip of the hood enabling direct visualization of the submucosal tissue. The tip of the hood also helps control the knife by gently pressing on and stabilizing the target tissue, which could move with cardiac beats and respiration.

In the esophageal ESD, the small-caliber-tip transparent (ST) hood is particularly useful, because it

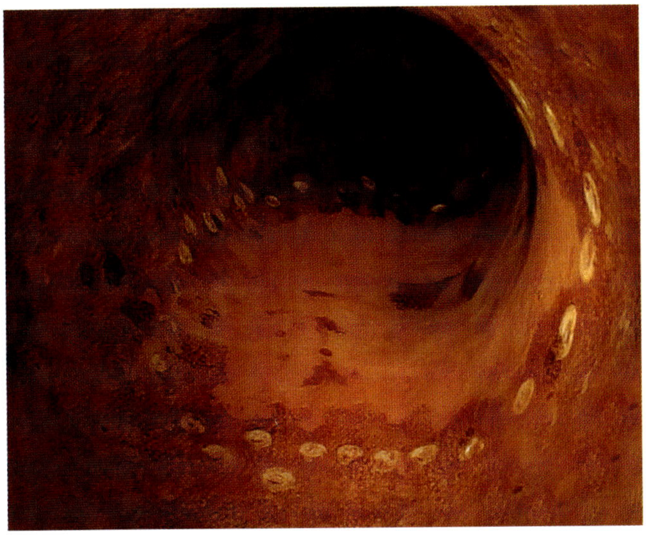

FIGURE 2-3 SCC lesion can be easily recognized as an unstained area with Lugol staining.

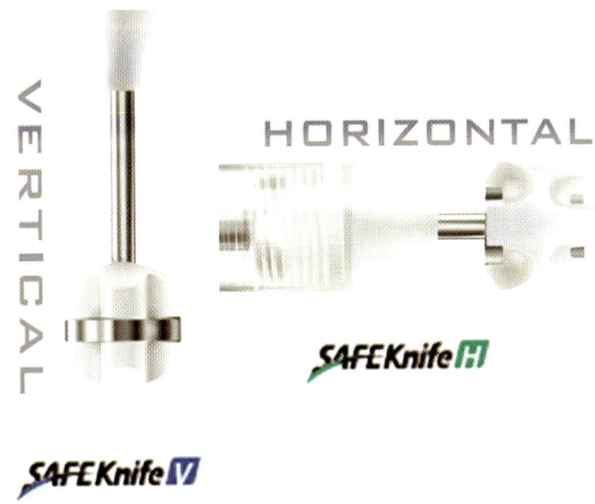

FIGURE 2-4 ESD Safe knives.

has a tapered aperture that allows the operator to open up the incision with ease and also to accurately adjust the depth of incision, which is made with the tip of the knife (Figure 2-6).[16] Recently, a new type, short ST hood has been introduced (Figure 2-7). This short ST hood has a bit wider opening (8 mm) than the traditional type (7 mm). Because of the wider opening and the shorter length, endoscopic view has been dramatically improved compared with the previous type. The shorter ST hood is suitable for most of the cases in the esophagus; however, the traditional type is particularly useful in cases with fibrosis in the submucosal tissue.

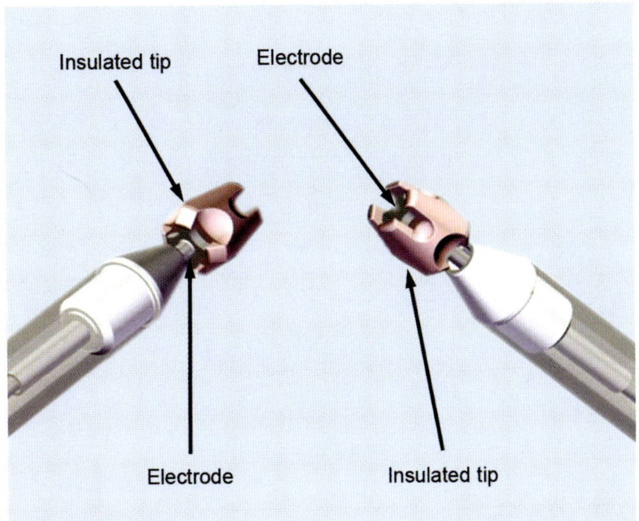

FIGURE 2-5 Electrodes of Safe knife H are arranged at the depressions between protrusions of the insulated tip at both the front and rear edges.

Strategy and Tips

As long as enough space and clear view for safe dissection are maintained, ESD is not that difficult. Enough space for safe dissection can be obtained by the thickness of the submucosal layer created by injection of a solution. For a long-lasting thickening of the submucosal layer, sodium hyaluronate is a suitable injection solution. In addition to the use of sodium hyaluronate, the strategy for mucosal incision and submucosal dissection is important to maintain the submucosal thickening. A circumferential mucosal incision all around the lesion at the beginning should be avoided unless the lesion is small enough. Instead of making a circumferential incision of the mucosa, a partial mucosal incision should be made. Submucosal dissection of that part of the mucosa should follow immediately after the partial mucosal incision. Mucosal incision and submucosal dissection should be repeated thereafter step by step. The length of the mucosal incision should be limited to the size of the area in which submucosal dissection can be performed within a short enough time frame to maintain sufficient submucosal thickening. If the mucosal incision is made for a large area, submucosal thickening might be lost before finishing the submucosal dissection of that area. Once submucosal thickening is lost, re-injection into the submucosal layer can be very difficult, and if a circumferential mucosal incision is already made all around the lesion, then the injected fluid can easily flow out from the mucosal incision.

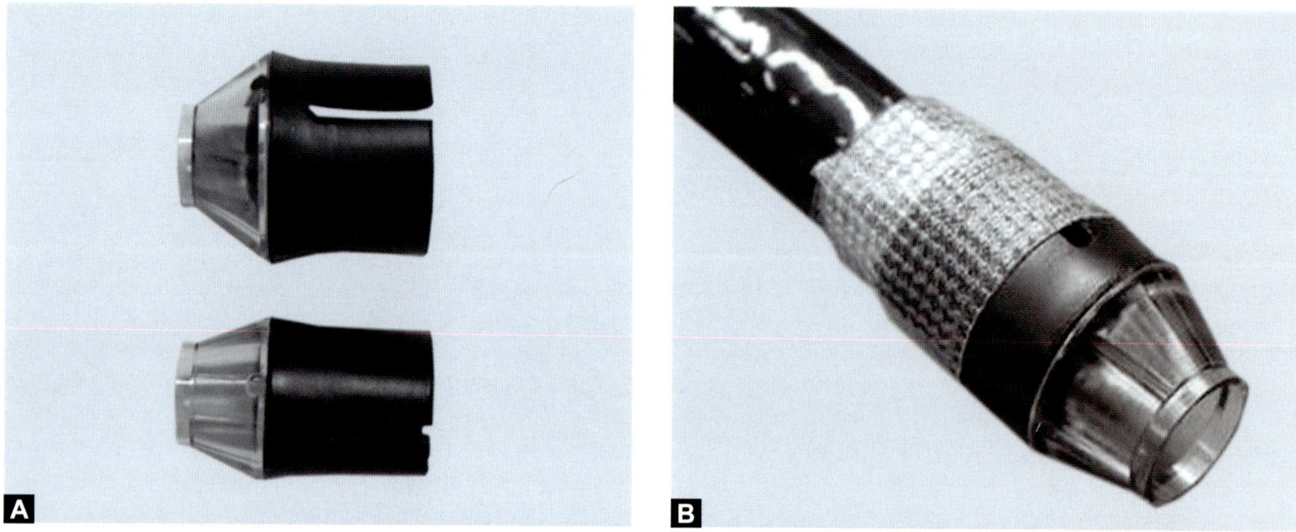

FIGURE 2-6 During esophageal ESD, the ST hood (DH-16GR, Fujifilm Corp., Tokyo, Japan) is particularly useful.

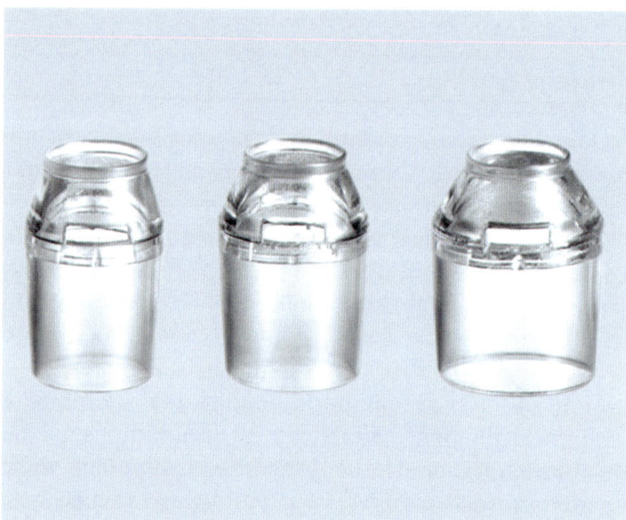

FIGURE 2-7 Short ST hood.

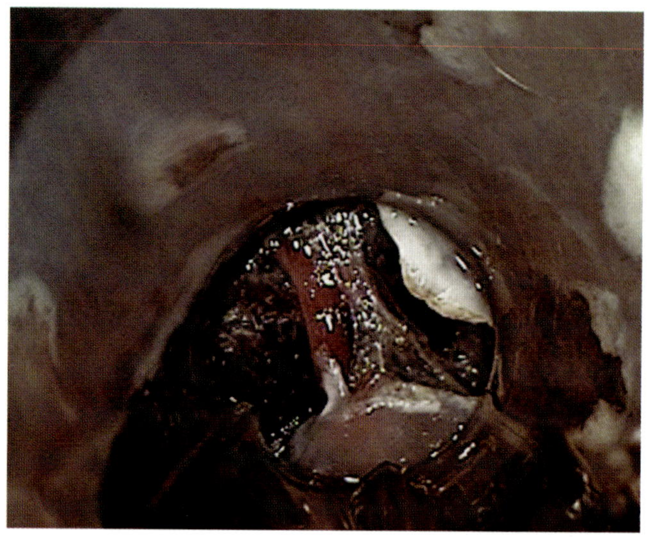

FIGURE 2-8 Dissection of the submucosa on both sides being performed to complete the resection.

In the esophagus, tunneling method is also a good strategy to maintain submucosal thickening and to provide stable control of the knife. With this method, after mucosal incision and submucosal dissection at the distal edge of the esophageal tumor, the mucosal incision and submucosal dissection are then performed from the proximal edge of the tumor. Submucosal dissection is continued to make a tunnel in the submucosal layer by inserting the tip of the endoscope with a transparent hood under the mucosal tumor. The tunneling dissection is continued to reach the mucosal incision at the distal edge. After penetration of the tunnel from the proximal edge to the distal edge of the tumor, the tunnel is widened on both sides laterally. Finally, the mucosa on both sides of the tumor is incised laterally, and then dissection of the submucosa on both sides is also performed to complete the resection (Figure 2-8). By making a submucosal tunnel, the endoscope tip is stabilized allowing precise control of the knife for dissection. It also opens the dissected wound with the hood at the endoscope tip providing a good safety margin for further dissection by stretching the submucosal tissue.[17] In the esophagus, tunneling method is easy to apply because the approaching angle to the lesion is always tangential

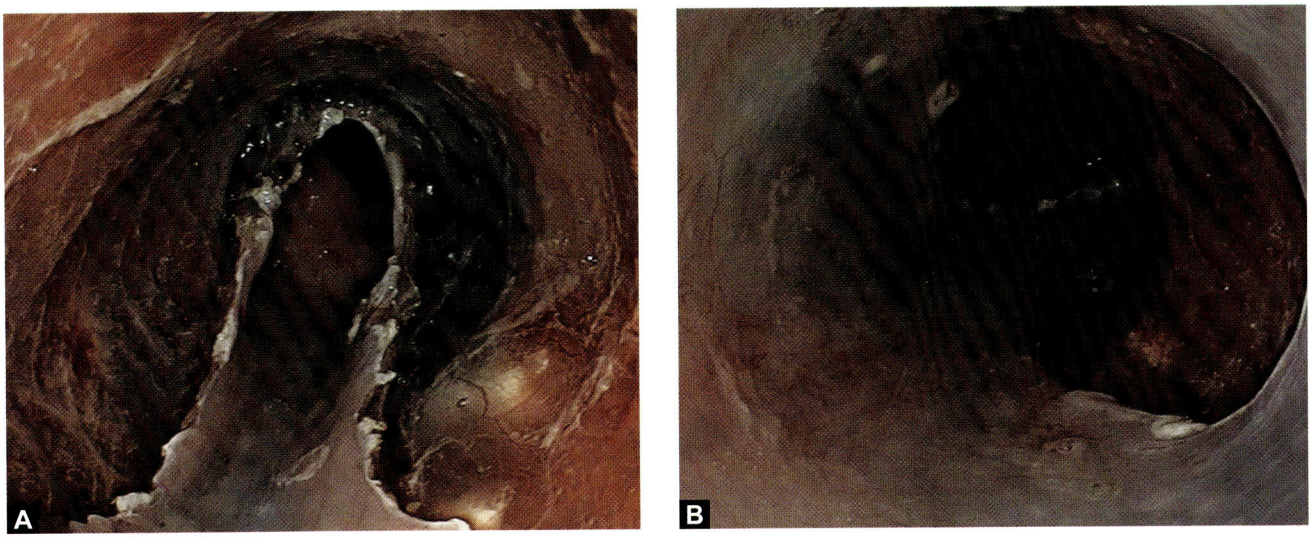

FIGURE 2-9 Blood vessels left behind during ESD.

due to its narrow lumen. The ST hood is suitable for the tunneling method.

Another important factor for a successful ESD is control of bleeding during the procedure. If bleeding cannot be managed properly, clear view of the operation field cannot be maintained either. Dissection of a tissue in a blind fashion could cause further bleeding and even perforation. Therefore, identification and coagulation of blood vessels are important to maintain a clear view. When blood vessels are found during the submucosal dissection, it is better to dissect submucosal tissue leaving the vessels to expose them (Figure 2-9). The same ESD knives can be used for coagulation of the vessels by selecting coagulation current, if the vessels are small. For large vessels, coagulation forceps with a soft coagulation mode should be used to prevent bleeding.

Outcomes

Short-term Outcome

Ono et al. reported the outcomes of their ESD for superficial esophageal squamous cell neoplasms.[18] The rates of en bloc resection and complete resection reported were 100 and 88%, respectively, for 107 lesions with the mean size of 22.9 (1–66) mm in 84 patients. Perforation accompanied by mediastinal emphysema was observed in 4 (4%) patients and no patient experienced massive bleeding in their series.

As per the authors' experience, the rates of en bloc resection and complete resection were 99 and 87%, respectively, for 90 lesions with the mean size of 39.7 ± 14.5 mm in 75 patients. Perforation accompanied by mediastinal emphysema was observed in 3 (4%) patients and postoperative bleeding was experienced in 1 (1%) patient. All the complications were successfully managed endoscopically or conservatively without requirement of surgical repair.

Long-term Outcome

During the median observation of 632 days (range 8–2,358), 15 (18%) patients experienced benign esophageal stricture with dysphagia, which was successfully managed by balloon dilation for a median of 2 sessions (range 1–20) in the series by Ono et al.[18] One local recurrence was observed in a patient, 6 months after the ESD. In 2 patients with intramucosal invasive carcinomas in the muscularis mucosa, distant metastases were observed 9 and 18 months after ESD. During the observation period, 3 patients died of esophageal carcinoma. The 5-year cause-specific survival rates of patients with intraepithelial neoplasm or invasive carcinoma limited to the lamina propria mucosa and patients with invasive carcinoma deeper than the lamina propria mucosa were 100 and 85%, respectively.

In an experience by the authors, ESD for 17 lesions (19%) caused benign stricture which was successfully managed by balloon dilation. Stricture ensues when the area of mucosal resection exceeds 3/4th of the luminal circumference. However, the rate of developing postoperative strictures declined after we had employed long-acting steroid injection at the ESD site for such extensive resections. No patient experienced local recurrence after ESD in the series.

CONCLUSION

Early SCC of the esophagus can often be cured by endoscopic treatment. To ensure good outcomes of the treatment, early detection of the disease and application of a complete resection technique are essential. Image enhanced endoscopy, such as NBI and FICE, magnifying endoscopy and chromoendoscopy with Lugol is useful for both early detection and detailed evaluation of the lesion for the selection of endoscopic treatment. ESD has markedly improved the reliability of therapeutic endoscopic procedures. ESD can provide a reliable complete resection of the lesion in en bloc fashion. Although ESD is a minimally invasive, reliable, and excellent endoscopic procedure, it can be risky with an increased rate of complications, if performed by a poorly trained operator. For ESD to be safe and reliable, it requires intensive learning and a thorough knowledge of its indications and techniques. Continuing improvement in devices and techniques as well as establishment of appropriate training will make ESD a standard endoscopic treatment for early SCC of the esophagus.

REFERENCES

1. Yamamoto H. Technology insight: endoscopic submucosal dissection of gastrointestinal neoplasms. *Nat Clin Pract Gastroenterol Hepatol.* 2007;4:511-20.
2. Muto M, Minashi K, Yano T, Saito Y, Oda I, Nonaka S, et al. Early detection of superficial squamous cell carcinoma in the head and neck region and esophagus by narrow band imaging: a multicenter randomized controlled trial. *J Clin Oncol.* 2010;28:1566-72.
3. Osawa H, Yoshizawa M, Yamamoto H, Kita H, Satoh K, Ohnishi H, et al. Optimal band imaging system can facilitate detection of changes in depressed-type early gastric cancer. *Gastrointest Endosc.* 2008;67:226-34.
4. Ishihara R, Inoue T, Uedo N, Yamamoto S, Kawada N, Tsujii Y, et al. Significance of each narrow-band imaging finding in diagnosing squamous mucosal high-grade neoplasia of the esophagus. *J Gastroenterol Hepatol.* 2010;25:1410-5.
5. Makuuchi H, Yoshida T, Ell C. Four-step endoscopic esophageal mucosal resection (EEMR) tube method of resection for early esophageal cancer. *Endoscopy.* 2004;36:1013-8.
6. Inoue H, Kawano T, Tani M, Takishita K, Iwai T. Endoscopic mucosal resection using a cap: techniques for use and preventing perforation. *Can J Gastroenterol.* 1999;13:477-80.
7. Tanabe S, Koizumi W, Mitomi H, Kitamura T, Tahara K, Ichikawa J, et al. Usefulness of EMR with an oblique aspiration mucosectomy device compared with strip biopsy in patients with superficial esophageal cancer. *Gastrointest Endosc.* 2004;59:558-63.
8. May A, Gossner L, Behrens A, Kohnen R, Vieth M, Stolte M, et al. A prospective randomized trial of two different endoscopic resection techniques for early stage cancer of the esophagus. *Gastrointest Endosc.* 2003;58:167-75.
9. Takeo Y, Yoshida T, Shigemitu T, Yanai H, Hayashi N, Okita K. Endoscopic mucosal resection for early esophageal cancer and esophageal dysplasia. *Hepatogastroenterology.* 2001;48:453-7.
10. Nomura T, Boku N, Ohtsu A, Muto M, Matsumoto M, Tajiri H, et al. Recurrence after endoscopic mucosal resection for superficial esophageal cancer. *Endoscopy.* 2000;32:277-80.
11. Eguchi T, Nakanishi Y, Shimoda T, Iwasaki M, Igaki H, Tachimori Y, et al. Histopathological criteria for additional treatment after endoscopic mucosal resection for esophageal cancer: analysis of 464 surgically resected cases. *Mod Pathol.* 2006;19:475-80.
12. Oyama T, Miyata Y, Shimaya S, Tomori A, Hotta K, Yoshida M. Diagnosis and long-term results and prognosis of m3 and sm1 esophageal cancer. Lymph node metastasis of m3, sm1 esophageal cancer. *Stomach Intest.* 2002;37:71-4.
13. Guidelines for the treatment of esophageal cancer. The Japan Esophageal Society; 2007.
14. Yamamoto H, Yube T, Isoda N, Sato Y, Sekine Y, Higashizawa T, et al. A novel method of endoscopic mucosal resection using sodium hyaluronate. *Gastrointest Endosc.* 1999;50:251-6.
15. Yamamoto H, Yahagi N, Oyama T, Gotoda T, Dio T, Hirasaki S, et al. Usefulness and safety of 0.4% sodium hyaluronate solution as a submucosal fluid "cushion" in endoscopic resection for gastric neoplasms: a prospective multicenter trial. *Gastrointest Endosc.* 2008;67:830-9.
16. Yamamoto H, Kawata H, Sunada K, Sasaki A, Nakazawa K, Miyata T, et al. Successful en-bloc resection of large superficial tumors in the stomach and colon using sodium hyaluronate and small-caliber-tip transparent hood. *Endoscopy.* 2003;35:690-4.
17. Yamamoto H. Endoscopic submucosal dissection for colorectal tumors. *Front Gastrointest Res.* 2010;27:287-95.
18. Ono S, Fujishiro M, Niimi K, Goto O, Kodashima S, Yamamichi N, et al. Long-term outcomes of endoscopic submucosal dissection for superficial esophageal squamous cell neoplasms. *Gastrointest Endosc.* 2009;70:860-6.

3 Barrett's Esophagus and Esophageal Adenocarcinoma: Wide Field Imaging Techniques

Jayan Mannath, Krish Ragunath

ABSTRACT

Barrett's esophagus (BE) is a well-known risk factor for esophageal adenocarcinoma. BE and associated dysplasia are routinely diagnosed by random biopsies using standard white light endoscopy (WLE). Newer imaging modalities have been developed over the last decade for effective management in the diagnosis and surveillance of BE. These include wide field imaging and point enhancement imaging techniques. Various examples of wide field imaging techniques include chromoendoscopy, autofluorescence imaging (AFI), and electronic chromoscopy. These imaging modalities have been used to improve the detection and delineation of dysplasia in BE with variable accuracy and efficiency than that of the standard WLE. In this chapter, we will be reviewing the utility of these imaging techniques in patients with BE.

INTRODUCTION

Barrett's esophagus (BE) is characterized by columnar lined mucosa containing specialized intestinal metaplasia (SIM), which develops as a consequence of gastroesophageal reflux disease (GERD). BE is associated with a small but significant risk of developing esophageal adenocarcinoma (EAC). SIM has thought to be an essential precursor for development of EAC; however, columnar epithelium without SIM was also found to be associated with increased cancer risk.[1] The perceived cancer risk in patients with BE is approximately 30–125 times higher than that of an age-matched population.[2] Malignant transformation in BE occurs in a step wise manner progressing through low-grade dysplasia (LGD), high-grade dysplasia (HGD), and finally cancer.[3,4] There is no convincing evidence to suggest that medical or surgical therapy for GERD would prevent development of EAC or dysplasia in BE, even though some observational studies reported benefit with the use of proton pump inhibitors.[5] In the absence of any preventive measures in the development of EAC, regular surveillance to identify early neoplasia is the most pragmatic approach. Various international gastroenterological societies advise on regular surveillance programs in patients with BE with a view to identify occurrence of early neoplasia.[6,7] The role for surveillance is strengthened by the fact that asymptomatic cancers discovered during surveillance are less advanced than those found in patients who present with cancer symptoms[8,9] and early lesions could be treated by endotherapy, avoiding morbidity and mortality associated with esophagectomy. During surveillance, in the absence of any obvious abnormalities in the Barrett's segment, random 4 quadrant biopsies are taken every 1–2 cm. The yield of dysplasia with such a labor intensive endoscopic biopsy protocol is suboptimal.[10,11] Furthermore, HGD and early cancer are often difficult to identify as many lesions will be flat and subtle with no obvious mucosal irregularity or nodules. It is important to examine the Barrett's segment by clearing off all the adherent mucus and mucolytic agents like N-acetylcysteine (NAC) should be considered in all cases to have a thorough mucosal examination.[12]

WIDE FIELD IMAGING TECHNIQUES

The use of special stains (chromoendoscopy) enhances the mucosal details seen at endoscopy with characteristic mucosal appearances, such as pit patterns in various parts of the gastrointestinal (GI) tract. This will help in targeting biopsies from suspicious areas and thus improve the yield of dysplasia during BE surveillance. Even though chromoendoscopy is cheap and effective, it is widely underused in the Western world compared to the Far East. Recent introduction of optical [(Narrow band imaging (NBI)] and electronic [(Fuji intelligent chromoendoscopy (FICE) and i-Scan)] image enhancement techniques have facilitated electronic chromoscopy, thus avoiding the need for dye spraying. These techniques are easy to use and can be switched on by the press of a button on the hand control of the endoscope.

Chromoendoscopy

Vital stains (absorptive stains), such as methylene blue (MB), acetic acid, and non-absorbed stains (contrast stains), such as indigo carmine have been studied in BE with variable results. Absorptive stains diffuse or are preferentially absorbed across epithelial cell membranes whereas contrast stains highlight surface characteristics or mucosal irregularities by permeating mucosal crevices.

Methylene Blue

MB is an absorptive dye, which is probably the most widely studied in BE. It is taken up by actively absorbing intestinal epithelial cells and dysplastic mucosa, but not by normal esophageal and gastric mucosa. During MB chromoendoscopy, SIM typically stains blue, whereas a lighter intensity and increased heterogeneity in the staining pattern predict high-grade dysplasia (HGD) and/or adenocarcinoma (Figure 3-1).

One of the earlier studies by Canto et al. investigated the MB staining patterns and the yield of SIM and dysplasia in Barrett's. The accuracy of SIM detection was 90%, and they found that light to absent staining and moderate to marked heterogeneity were significantly associated with HGD or cancer.[13] Further, various studies compared the yield of MB directed target biopsies to random biopsies in detection of dysplasia and SIM. Some of the studies demonstrated significantly higher yield of SIM with MB chromoendoscopy with sensitivities ranging from 80 to 98%,[14-16] while others showed much lower sensitivities.[17-19] Differences in the concentration of MB, the volume used, and the time of contact could all be the reasons for this variability in results. The results for detecting dysplasia are even more inconsistent. A recent meta-analysis included 9 studies comparing MB directed biopsies to random biopsies. They found that there was no significant incremental yield of SIM and dysplasia with MB chromoendoscopy.[20] The yield of SIM with MB was 75 vs. 70% for random biopsies, and that for dysplasia was 43 and 32%, respectively, for MB targeted biopsies and random biopsies. Subanalysis showed a modest 7% incremental yield for detecting HGD and cancer.[20] Even among experts, there is a controversy regarding the ideal way to target the biopsies after MB chromoendoscopy. The staining patterns for SIM and dysplasia are also controversial, which has made this technique less frequently used in the present era. MB staining is generally concerned safe; however, a concern has been raised regarding the potential to induce oxidative

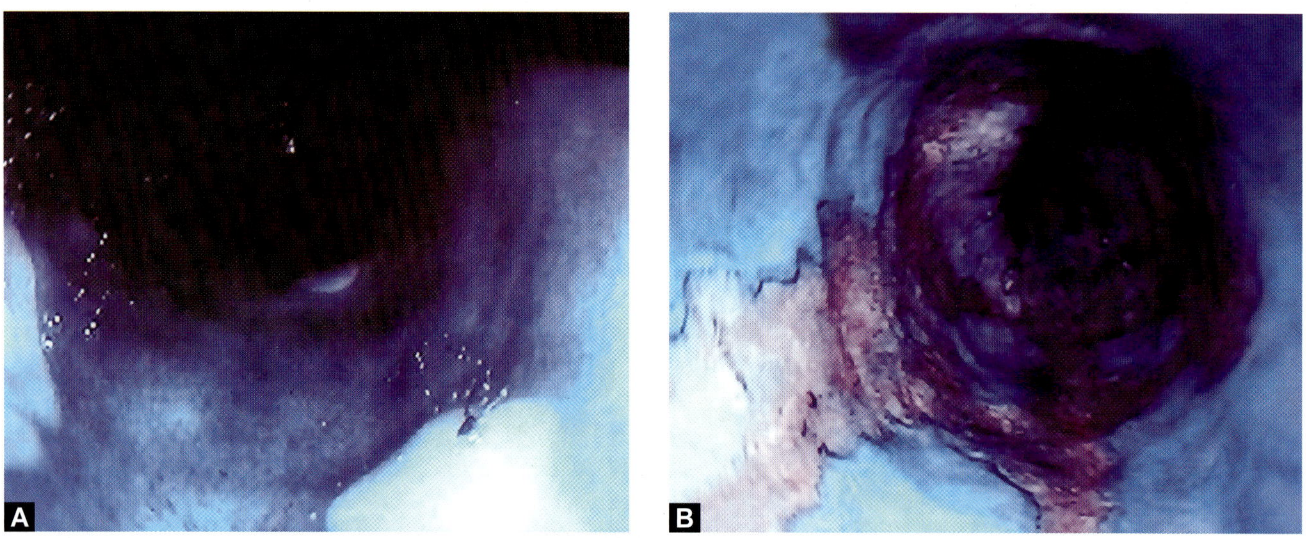

FIGURE 3-1 Methylene blue chromoendoscopy. **A,** Uniform dark blue staining of nondysplastic Barrett's mucosa. **B,** Typical irregular patchy staining of multifocal high-grade dysplasia.

damage to DNA in tissues exposed to methylene plus white light.[21] This theoretical risk of increasing neoplastic transformation has not been proven by clinical studies.

Indigo Carmine

Unlike the vital stains, indigo carmine is not absorbed by GI epithelium, and it pools in crevices between epithelial cells highlighting the mucosal architecture, particularly when used with high-magnification or high-resolution endoscopy (HRE) (Figure 3-2). Sharma et al. found that magnification endoscopy with indigo carmine spray is useful in identifying intestinal metaplasia and dysplasia in BE. All patients with HGD had irregular/distorted pit patterns on inspection. Ridged/villous patterns were suggestive of intestinal metaplasia. However, LGD patients also had ridged pattern and could not be differentiated from intestinal metaplasia alone.[22] When compared to HRE, indigo carmine chromoendoscopy (ICC) could detect only a limited number of additional dysplastic lesions, and did not alter the sensitivity of detecting dysplasia in a later study.[23] Similar results were obtained by Curvers et al. who did not find any improvement in interobserver variability and yield of

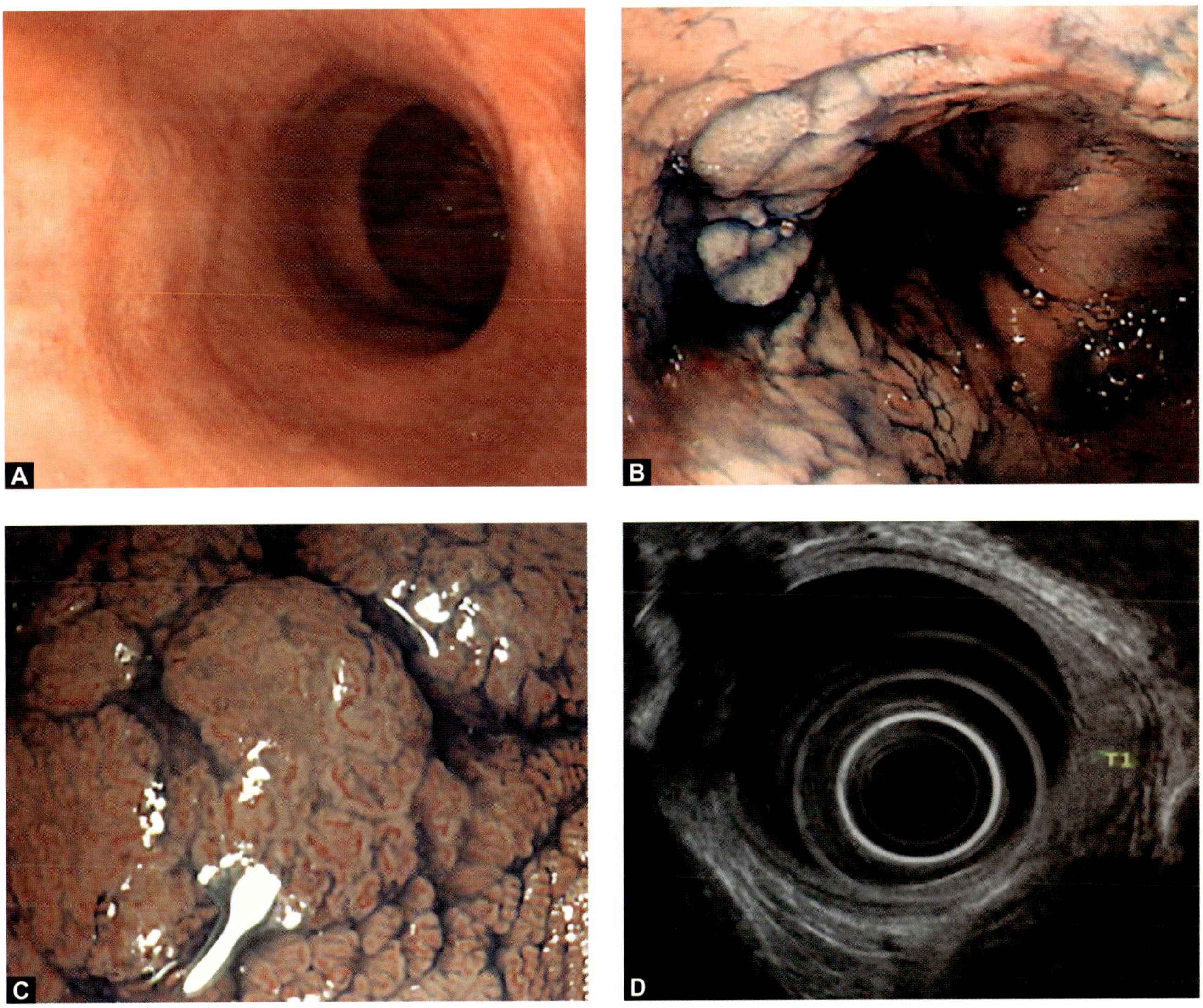

FIGURE 3-2 Indigo carmine chromoendoscopy. **A,** High-resolution white light endoscopy showing long segment of Barrett's esophagus. **B,** Indigo carmine dye spray revealing a flat elevated lesion close to the gastroesophageal junction. **C,** High-magnification view of the flat lesion showing distorted villous pit pattern typical of neoplasia. **D,** High frequency radial endoscopic ultrasound scan revealing a T1 tumor.

dysplasia when magnification ICC was compared with magnified high-resolution images.[24] HRE with high-definition systems and magnification is able to provide sufficient mucosal details compared to the previous generation of endoscopes, which could explain these results.

Acetic Acid

Acetic acid chromoendoscopy has been found to be useful in delineating remnant Barrett's islands after multipolar electrocoagulation therapy in one of the earliest published studies. They used 1.5% acetic acid spray, which produces a whitish discoloration of the esophageal and gastric mucosa. This appearance is due to the acetowhite reaction, which has been used in detecting cervical dysplasia for many years. The columnar epithelium of BE adopts a reddish color after 2–3 minutes,[25] which is easy to distinguish from normal mucosa. Use of magnification endoscopy in this context could help identify the pit patterns of the Barrett's epithelium, and various recognized patterns like round, linear, villous, gyrus, and distorted are described (Figure 3-3). A prospective study in 64 patients found this combined technique to yield significantly higher SIM and dysplasia in targeted biopsies.[26] However, the overall accuracy of magnification enhanced endoscopy

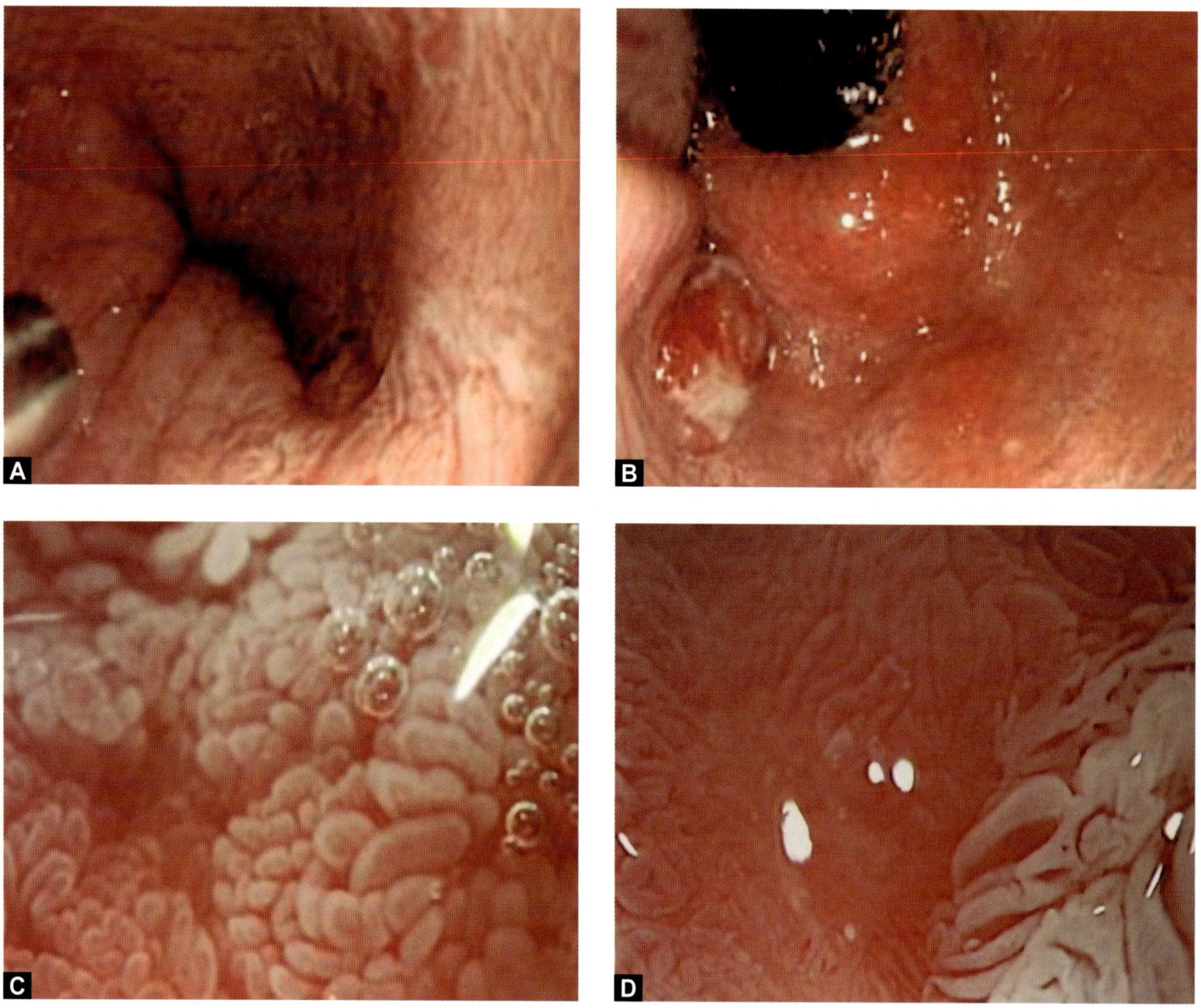

FIGURE 3-3 Acetic acid chromoendoscopy. **A,** Note the acetowhite reaction. **B,** Erythematous neoplastic lesion on retroversion. **C,** High-magnification view in the nondysplastic Barrett's mucosa showing ridge/villous pit pattern typical of intestinal metaplasia. **D,** High-magnification view of the neoplastic area showing distorted pit pattern.

using acetic acid in the diagnosis of BE is variable ranging from 50 to 90%.[27-29] The role of high-resolution acetic acid enhanced endoscopy without magnification was studied in a large cohort. In 701 patients enrolled, 406 patients had a history of Barrett's dysplasia/early cancer (high-risk group), whereas, 295 patients belonged to the low-risk group with no previous history of dysplasia. Majority of the dysplastic lesions were identified by acetic acid enhanced endoscopy and use of 4 quadrant random biopsies did not add significant yield. The sensitivity and specificity rates of acetic acid enhanced endoscopic imaging with targeted biopsies were 96.7 and 66.5%, with a positive and negative predictive value of 30.4 and 99.3%, respectively.[30] Similarly, another prospective study in 190 patients revealed a higher sensitivity and specificity (95.5 and 80%, respectively) for dysplasia detection when acetic acid endoscopy is compared to white light endoscopy (WLE).[31] Thus, acetic acid remains an inexpensive and useful tool for detection of dysplasia in BE.

NARROW BAND IMAGING

NBI, which was first described in 2004 by Gono et al.,[32] is a filter technology that works on the principle of narrowing the band widths of the emitted blue (440–460 nm) and green light (540–560 nm). The relative contribution of blue light has been increased, which is absorbed by hemoglobin, and narrowing the bandwidths of blue and green light enables the superficial mucosal details to be visualized better. NBI is user-friendly and provides uniform visualization of the endoscopic field without the need for any additional dyes.

In a prospective tandem endoscopy study of 65 patients, higher grades of dysplasia were detected by NBI compared to WLE and NBI directed target biopsies yielded more dysplasia than WLE directed biopsies.[33] Kara et al. compared the dysplasia detection rates of HRE, ICC, and NBI with magnification. Targeted biopsies with HRE alone had a sensitivity of 79% in detecting HGD. The addition of chromoscopy and NBI did not improve the yield significantly.[23] The current evidence does not show any additional advantage of NBI in identifying more number of patients with dysplasia compared to WLE.

NBI with magnification, however, could help in assessing the mucosal vascular and pit patterns of any suspicious areas detected in the Barrett's segment. Various studies have identified different pit and capillary patterns in BE.[34-36] Regular pit patterns include round, linear, tubular/ridged, and villous type. Irregular and absent pit patterns are also reported. Microvascular patterns are classified as either regular or irregular (Figure 3-4). Sensitivity and specificity of the irregular microvascular and pit patterns for prediction of HGD was as high as 90 and 100%, respectively in an earlier observational study.[34] Similarly, the villous/ridged/absent pit patterns were thought be highly suggestive of SIM and the round patterns associated with columnar lined epithelium.[36]

NBI is widely available for clinical use, and magnification endoscopes are commercially available. The role of NBI in detecting dysplastic lesions remains controversial, but there are a number of studies, which have used NBI to characterize the suspicious lesions.[34-38] These studies have shown good overall accuracy in diagnosing the lesions, especially so in cases of HGD and early cancer, which are depicted by irregular pit patterns and/or vascular patterns. This would help in reducing the number of random biopsies and in targeting lesions. By adopting a standardized pit pattern and vascular classification, it would be possible to improve the diagnostic accuracy of NBI with magnification in diagnosing dysplasia and SIM.

AUTOFLUORESCENCE ENDOSCOPY

The phenomenon of autofluorescence occurs when a light of shorter wavelength interacts with a tissue containing endogenous fluorophores, which, in turn, emits light of longer wavelength. A number of biological substances in the GI tract, such as collagen, elastin, nicotinamide, and flavins can act as endogenous fluorophores. The emergence of high-resolution video-endoscopy with a second charged couple device (CCD) for autofluorescence imaging (AFI) has made it possible to obtain pseudocolor images with significant improvement in the quality of images. AFI offers an easy way to distinguish between normal and dysplastic tissue by combining an autofluorescence image on irradiating with a blue light of wavelength of 390–470 nm. The image of green reflected light depicts the absorbed light of hemoglobin, so that normal tissue appears pale green and dysplastic tissue appears magenta.

One of the earliest studies in BE used a fiber-based laser-induced fluorescence system, which could be passed through the accessory channel of the endoscopes. Panjehpour et al. studied this system in 36 patients with BE. They found that 96% of nondysplastic Barrett's was classified as benign and 90% HGD as premalignant.[39] 5-aminolevulinic acid induced protoporphyrin IX fluorescence was found to identify areas of HGD with a modest sensitivity of 70% in a later study.[40] *In vitro* studies on

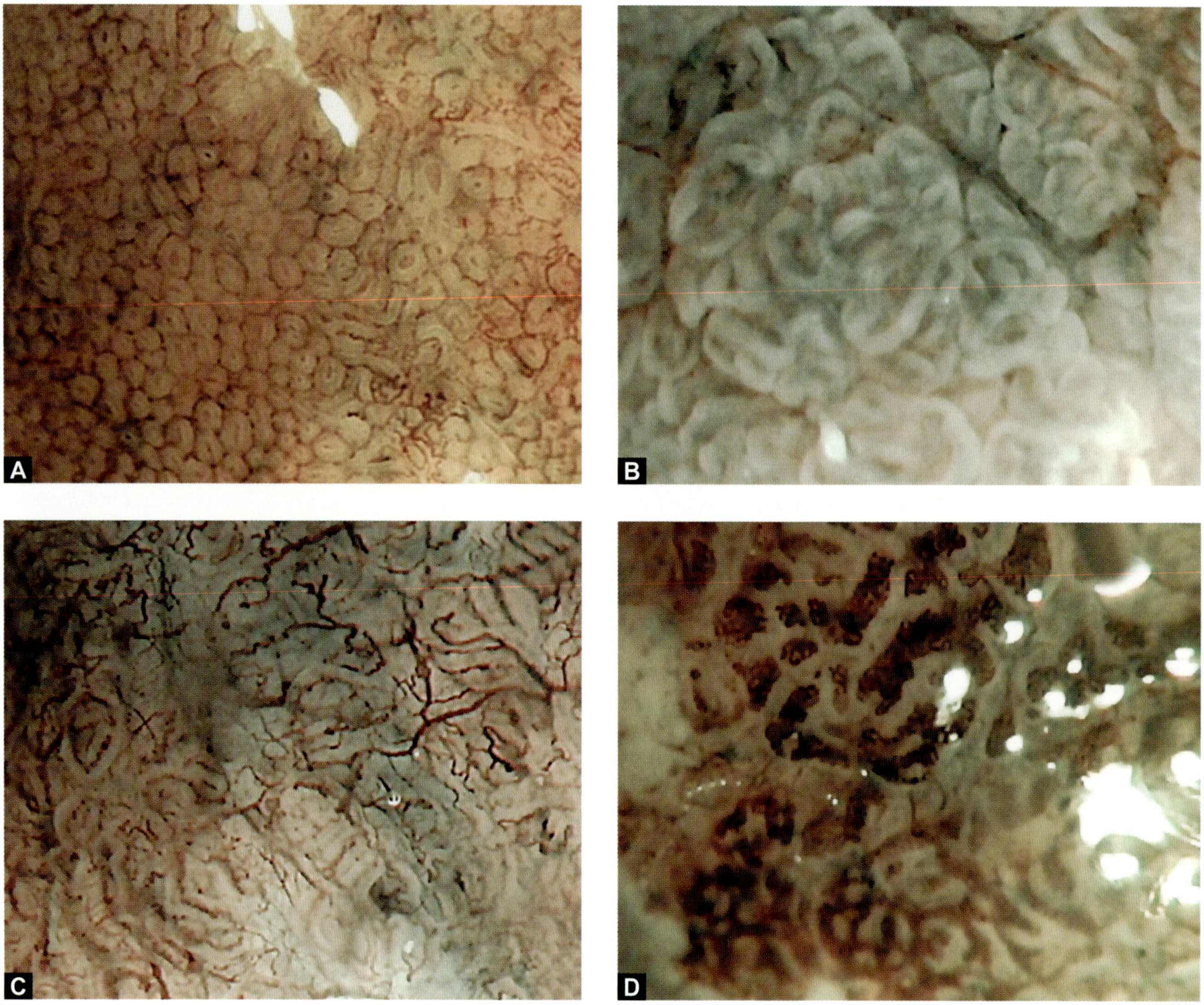

FIGURE 3-4 Magnification view of narrow band imaging patterns described in Barrett's esophagus. **A,** Round/circular patterns. **B,** Gyrous/cerebriform patterns. **C,** Absent pit patterns. **D,** Irregular vascular and pit patterns.

surgical specimens showed that the highest fluorescence ratio was obtained in areas of adenocarcinoma, compared to dysplastic and nondysplastic Barrett's.[41] The next generation of light-induced fluorescence endoscopes (LIFE) was investigated by Kara et al. in a randomized crossover trial. The sensitivity of dysplasia detection using WLE targeted biopsies was better than that of AFI in this study (85 vs. 69%).[42] Thus, AFI did not improve dysplasia detection rates using this system. This resulted in introduction of a video autofluorescence endoscope, which was studied in 2005 by the same group. Twenty-two patients with HGD were examined with AFI and WLE. AFI detected additional lesions in 3 patients compared to WLE. The use of AFI was found to be feasible and promising in detecting dysplasia.[43]

One of the disadvantages observed with AFI was the high false-positive rates for AFI, and it was hypothesized that this could be improved by additional NBI use. Twenty patients with suspected HGD were observed with AFI and suspected areas were examined closely with NBI. All the 28 lesions in this cohort were picked up by AFI; however, there was a false-positive rate of 40%. This was reduced to 10% by the use of NBI, thus, making a combined approach more specific.[44] In a randomized trial comparing AFI and WLE in Barrett's surveillance patients, AFI was found to improve

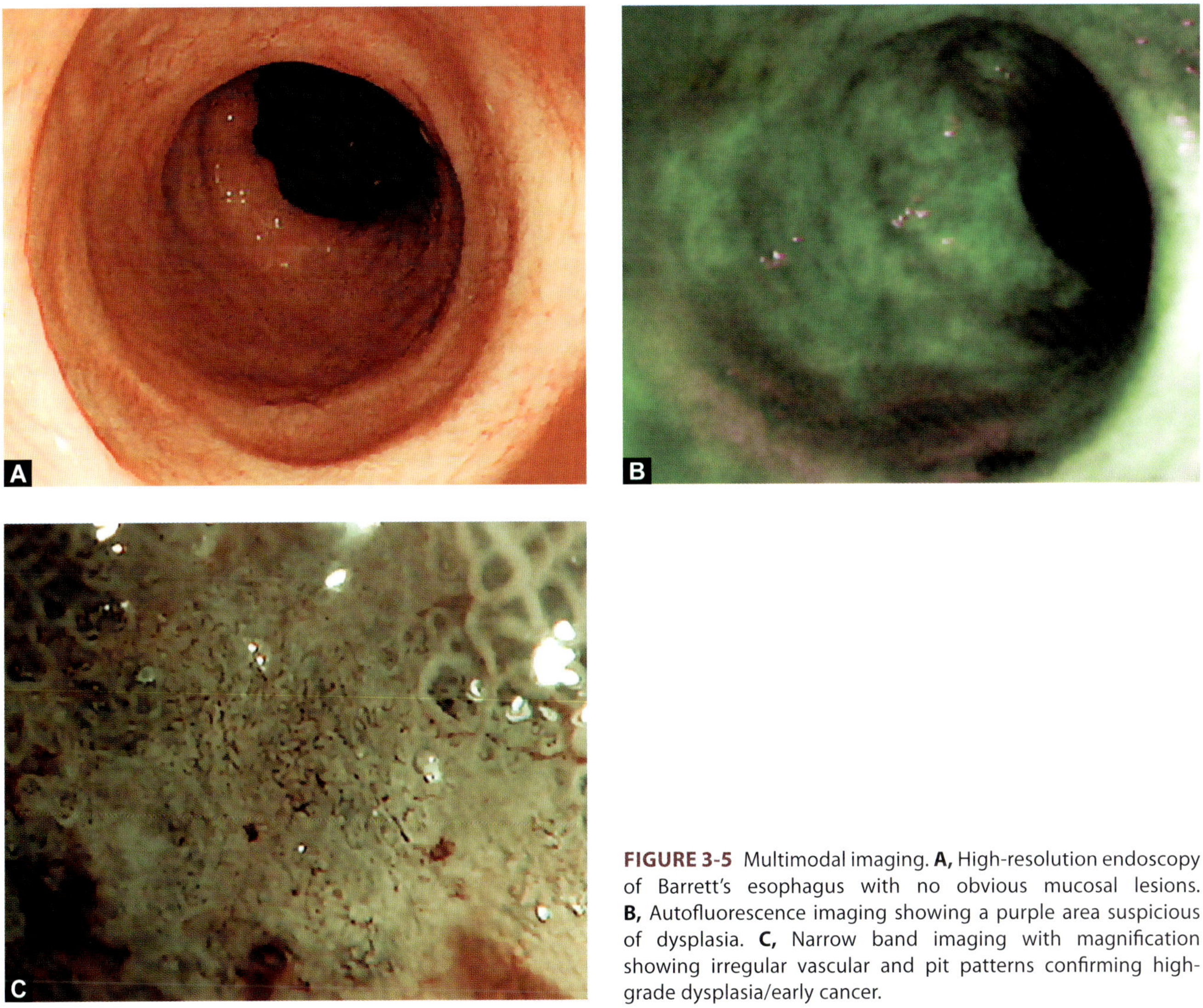

FIGURE 3-5 Multimodal imaging. **A,** High-resolution endoscopy of Barrett's esophagus with no obvious mucosal lesions. **B,** Autofluorescence imaging showing a purple area suspicious of dysplasia. **C,** Narrow band imaging with magnification showing irregular vascular and pit patterns confirming high-grade dysplasia/early cancer.

dysplasia detection rates. However, this did not suggest replacing the standard 4 quadrant biopsy protocols, as, in 11/19 patients, dysplasia was detected only on random sampling.[45] Most of the studies have found that AFI has a high sensitivity in detecting dysplastic lesions at the expense of increased false-positive rates. Thus, AFI is best used as a red-flag technique during BE surveillance.

MULTIMODAL IMAGING

The combined use of WLE, AFI, and NBI is possible with commercially available endoscopes with magnification (Figure 3-5). Earlier studies have shown that abnormal areas detected by AFI could be closely examined with NBI and magnification to characterize these further and target biopsies. The value of this so called 'endoscopic trimodal imaging' (ETMI) was investigated in a multicenter study. AFI was superior to WLE in detecting dysplastic lesions, but the false-positivity was high as reported before (81%). This was reduced to 26% after inspection with NBI.[37] A recent study investigated the role of ETMI compared to standard videoendoscopy (SVE) in a randomized cross-over fashion, 87 patients underwent both ETMI and SVE. This study showed that ETMI significantly improved targeted detection of HGD/early cancer in BE, which was due to higher pick-up by AFI. However, NBI was shown to have limited value in subsequent characterization of detected lesions.[46] NBI misclassified 11 areas of HGD/early cancer as nonsuspicious. This was contrary to earlier observations where NBI was found to have a very high sensitivity and specificity in characterizing lesions detected by AFI or WLE.[47] Thus, on balance, trimodal imaging seems to improve the dysplasia detection rates in BE. However, at this stage, ETMI cannot replace random biopsies in BE for detection of lesions. These studies were done in high-risk population, and the value of ETMI needs to be determined in general surveillance population by large randomized trials.

FUJI INTELLIGENT CHROMOENDOSCOPY AND i-SCAN

These techniques are based on a new computed spectral estimation technology. FICE and i-Scan transform an ordinary endoscopic image taken from the video processor and arithmetically processes the reflected photons to reconstitute virtual images by increasing the relative intensity of narrowed blue light to a maximum and by decreasing narrowed red and green light to a minimum. This leads to better delineation of micro-vasculature and mucosal pit patterns due to the differential absorption of light by hemoglobin in the mucosa. A recent study has found that BE can be easily diagnosed with FICE compared to standard endoscopy, with a clear demarcation between the Barrett's segment and gastric mucosa.[48] A randomized cross-over trial by Pohl et al. compared the accuracy of FICE to acetic acid chromoscopy in detection of HGD/early cancer and found that FICE is comparable to acetic acid chromoscopy.[49] i-Scan was studied in patients with reflux symptoms and was noted to help in identifying reflux associated lesions.[50] More studies are necessary in BE to assess the utility of these new techniques.

CONCLUSION

Various wide field imaging techniques are found to be useful to improve the detection of dysplasia in BE. Chromoendoscopy is inexpensive, and recent studies have highlighted the value of acetic acid even in the current era of high-definition WLE. Newer imaging techniques, such as AFI, NBI, and FICE are promising, and ETMI has found to improve the targeted yield of dysplasia. NBI with magnification is also useful in characterizing the suspicious lesions. None of these techniques have produced substantial evidence to replace the current practice of random 4 quadrant biopsies. Nonetheless, a thorough examination of BE using a high-definition WLE with the use of mucolytics should be considered the bare minimum standard for routine Barrett's surveillance.

REFERENCES

1. Kelty CJ, Gough MD, Van Wyk Q, Stephenson TJ, Ackroyd R. Barrett's oesophagus: intestinal metaplasia is not essential for cancer risk. *Scand J Gastroenterol.* 2007;42:1271-4.
2. Stein HJ, Siewert JR. Barrett's esophagus: pathogenesis, epidemiology, functional abnormalities, malignant degeneration, and surgical management. *Dysphagia.* 1993;8:276-88.
3. Hameeteman W, Tytgat GN, Houthoff HJ, van den Tweel JG. Barrett's esophagus: development of dysplasia and adenocarcinoma. *Gastroenterology.* 1989;96:1249-56.
4. van Sandick JW, van Lanschot JJ, Kuiken BW, Tytgat GN, Offerhaus GJ, Obertop H. Impact of endoscopic biopsy surveillance of Barrett's oesophagus on pathological stage and clinical outcome of Barrett's carcinoma. *Gut.* 1998;43:216-22.
5. El-Serag HB, Aguirre TV, Davis S, Kuebeler M, Bhattacharyya A, Sampliner RE. Proton pump inhibitors are associated with reduced incidence of dysplasia in Barrett's esophagus. *Am J Gastroenterol.* 2004;99:1877-83.
6. Sampliner RE. Practice guidelines on the diagnosis, surveillance, and therapy of Barrett's esophagus. The Practice Parameters Committee of the American College of Gastroenterology. *Am J Gastroenterol.* 1998;93:1028-32.
7. Wang KK, Sampliner RE. Updated guidelines 2008 for the diagnosis, surveillance and therapy of Barrett's esophagus. *Am J Gastroenterol.* 2008;103:788-97.
8. Corley DA, Levin TR, Habel LA, Weiss NS, Buffler PA. Surveillance and survival in Barrett's adenocarcinomas: a population-based study. *Gastroenterology.* 2002;122:633-40.
9. Streitz JM Jr, Andrews CW Jr, Ellis FH Jr. Endoscopic surveillance of Barrett's esophagus. Does it help? *J Thorac Cardiovasc Surg.* 1993;105:383-7.
10. Falk GW, Rice TW, Goldblum JR, Richter JE. Jumbo biopsy forceps protocol still misses unsuspected cancer in Barrett's esophagus with high-grade dysplasia. *Gastrointest Endosc.* 1999;49:170-6.
11. Kim SL, Waring JP, Spechler SJ, Sampliner RE, Doos WG, Krol WF, et al. Diagnostic inconsistencies in Barrett's esophagus. Department of Veterans Affairs Gastroesophageal Reflux Study Group. *Gastroenterology.* 1994;107:945-9.
12. Chang CC, Chen SH, Lin CP, Hsieh CR, Lou HY, Suk FM, et al. Premedication with pronase or N-acetylcysteine improves visibility during gastroendoscopy: an endoscopist-blinded, prospective, randomized study. *World J Gastroenterol.* 2007;13:444-7.
13. Canto MI, Setrakian S, Willis JE, Chak A, Petras RE, Sivak MV. Methylene blue staining of dysplastic and nondysplastic Barrett's esophagus: an in vivo and ex vivo study. *Endoscopy.* 2001;33:391-400.
14. Canto MI, Setrakian S, Petras RE, Blades E, Chak A, Sivak MV Jr. Methylene blue selectively stains intestinal metaplasia in Barrett's esophagus. *Gastrointest Endosc.* 1996;44:1-7.

15. Kiesslich R, Hahn M, Herrmann G, Jung M. Screening for specialized columnar epithelium with methylene blue: chromoendoscopy in patients with Barrett's esophagus and a normal control group. *Gastrointest Endosc.* 2001; 53:47-52.
16. Ragunath K, Krasner N, Raman VS, Haqqani MT, Cheung WY. A randomized, prospective cross-over trial comparing methylene blue-directed biopsy and conventional random biopsy for detecting intestinal metaplasia and dysplasia in Barrett's esophagus. *Endoscopy.* 2003;35:998-1003.
17. Gangarosa LM, Halter S, Mertz H. Methylene blue staining and endoscopic ultrasound evaluation of Barrett's esophagus with low-grade dysplasia. *Dig Dis Sci.* 2000;45:225-9.
18. Sharma P, Topalovski M, Mayo MS, Weston AP. Methylene blue chromoendoscopy for detection of short-segment Barrett's esophagus. *Gastrointest Endosc.* 2001;54:289-93.
19. Wo JM, Ray MB, Mayfield-Stokes S, Al-Sabbagh G, Gebrail F, Slone SP, et al. Comparison of methylene blue-directed biopsies and conventional biopsies in the detection of intestinal metaplasia and dysplasia in Barrett's esophagus: a preliminary study. *Gastrointest Endosc.* 2001;54:294-301.
20. Ngamruengphong S, Sharma VK, Das A. Diagnostic yield of methylene blue chromoendoscopy for detecting specialized intestinal metaplasia and dysplasia in Barrett's esophagus: a meta-analysis. *Gastrointest Endosc.* 2009;69: 1021-8.
21. Olliver JR, Wild CP, Sahay P, Dexter S, Hardie LJ. Chromoendoscopy with methylene blue and associated DNA damage in Barrett's oesophagus. *Lancet.* 2003;362: 373-4.
22. Sharma P, Weston AP, Topalovski M, Cherian R, Bhattacharyya A, Sampliner RE. Magnification chromoendoscopy for the detection of intestinal metaplasia and dysplasia in Barrett's oesophagus. *Gut.* 2003;52:24-7.
23. Kara MA, Peters FP, Rosmolen WD, Krishnadath KK, ten Kate FJ, Fockens P, et al. High-resolution endoscopy plus chromoendoscopy or narrow-band imaging in Barrett's esophagus: a prospective randomized crossover study. *Endoscopy.* 2005;37:929-36.
24. Curvers W, Baak L, Kiesslich R, van Oijen A, Rabenstein T, Ragunath K, et al. Chromoendoscopy and narrow-band imaging compared with high-resolution magnification endoscopy in Barrett's esophagus. *Gastroenterology.* 2008; 134:670-9.
25. Guelrud M, Herrera I. Acetic acid improves identification of remnant islands of Barrett's epithelium after endoscopic therapy. *Gastrointest Endosc.* 1998;47:512-5.
26. Fortun PJ, Anagnostopoulos GK, Kaye P, James M, Foley S, Samuel S, et al. Acetic acid-enhanced magnification endoscopy in the diagnosis of specialized intestinal metaplasia, dysplasia and early cancer in Barrett's oesophagus. *Aliment Pharmacol Ther.* 2006;23:735-42.
27. Hoffman A, Kiesslich R, Bender A, Neurath MF, Nafe B, Herrmann G, et al. Acetic acid-guided biopsies after magnifying endoscopy compared with random biopsies in the detection of Barrett's esophagus: a prospective randomized trial with crossover design. *Gastrointest Endosc.* 2006;64:1-8.
28. Meining A, Rösch T, Kiesslich R, Muders M, Sax F, Heldwein W. Inter- and intra-observer variability of magnification chromoendoscopy for detecting specialized intestinal metaplasia at the gastroesophageal junction. *Endoscopy.* 2004;36:160-4.
29. Toyoda H, Rubio C, Befrits R, Hamamoto N, Adachi Y, Jaramillo E. Detection of intestinal metaplasia in distal esophagus and esophagogastric junction by enhanced-magnification endoscopy. *Gastrointest Endosc.* 2004;59: 15-21.
30. Pohl J, Pech O, May A, Manner H, Fissler-Eckhoff A, Ell C. Incidence of macroscopically occult neoplasias in Barrett's esophagus: are random biopsies dispensable in the era of advanced endoscopic imaging? *Am J Gastroenterol.* 2010;105:2350-6.
31. Longcroft-Wheaton G, Duku M, Mead R, Poller D, Bhandari P. Acetic acid spray is an effective tool for the endoscopic detection of neoplasia in patients with Barrett's esophagus. *Clin Gastroenterol Hepatol.* 2010;8: 843-7.
32. Gono K, Obi T, Yamaguchi M, Ohyama N, Machida H, Sano Y, et al. Appearance of enhanced tissue features in narrow-band endoscopic imaging. *J Biomed Opt.* 2004;9: 568-77.
33. Wolfsen HC, Crook JE, Krishna M, Achem SR, Devault KR, Bouras EP, et al. Prospective, controlled tandem endoscopy study of narrow band imaging for dysplasia detection in Barrett's esophagus. *Gastroenterology.* 2008; 135:24-31.
34. Anagnostopoulos GK, Yao K, Kaye P, Hawkey CJ, Ragunath K. Novel endoscopic observation in Barrett's oesophagus using high resolution magnification endoscopy and narrow band imaging. *Aliment Pharmacol Ther.* 2007;26:501-7.
35. Kara MA, Ennahachi M, Fockens P, ten Kate FJ, Bergman JJ. Detection and classification of the mucosal and vascular patterns (mucosal morphology) in Barrett's esophagus by using narrow band imaging. *Gastrointest Endosc.* 2006;64:155-66.
36. Singh R, Anagnostopoulos GK, Yao K, Karageorgiou H, Fortun PJ, Shonde A, et al. Narrow-band imaging with magnification in Barrett's esophagus: validation of a simplified grading system of mucosal morphology patterns against histology. *Endoscopy.* 2008;40:457-63.
37. Curvers WL, Singh R, Song LM, Wolfsen HC, Ragunath K, Wang K, et al. Endoscopic tri-modal imaging for detection of early neoplasia in Barrett's oesophagus: a multi-centre feasibility study using high-resolution endoscopy, autofluorescence imaging and narrow band imaging incorporated in one endoscopy system. *Gut.* 2008;57: 167-72.
38. Sharma P, Bansal A, Mathur S, Wani S, Cherian R, McGregor D, et al. The utility of a novel narrow band imaging endoscopy system in patients with Barrett's esophagus. *Gastrointest Endosc.* 2006;64:167-75.

39. Panjehpour M, Overholt BF, Vo-Dinh T, Haggitt RC, Edwards DH, Buckley FP 3rd. Endoscopic fluorescence detection of high-grade dysplasia in Barrett's esophagus. *Gastroenterology.* 1996;111:93-101.
40. Brand S, Wang TD, Schomacker KT, Poneros JM, Lauwers GY, Compton CC, et al. Detection of high-grade dysplasia in Barrett's esophagus by spectroscopy measurement of 5-aminolevulinic acid-induced protoporphyrin IX fluorescence. *Gastrointest Endosc.* 2002;56:479-87.
41. von Holstein CS, Nilsson AM, Andersson-Engels S, Willen R, Walther B, Svanberg K. Detection of adenocarcinoma in Barrett's oesophagus by means of laser induced fluorescence. *Gut.* 1996;39:711-6.
42. Kara MA, Smits ME, Rosmolen WD, Bultje AC, ten Kate FJ, Fockens P, et al. A randomized crossover study comparing light-induced fluorescence endoscopy with standard videoendoscopy for the detection of early neoplasia in Barrett's esophagus. *Gastrointest Endosc.* 2005;61:671-8.
43. Kara MA, Peters FP, Ten Kate FJ, Van Deventer SJ, Fockens P, Bergman JJ. Endoscopic video autofluorescence imaging may improve the detection of early neoplasia in patients with Barrett's esophagus. *Gastrointest Endosc.* 2005;61:679-85.
44. Kara MA, Peters FP, Fockens P, ten Kate FJ, Bergman JJ. Endoscopic video-autofluorescence imaging followed by narrow band imaging for detecting early neoplasia in Barrett's esophagus. *Gastrointest Endosc.* 2006;64:176-85.
45. Borovicka J, Fischer J, Neuweiler J, Netzer P, Gschossmann J, Ehmann T, et al. Autofluorescence endoscopy in surveillance of Barrett's esophagus: a multicenter randomized trial on diagnostic efficacy. *Endoscopy.* 2006;38:867-72.
46. Curvers WL, Herrero LA, Wallace MB, Wong Kee Song LM, Ragunath K, Wolfsen HC, et al. Endoscopic tri-modal imaging is more effective than standard endoscopy in identifying early-stage neoplasia in Barrett's esophagus. *Gastroenterology.* 2010;139:1106-14.
47. Mannath J, Subramanian V, Hawkey CJ, Ragunath K. Narrow band imaging for characterization of high grade dysplasia and specialized intestinal metaplasia in Barrett's esophagus: a meta-analysis. *Endoscopy.* 2010;42: 351-9.
48. Osawa H, Yamamoto H, Yamada N, Yoshizawa M, Sunada K, Kita H, et al. Diagnosis of endoscopic Barrett's esophagus by transnasal flexible spectral imaging color enhancement. *J Gastroenterol.* 2009;44:1125-32.
49. Pohl J, May A, Rabenstein T, Pech O, Nguyen-Tat M, Fissler-Eckhoff A, et al. Comparison of computed virtual chromoendoscopy and conventional chromoendoscopy with acetic acid for detection of neoplasia in Barrett's esophagus. *Endoscopy.* 2007;39:594-8.
50. Hoffman A, Basting N, Goetz M, Tresch A, Mudter J, Biesterfeld S, et al. High-definition endoscopy with i-Scan and Lugol's solution for more precise detection of mucosal breaks in patients with reflux symptoms. *Endoscopy.* 2009;41:107-12.

4 Barrett's Esophagus and Esophageal Adenocarcinoma: Endomicroscopy and Spectroscopy

Michael B Wallace, Ralf Kiesslich

ABSTRACT

Numerous endoscopic imaging modalities have been developed and introduced into clinical practice to enhance the screening and surveillance of Barrett's esophagus (BE). In the past, detection of dysplasia and carcinoma of the esophagus has been dependent on random and, to a lesser extent, on directed biopsies taken during standard white light endoscopy (WLE). Recent important developments in biomedical optics have improved the visualization of esophageal epithelium to a point where cellular details can be directly imaged *in vivo* during endoscopy, allowing diagnosis to be made in gastrointestinal endoscopy unit and, thereby, avoiding the cost, risk, and time delay involved in tissue biopsy. Chromoendoscopy, wide-field imaging enhancement methods [i.e., narrow band imaging (NBI), Fujinon intelligent chromoendoscopy (FICE), and i-Scan], and point enhancement, such as confocal laser endomicroscopy (CLE) and spectroscopy are some of the examples of enhanced technologies, which are being used in daily practice. In this chapter, we will review and highlight these endoscopic-based imaging techniques for detection of esophageal dysplasia and carcinoma from perspective of routine clinical practice.

WHITE LIGHT ENDOSCOPIC IMAGING

Standard videoendoscopy magnifies the image to approximately 5–10 times normal and gives image resolution of 100,000–300,000 pixels. Image resolution, i.e., the ability to discriminate between two adjacent points, achieved with standard videoendoscope, is not sufficient to make specific pathological diagnoses in most cases. Hence, mucosal biopsies are required, even though the vast majority of random biopsies do not yield neoplasia. Random biopsy sampling is associated with increased cost, more time consumption, delay and extraprocedures between diagnosis and treatment, sampling errors, and high interobserver variability in histopathological diagnosis.[1] Techniques are needed that would easily differentiate normal from abnormal mucosa to guide, and if possible, eliminate the need for random biopsies. High-resolution endoscopes (HRE) are newer class of endoscopes, which are better in detecting microscopic mucosal abnormalities due to their ability to produce images with higher magnification of up to 100 times normal and increased spatial resolution of 600,000–1,000,000 pixels. Some are equipped with a movable lens resulting in optical zoom. These qualities allow more detailed examination of the mucosal, glandular, and vascular structures.

CHROMOENDOSCOPY

Chromoendoscopy involves endoscopic examination of gastrointestinal mucosa after applying a dye solution to the surface. These dyes enhance the appearance of otherwise nonperceivable mucosal changes. This technique guides the endoscopist to take target biopsies from suspicious areas. Different dye solutions are used, including Lugol's iodine solution, methylene blue (MB), indigo carmine, crystal violet, and acetic acid. Lugol's solution consists of 0.5–3% aqueous solution of potassium iodide and iodine, and is taken up by glycogen containing cells. It is used primarily for detecting dysplasia in patients with increased risk of squamous cell carcinoma (history of smoking, alcoholism, oropharyngeal cancer, and lye ingestion). Iodine generally stains normal squamous mucosa, leaving neoplastic regions pale/unstained (Figure 4-1). On the other hand, MB, indigo carmine, and acetic acid are more useful in detection of

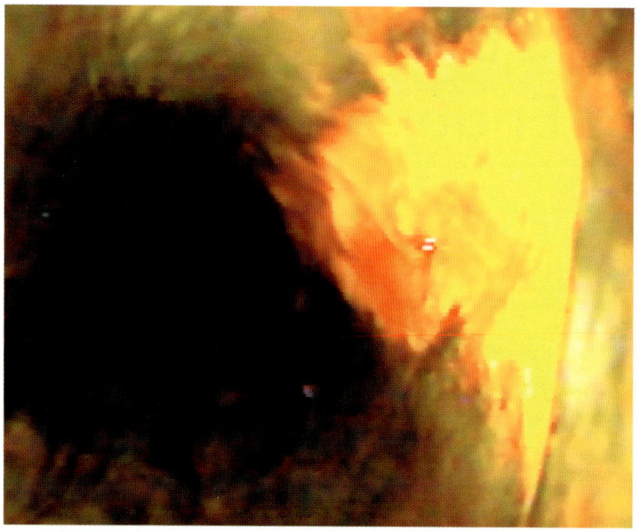

FIGURE 4-1 Lugol's iodine staining of an early squamous cell carcinoma. Note the unstained area at 3 o'clock corresponding to the neoplasia. Normal squamous esophagus stains a chocolate-brown color.

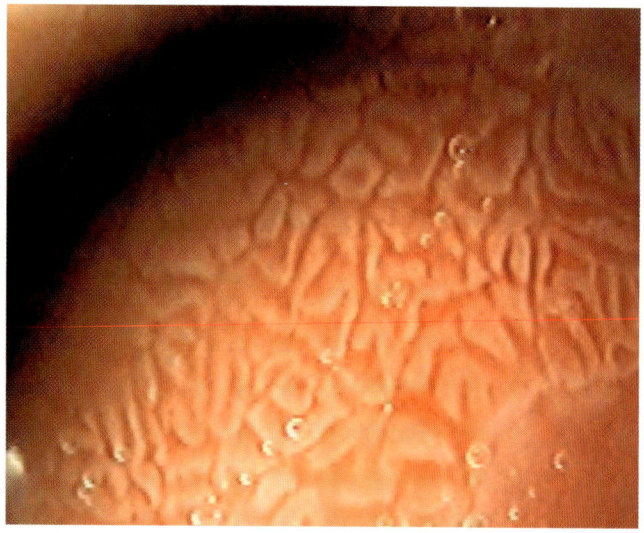

FIGURE 4-2 Acetic acid chromoendoscopy of the distal esophagus showing the ridged/villous pattern suggestive of specialized intestinal metaplasia.

glandular abnormalities, as seen in Barrett's esophagus (BE) associated neoplasia. After staining with these agents, different mucosal patterns become visible during endoscopy. Various studies have been done to classify and detect dysplasia and early carcinoma based on these patterns. Guelrud et al. used acetic acid to stain the esophageal mucosa and observed four pit patterns (round, reticular, villous, and ridged) (Figure 4-2). Villous and ridged patterns were found to be associated with intestinal metaplasia.[2] Sharma et al. studied the mucosal changes in 80 patients of BE after application of indigo carmine, and observed three mucosal patterns, namely, ridged/villous, circular, and irregular/distorted. The irregular or distorted pattern was found to be associated with Barrett's high-grade dysplasia (HGD) or superficial adenocarcinoma in six patients.[3] In the same study, the presence of the ridged or villous pattern had 97% sensitivity, 76% specificity, and 92% positive predictive value for prediction of intestinal metaplasia. However, in subsequent studies, these results could not be reproduced, and no detection benefit for either Barrett's metaplasia or dysplasia could be established with chromoendoscopy.[4,5] Other studies using acetic acid and cresyl violet stain also produced variable results.[6-8] The probable reasons for these conflicting observations could be the differences in technique, operator experience, and a patient population with the prevalence of BE.[9,10] This was further substantiated in a European study in which four expert gastrointestinal endoscopists, blinded to the histology, analyzed magnification chromoendoscopy images of BE, using acetic acid or MB. The interobserver agreement was only fair (kappa = 0.40) for all parameters studied, including the mucosal patterns, MB positive staining, and the presence of specialized intestinal metaplasia (SIM).[11]

Ngamruengphong et al. performed a meta-analysis of 9 studies for assessment of the diagnostic yield of techniques of chromoendoscopy compared with conventional 4-quadrant random biopsy in detection of SIM and dysplasia in patients with BE. A total of 450 patients with BE were reported in 9 studies included in the meta-analysis. Data on yield of both modalities were extracted and analyzed to estimate weighted incremental yield and 95% CIs of MB over random biopsy using Cochrane's Q chi (2) test. There was no significant incremental yield with MB over random biopsy for detection of SIM (incremental yield 4%; 6 studies, n = 251), dysplasia (incremental yield 9%; 9 studies, n = 450), and HGD and/or early cancer (incremental yield 5%; 8 studies, n = 405). This meta-analysis shows that the technique of MB chromoendoscopy has only a comparable yield with random biopsies for the detection of SIM and dysplasia during endoscopic evaluation of patients with BE.[12]

Ormeci et al. compared the convention endoscopy with chromoendoscopy in 109 patients using MB. The sensitivity of chromoendoscopy for Barrett's epithelium was superior to that of conventional endoscopy (87% as compared to 66%; $p < 0.05$). However, there was no statistical difference between the two methods in the diagnosis of esophageal carcinoma ($p > 0.05$). They concluded that chromoendoscopy is useful for delineating Barrett's epithelium, and for indicating the correct location for securing biopsies where dysplasia or early esophageal cancer is suspected.[13]

Safety issues regarding the use of MB have also been raised, as these may cause DNA damage when used with white light illumination.[14] These concerns along with high cost, procedure time, and unreliable detection of mucosal abnormalities prevented the widespread application of vital dye staining chromoendoscopy technique in clinical practice.[11]

NARROW BAND IMAGING

The working principle of narrow band imaging (NBI) is based on the use of light filters, which reduce the red and green light and increase the amount of blue light that illuminates the tissue. The resultant blue excitation light with narrow band width has limited optical scattering and shallow penetration depth. It improves the imaging of mucosal and glandular changes and efficiently visualizes abnormal vascular patterns. As blue light is readily taken up by hemoglobin, NBI successfully detects the increased density of abnormal microvessels that is associated with dysplasia and carcinoma (Figure 4-3).[15]

This technology was first introduced by Gono et al. in 1999, as a combined effort of the Japanese National Cancer Center Hospital East and a team of bio-optical physicists from Olympus Corporation (Tokyo, Japan).[16] There are two versions of NBI system. One based on the 3-color chip in Olympus Exera II system, which is predominately used in North America and Europe. It is equipped with several diminutive band pass color filters, which allows the green light of 530–550 nm band width and blue light of 390–445 nm band width to pass through and activate each pixel on trichromatic charged couple device (CCD). The other system is Lucera system, which utilizes a monochromatic CCD system and cycling color filter wheel to generate a color image. Lucera is used predominantly in Japan. Both the systems allow switching between high-resolution white light and NBI modes with the help of a switch on the handle of endoscope. Although they have slight technical differences, both systems are functionally similar.

NBI has shown several advantages over the vital dye chromoendoscopy in terms of applicability, cost, time consumption, tidiness, and precision. It is widely available commercially and has received regulatory approval. It is one of the most extensively studied advanced endoscopic imaging techniques for the detection of esophageal dysplasia and superficial carcinoma. Mucosal and vascular patterns seen in BE have been the basis of many single center studies. Kara et al. studied these patterns in BE patients and observed the association of regular mucosal and vascular patterns with intestinal metaplasia, while irregular mucosa and abnormal blood vessels were present in Barrett's HGD.[17,18] In another study, Kara et al. compared HRE with indigo carmine chromoendoscopy to NBI in 14 patients with Barrett's HGD. The aim of the

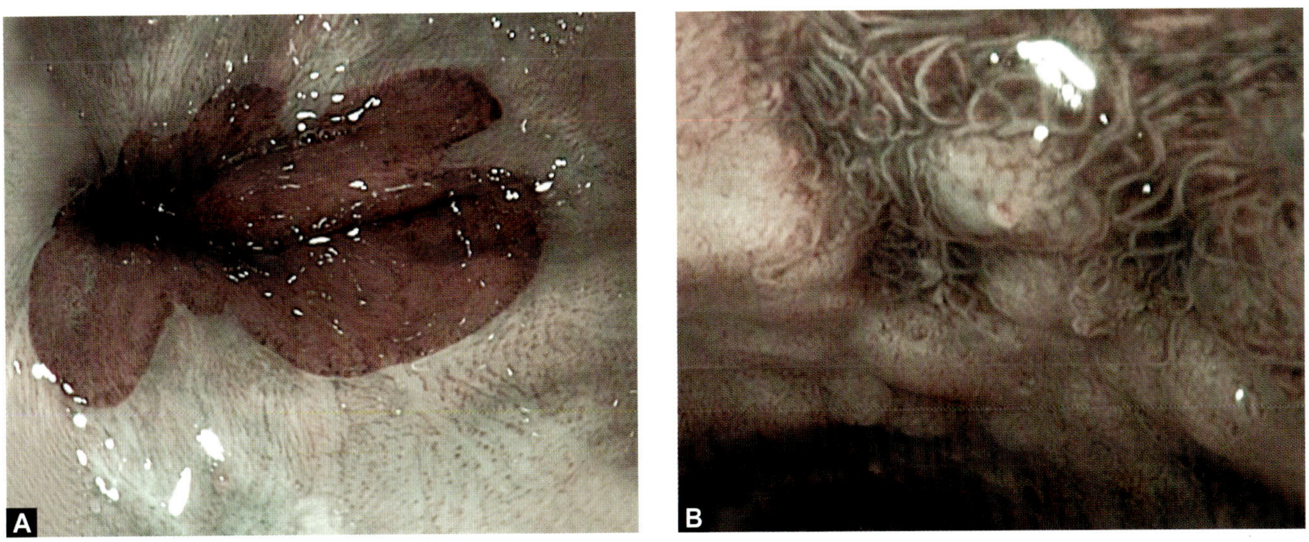

FIGURE 4-3 Short segment Barrett's esophagus. **A,** Narrow band imaging. Note the regular villiform mucosal and vascular pattern. **B,** Focal depressed high-grade dysplasia with narrow band imaging. Note the irregular dilated vessels and mucosal pattern and depression of mucosa.

study was to compare and correlate the findings with the combinations of these techniques for the detection of Barrett's HGD or superficial carcinoma. Eleven patients of HGD (79%) were detected with HRE alone, while NBI found HGD in 12 patients (86%). Indigo carmine was able to detect HGD in 13 patients (93%), while one patient with HGD (7%) was found with random biopsies and could not be detected with any imaging modality. NBI found an additional 4 HGD lesions in 3 of these 12 patients. White light resolution endoscopy detected all cases of HGD, showing better efficacy for primary detection than NBI. However, NBI was more useful for detailed inspection of suspicious lesions. As a historical comparison, a previous study performed by this group detected HGD in 62% of patients using targeted standard resolution endoscopy (SRE) biopsies, and in 85% of patients with SRE targeted plus random quadrantic biopsies.[19,20]

Anagnostopoulos et al. studied mucosal and vascular features of Barrett's disease in 50 patients with 344 lesions using high-resolution magnification endoscopy and NBI. The sensitivity, specificity, and positive and negative predictive values of regular mucosal and vascular patterns for intestinal metaplasia were 100, 79, 94, and 100%, respectively, while the same for HGD in these patients were 90, 100, 99, and 100%, respectively.[17]

Curvers et al. performed a blinded study involving 14 patients with 22 suspicious lesions, including 8 lesions of HGD, 1 lesion with low-grade dysplasia (LGD), 1 lesion indefinite for dysplasia, and 12 areas of nondysplastic Barrett's disease. They performed HRE with vital dye staining techniques, using acetic acid and indigo carmine as well as NBI. In a blinded fashion, seven community and five expert gastrointestinal endoscopists evaluated standard images from these lesions for any association of glandular and vascular patterns with dysplasia. The detection rate for dysplasia or neoplasia, with high-resolution white light endoscopy (WLE-Z), was 86% overall (90% for experts and 84% for non-experts). Interestingly, the addition of vital dye staining or NBI did not improve the diagnostic yield.[21]

In a prospective blinded tandem study, Wolfsen et al. compared SRE and HRE-NBI in 65 patients with BE. With HRE-NBI, dysplasia was detected in 37 patients (57%), while SRE with targeted plus random biopsies detected dysplasia in 28 patients (43%), which was statistically significant ($p < 0.001$). NBI with targeted biopsy also found incrementally higher grades of dysplasia in 12 patients (18%), compared to SRE with targeted plus random biopsies ($p < 0.001$). This study also showed greater efficiency of HRE-NBI, as less NBI directed biopsies (mean 4.7 biopsies per case; $p < 0.001$) were needed to detect dysplasia as compared to SRE with targeted plus random biopsies (mean 8.5 biopsies per case). This outcome illustrates the importance of HRE in combination with NBI for the surveillance evaluation of BE patients.[22-24]

Herrero et al. evaluated a simplified NBI classification of mucosal morphology to assess interobserver and intraobserver agreement and the correlation with histology. Two hundred NBI images were evaluated twice by four NBI-experienced and four non-experienced endoscopists at two referral centers. Endoscopists assessed each image for: quality, suspicion for dysplasia, and regularity of mucosal and vascular patterns. Overall interobserver agreement was seen to be 'moderate' (kappa 0.42–0.44), while overall intraobserver agreement was 'moderate' to 'substantial' (kappa 0.60–0.62). The endoscopist correctly identified 71% of the images containing high-grade intraepithelial neoplasia/early cancer and 68% of nondysplastic images were correctly identified as not suspicious. There were no significant differences in agreement between expert and nonexpert endoscopists suggesting a short learning curve. However, the low rate of identification of HGD/early cancer (71%) raises serious questions regarding the ability of NBI to replace histological sampling.[25]

Singh et al. conducted a prospective single-center study involving 21 patients with BE to evaluate whether there is any appreciable difference in imaging characteristics between WLE-Z and NBI, and if this translates into superior prediction of histology. Mucosal patterns (pit pattern and microvascular morphology) were evaluated for their image quality on a visual analogue scale of 1–10 by five expert endoscopists, who then predicted mucosal changes based on pit and microvascular patterns. It was found that NBI-Z is superior to WLE-Z in the prediction of histology in BE, as the overall pit and microvasculature quality was significantly higher ($p < 0.001$). Furthermore, NBI was also observed to be superior to WLE-Z for prediction of dysplasia [chi (2) = 10.3, $p < 0.05$]. The overall kappa agreement among the five endoscopists was 0.59 and 0.31 ($p < 0.001$) showing good reproducibility.[26]

Overall, NBI, when used in combination with HRE appears to be a valuable tool, which increases detection of neoplasia. This tool and similar methods, such as FICE or i-Scan are now widely used in referral centers for Barrett's neoplasia. The most valuable application appears to be a guide to target biopsies. Although promising, the data does not yet support complete replacement of random biopsy.

CONFOCAL LASER ENDOMICROSCOPY

A major milestone in the field of endoscopic-based enhanced imaging technology is the development of confocal laser endomicroscopy (CLE). This technology enables realtime *in vivo* microscopic imaging of esophageal mucosa. The basic principle of CLE involves stimulation of mucosal cells with laser excitation light after tissues have been exposed to topical or intravenous fluorescent contrast agents, such as acriflavine or fluorescein. The incident light and reflected light are transmitted through a pinhole to eliminate out of focus light coming from tissue above or below the tissue plane of interest. A black and white cross-sectional image of the mucosa is generated. There are two systems, which have been developed based on this technology. The endoscope-integrated system (Figure 4-4) has been developed by OptiScan and integrated into Pentax endoscopes. The eCLE system consists of an endoscope with integrated confocal laser system. It permits magnification beyond 1,000 times the normal, with cellular and subcellular resolution of epithelial, glandular, and vascular architecture to a depth from 0 to 250 microns (level of the lamina propria). eCLE has several advantages and disadvantages relative to probe-based CLE (pCLE discussed below). The image for eCLE is more stable, since the suction channel immediately adjacent to the imaging window can be used to hold the tissue in direct contact. The ability to scan through variable depths (z-axis) and slightly higher resolution (<1 vs. 1 micron) are the further

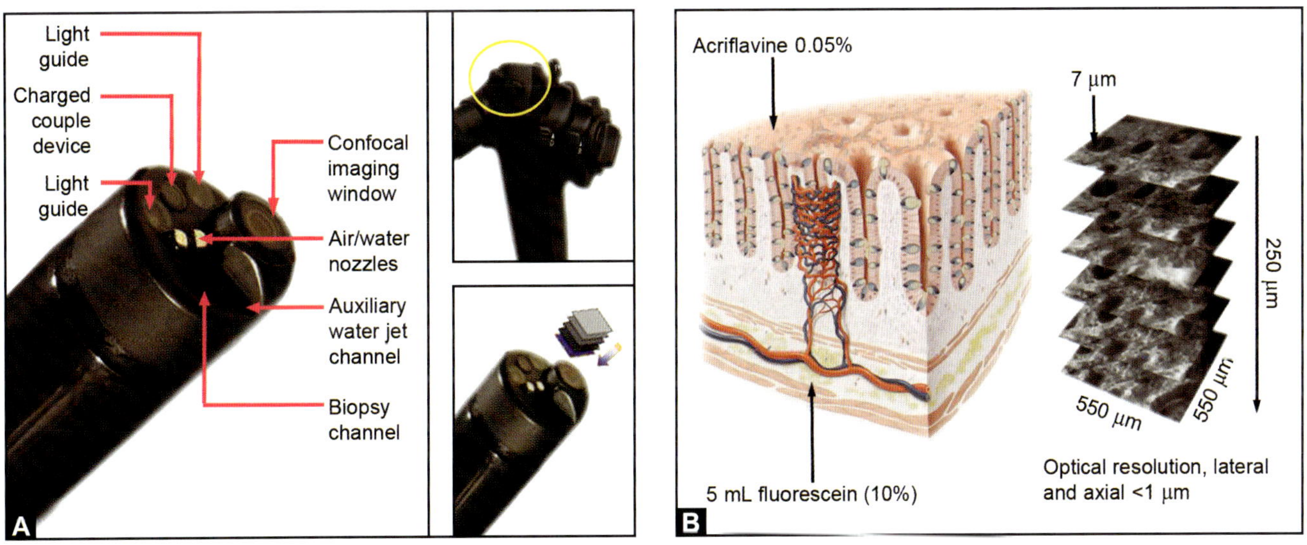

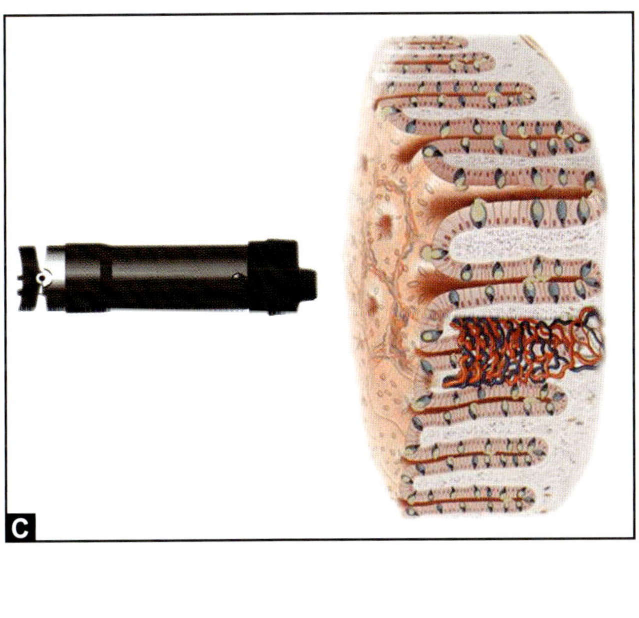

FIGURE 4-4 Integrated endoscopic confocal laser endomicroscopy system (eCLE, Pentax Corp, Japan). **A,** View of endoscope tip with integrated CLE optics. **B,** Representation of vertical "slices" as the eCLE system scans in the z-axis plane. **C,** Orientation of the eCLE system relative to the mucosa providing images parallel to the surface, unlike traditional histology which is perpendicular to the surface.

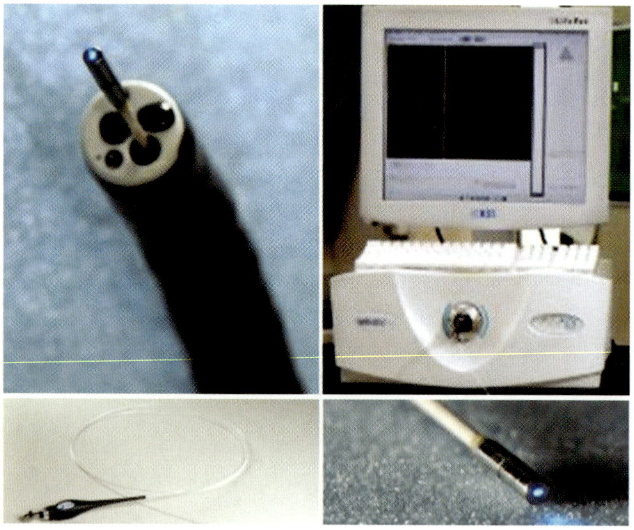

FIGURE 4-5 Probe-based confocal laser endomicroscopy (pCLE, Mauna Kea Technologies, France).

advantages. However, a limitation is the requirement of a dedicated confocal endoscope made by a single endoscope manufacturer. Thus, the decision to use confocal imaging in a particular case requires purchase of specific endoscopes, and use of these endoscopes in each case makes this system cumbersome in clinical practice. Initial studies using this system have reported very high accuracy (85–97%) for the detection of HGD in BE.[27-31]

The other confocal laser endomicroscopy system has been developed by Mauna Kea Technologies, France, which is based on a miniature laser probe (pCLE, figure 4-5). This probe is thin enough to be passed through the accessory channel of any endoscope, making it more practical and easy to use in clinical practice. This system also provides magnification of more than 1,000 times the normal for realtime endoscopic microscopy at fixed depths from 50 to 120 microns, depending on which probe is selected.[32] It has a smaller field of view (250 microns), which is partially overcome by post-procedure image reconstruction through a process called video mosaicking.[33] Both the systems utilize application of intravenous fluorescein or topical contrast agent, such as acriflavine or cresyl violet.

Pohl et al. conducted a prospective two-center, two-phase trial using a lower resolution, wider field (Z probe) pCLE during standard HRE to establish pCLE criteria for detection of Barrett's neoplasia, and subsequently to test these criteria on 296 biopsy sites in 38 consecutive patients with BE. pCLE showed a high negative predictive value for the diagnosis of endoscopically invisible neoplasia in BE. In a per biopsy analysis, sensitivity and specificity for two independent investigators were 75 and 88.8%; 75 and 91%, respectively, translating at best into a positive predictive value of 44.4% and a negative predictive value of 98.8%. Interobserver agreement was good (kappa 0.6).[34]

Wallace et al. evaluated the accuracy and inter-observer agreement of 9 international endoscopists in using the high definition (UHD) pCLE probe in patients with BE associated dysplasia. Forty BE sites were imaged with pCLE using high-definition probe-UHD and corresponding biopsies were obtained at 3 different centers from the US and Europe. The overall accuracy of pCLE for the diagnosis of HGD of the nine experts was 91%: sensitivity 88% and specificity 94% (75–100%). Of the 9 endoscopists, the 3 most experienced endomicroscopists had an overall accuracy of 97%: sensitivity 94% and specificity of 100%. The interobserver agreement for all 9 experts was very good (intraclass correlation coefficient 0.72; 95% CI 0.57–0.85).[35]

A large multicenter prospective trial comparing HRE with NBI to HE-NBI with pCLE by Sharma et al. has been presented in preliminary form at the Digestive Disease Week, 2010.[30] The study, called detection of neoplastic tissue in BE with *in vivo* probe-based confocal endoscopy (DON'T BIOPCE) showed that pCLE was significantly more sensitive (68 vs. 34%) and similarly specific (88 vs. 93%) than high-definition white light. Adding pCLE to WLE and NBI increased the sensitivity from 75 vs. 45% with similar specificity (84 vs. 88%). If used to replace random biopsy, the combination of WLE, NBI, and pCLE approach would allow a 39% reduction in biopsies and no patients would be missed with HGD.

A more recent single center study from Meining et al. evaluating pCLE alone (blinded to the endoscopic image) showed substantially lower accuracy using realtime interpretation of images in a low prevalence (typically surveillance) population.[31] The study raised concern about use of pCLE in a surveillance population. However, the image interpretation in routine clinical use is likely to combine imaging methods as was seen in the DON'T BIOPCE study (which included the same investigators).

Dunbar et al. designed a prospective double-blind randomized crossover study to evaluate the difference in diagnostic yields of eCLE with targeted biopsy and standard endoscopy with a 4-quadrant random biopsy in endoscopically unapparent BE-associated neoplasia. Thirty-nine patients of BE completed the study; 16 of which were suspected to have HGD, and 23 underwent surveillance for BE. CLE with targeted biopsy significantly improved the diagnostic yield for endoscopically unapparent BE neoplasia (33.7%) compared to a standard endoscopy with a random-biopsy protocol (17%) ($p < 0.01$). eCLE with targeted biopsy also resulted in 59% reduction in the number of biopsies needed per patient compared to standard endoscopy with a random biopsy protocol (9.8 vs. 23.8 biopsies) and allows some patients without neoplasia to completely forgo mucosal biopsy. Two-thirds of patients in the surveillance group did not need any mucosal biopsies at all during CLE examination.[36]

Kiesslich et al. evaluated the ability of CLE for detection of BE and associated neoplasia during ongoing HRE in 63 patients. Endomicroscopy allowed distinguishing between different types of epithelial cells and detected cellular and vascular changes in Barrett's epithelium. BE and associated neoplasia could be predicted with a sensitivity of 98.1 and 92.9%, specificity of 94.1 and 98.4%, respectively (accuracy of 96.8 and 97.4%). The mean kappa value for interobserver agreement for the prediction of histopathological diagnosis was very high (0.843) as was the intraobserver agreement (kappa 0.892).[27]

Overall, CLE appears to be highly promising as a method to guide biopsy and immediate treatment in high-risk populations, such as those referred for suspected dysplasia. In this setting, CLE can be used as an adjunct to HRE and other wide field image enhancement methods to localize regions for resection or targeted biopsy. Limited data do not yet support the routine use of CLE methods in low prevalence screening or surveillance populations.

AUTOFLUORESCENCE IMAGING

Autofluorescence imaging (AFI) is a technique that differentiates tissue types (normal vs. abnormal) based on their differences in fluorescence emission. The exposure of the tissue with light of a shorter wavelength leads to emission of a longer wavelength of light due to the excitation of endogenous biological substances (fluorophores). In the gastrointestinal tract, AFI can detect differences in the autofluorescence as a result of subtle changes in the concentration of these specific chemicals occurring as a result neoplastic proliferation. The molecules, which lead to tissue autofluorescence include nicotinamide adenine dinucleotide in reduced form, collagen, flavin, elastin, aromatic amino acids, and porphyrins. AFI uses blue light illumination to excite the tissue, producing a low-intensity autofluorescence that is detected through highly sensitive CCDs, along with reflectance imaging detected through nonintensified CCD.[37] The malignant transformation of tissue leads to emission of relatively longer wavelengths of light (shift from green toward the red end of the spectrum) due in to loss of collagen rich green fluorescing surface epithelium and increased concentrations of intrinsic biochemicals (porphyrins) with red fluorescence.[38,39] Earlier studies in which AFI was used with fiberoptic scopes were unable to show any differences when compared with WLE due to relative poor white light images.[20,40,41] However, in an uncontrolled study of 60 patients with BE, Kara et al. detected HGD in 22 patients. In six of these patients, WLE was unable to detect dysplastic lesions, but AFI did find those lesions. Therefore, AFI detected a significant number of patients with HGD, increasing the target detection rate from 63 to 91%. However, AFI testing was associated with a 51% false-positive rate, as 41 of 81 suspicious areas by AFI did not have dysplasia at biopsy, showing its poor specificity.[42]

An international multicentre study by Curvers et al. showed that the addition of AFI to HRE did increase the detection of both the number of lesions and the number of patients with early neoplasia in patients with BE. In this study, the false-positive rate of AFI was reduced by detailed inspection with NBI.[21] A multicenter randomized crossover trial of 130 patients compared the diagnostic accuracy of surveillance with AFI-guided plus 4-quadrant biopsies to the conventional approach. The investigators suggested that AFI-guided approach improved the diagnostic yield for neoplasia in comparison with the conventional approach using 4-quadrant biopsies. However, it was concluded that due to decreased sensitivity, AFI alone was not suitable for replacing the standard 4-quadrant biopsy protocol.[43]

SPECTROSCOPY

Unlike imaging-based methods, spectroscopy provides quantitative objective measures of how light interacts with tissue. Using a wide variety of light interactions, such as reflectance, scattering, and Raman, tissue properties can be determined and disease states, such as dysplasia can be inferred. Spectroscopy has the advantage of eliminating the need for image interpretation and inter-observer disagreement. A disadvantage is that it requires some trust in the system to interpret tissue (akin to flying an airplane by the "instruments"), whereas, most endoscopists prefer to base decision on live images and biopsy interpretation.

Light-scattering spectroscopy is a novel technique which uses the variation in scattered light across a full spectrum to obtain information about the size as well as number of nuclei of cellular layer.[38] This may detect mucosal abnormalities in realtime, using molecular and microstructural information in light-tissue interactions.[44] This technique has been reported to be very promising with high accuracy in detecting dysplasia in BE.[45,46] Epithelial cell nuclei are the primary targets of reflected light that is singly scattered, before it is collected by the probe. This imaging modality is a great breakthrough in technology, although more data and controlled studies are warranted for validation.

Reflectance spectroscopy quantitatively measures the color and intensity of reflected light after tissue illumination to differentiate normal from abnormal mucosa. Hemoglobin is the primary molecule that absorbs light and, on the basis of tissue oxygenation, provides information about the angiogenesis and dysplasia. Raman spectroscopy is a type of spectroscopy, which detects scattered light that has been slightly changed in wavelength (inelastic scattering) as a result of energy transfer between light and mucosa molecules. These shifts correspond to specific vibrations of molecular bonds. During this process, some of the energy is transferred to the molecules, so the light emitted back from the tissue is reduced in energy and has a longer wavelength. Raman spectra form multiple peaks and bands that produce detailed tissue characterization. However, due to weak Raman signal, near infrared light is typically used for excitation and sophisticated detection instruments, and signal processing computers are required. Raman spectroscopy has recently been applied to the detection of Barrett's-associated dysplasia with promising results.[47,48]

Studies by Mayinger et al.[49] and Bourg-Heckly et al.[50] reported high levels of accuracy in the identification of HGD in BE and early cancer by the use fluorescence spectroscopy.[50] von Holstein et al.[51] and Brand et al.[52] used exogenous fluorophores [photosensitizer porfimer sodium and photosensitizer 5-aminolevulinic acid (5-ALA)] to distinguish normal and dysplastic tissue in an *in vitro* study of esophagectomy specimens. Ortner et al. were able to enhance the features of dysplastic BE by combining time-resolved fluorescence spectroscopy and topical application of 5-ALA.[53] Trimodal spectroscopy is a novel technique, and few data are available. In their study, Georgakoudi et al. used trimodal spectroscopy and showed sensitivity and specificity to distinguish HGD from non-HGD in BE to be 100% and dysplastic vs. nondysplastic BE to be 93 and 100%, respectively.[45]

Spectroscopy methods, although very promising, are still not commercialized for routine use and, thus, should be considered investigational.

CONCLUSION AND THE FUTURE OF IMAGING FOR BARRETT'S ESOPHAGUS

Of the currently available enhancement modalities, HRE, NBI, and chromoendoscopy have shown clinical benefits: relatively practical, easy applicability, and widespread commercial availability of the equipment. These are widely used in routine clinical practice, especially in academic referral endoscopy centers and have been approved by FDA in the United States. FICE, spectroscopy, optical coherence tomography, and i-Scan have also passed regulatory approval and are currently under investigation for their clinical usefulness. CLE imaging is rapidly emerging as a useful tool in practice and is being aggressively studied.

Unresolved issues that need to be addressed involving some of these technologies include commercial availability, securing reimbursement for the required additional time, and imaging equipment as well as clarifying the medical-legal issues associated with image interpretation. In the long-term, the future of imaging for detection of dysplasia and early carcinoma is likely to be associated with the development of molecular targeting probes (such as monoclonal antibodies) that have been conjugated to dyes or nanoparticles. These sensitive and specific devices will serve as diagnostic molecular beacons as well as a delivery system for therapeutic agents.[44]

REFERENCES

1. Spechler SJ, Goyal RK. The columnar-lined esophagus, intestinal metaplasia, and Norman Barrett. *Gastroenterology.* 1996;110:614-21.
2. Guelrud M, Herrera I, Essenfeld H, Castro J. Enhanced magnification endoscopy: a new technique to identify specialized intestinal metaplasia in Barrett's esophagus. *Gastrointest Endosc.* 2001;53:559-65.
3. Sharma P, Weston AP, Topalovski M, Cherian R, Bhattacharyya A, Sampliner RE. Magnification chromoendoscopy for the detection of intestinal metaplasia and dysplasia in Barrett's oesophagus. *Gut.* 2003;52:24-7.
4. Lim CH, Rotimi O, Dexter SP, Axon AT. Randomized crossover study that used methylene blue or random 4-quadrant biopsy for the diagnosis of dysplasia in Barrett's esophagus. *Gastrointest Endosc.* 2006;64:195-9.
5. Wo JM, Ray MB, Mayfield-Stokes S, Al-Sabbagh G, Gebrail F, Slone SP, et al. Comparison of methylene blue-directed biopsies and conventional biopsies in the detection of intestinal metaplasia and dysplasia in Barrett's esophagus: a preliminary study. *Gastrointest Endosc.* 2001;54:294-301.
6. Amano Y, Kushiyama Y, Ishihara S, Yuki T, Miyaoka Y, Yoshino N, et al. Crystal violet chromoendoscopy with mucosal pit pattern diagnosis is useful for surveillance of

short-segment Barrett's esophagus. *Am J Gastroenterol.* 2005;100:21-6.

7. Ferguson DD, DeVault KR, Krishna M, Loeb DS, Wolfsen HC, Wallace MB. Enhanced magnification-directed biopsies do not increase the detection of intestinal metaplasia in patients with GERD. *Am J Gastroenterol.* 2006;101:1611-6.
8. Hoffman A, Kiesslich R, Bender A, Neurath MF, Nafe B, Herrmann G, et al. Acetic acid-guided biopsies after magnifying endoscopy compared with random biopsies in the detection of Barrett's esophagus: a prospective randomized trial with crossover design. *Gastrointest Endosc.* 2006;64:1-8.
9. Armstrong D. Review article: towards consistency in the endoscopic diagnosis of Barrett's oesophagus and columnar metaplasia. *Aliment Pharmacol Ther.* 2004;20:40-7.
10. Canto MI. Chromoendoscopy and magnifying endoscopy for Barrett's esophagus. *Clin Gastroenterol Hepatol.* 2005; 3:S12-5.
11. Canto MI, Kalloo A. Chromoendoscopy for Barrett's esophagus in the twenty-first century: to stain or not to stain? *Gastrointest Endosc.* 2006;64:200-5.
12. Ngamruengphong S, Sharma VK, Das A. Diagnostic yield of methylene blue chromoendoscopy for detecting specialized intestinal metaplasia and dysplasia in Barrett's esophagus: a meta-analysis. *Gastrointest Endosc.* 2009;69:1021-8.
13. Ormeci N, Savas B, Coban S, Palabiyikoðlu M, Ensari A, Kuzu I, et al. The usefulness of chromoendoscopy with methylene blue in Barrett's metaplasia and early esophageal carcinoma. *Surg Endosc.* 2008;22:693-700.
14. Olliver JR, Wild CP, Sahay P, Dexter S, Hardie LJ. Chromoendoscopy with methylene blue and associated DNA damage in Barrett's oesophagus. *Lancet.* 2003;362:373-4.
15. Sharma P, Bansal A, Mathur S, Wani S, Cherian R, McGregor D, et al. The utility of a novel narrow band imaging endoscopy system in patients with Barrett's esophagus. *Gastrointest Endosc.* 2006;64:167-75.
16. Gono K, Obi T, Yamaguchi M, Ohyama N, Machida H, Sano Y, et al. Appearance of enhanced tissue features in narrow-band endoscopic imaging. *J Biomed Opt.* 2004;9:568-77.
17. Anagnostopoulos GK, Yao K, Kaye P, Hawkey CJ, Ragunath K. Novel endoscopic observation in Barrett's oesophagus using high resolution magnification endoscopy and narrow band imaging. *Aliment Pharmacol Ther.* 2007;26:501-7.
18. Kara MA, Ennahachi M, Fockens P, ten Kate FJ, Bergman JJ. Detection and classification of the mucosal and vascular patterns (mucosal morphology) in Barrett's esophagus by using narrow band imaging. *Gastrointest Endosc.* 2006;64:155-66.
19. Kara MA, Peters FP, Rosmolen WD, Krishnadath KK, ten Kate FJ, Fockens P, et al. High-resolution endoscopy plus chromoendoscopy or narrow-band imaging in Barrett's esophagus: a prospective randomized crossover study. *Endoscopy.* 2005;37:929-36.
20. Kara MA, Smits ME, Rosmolen WD, Bultje AC, Ten Kate FJ, Fockens P, et al. A randomized crossover study comparing light-induced fluorescence endoscopy with standard videoendoscopy for the detection of early neoplasia in Barrett's esophagus. *Gastrointest Endosc.* 2005;61:671-8.
21. Curvers WL, Singh R, Song LM, Wolfsen HC, Ragunath K, Wang K, et al. Endoscopic tri-modal imaging for detection of early neoplasia in Barrett's oesophagus: a multi-centre feasibility study using high-resolution endoscopy, autofluorescence imaging and narrow band imaging incorporated in one endoscopy system. *Gut.* 2008;167:72.
22. Sharma P, Bansal A. Toward better imaging of Barrett's esophagus—see more, biopsy less! *Gastrointest Endosc.* 2006;64:188-92.
23. Gheorghe C. Narrow-band imaging endoscopy for diagnosis of malignant and premalignant gastrointestinal lesions. *J Gastrointestin Liver Dis.* 2006;15:77-82.
24. Wolfsen HC, Crook JE, Krishna M, Achem SR, Devault KR, Bouras EP, et al. Prospective, controlled tandem endoscopy study of narrow band imaging for dysplasia detection in Barrett's Esophagus. *Gastroenterology.* 2008;135:24-31.
25. Herrero LA, Curvers WL, Bansal A, Wani S, Kara M, Schenk E, et al. Zooming in on Barrett oesophagus using narrow-band imaging: an international observer agreement study. *Eur J Gastroenterol Hepatol.* 2009;21:1069-75.
26. Singh R, Karageorgiou H, Owen V, Garsed K, Fortun PJ, Fogden E, et al. Comparison of high-resolution magnification narrow-band imaging and white-light endoscopy in the prediction of histology in Barrett's oesophagus. *Scand J Gastroenterol.* 2009;44:85-92.
27. Kiesslich R, Gossner L, Goetz M, Dahlmann A, Vieth M, Stolte M, et al. In vivo histology of Barrett's esophagus and associated neoplasia by confocal laser endomicroscopy. *Clin Gastroenterol Hepatol.* 2006;4:979-87.
28. Polglase AL, McLaren WJ, Skinner SA, Kiesslich R, Neurath MF, Delaney PM. A fluorescence confocal endomicroscope for in vivo microscopy of the upper- and the lower-GI tract. *Gastrointest Endosc.* 2005;62:686-95.
29. Wallace MB, Sharma P, Lightdale C, Wolfsen H, Coron E, Buchner A, et al. Preliminary accuracy and interobserver agreement for the detection of intraepithelial neoplasia in Barrett's esophagus with probe-based confocal laser endomicroscopy. *Gastrointest Endosc.* 2010;72:19-24.
30. Sharma P, Meining A, Coron E, Lightdale CJ, Wolfsen HC, Bansal A, et al. Detection of neoplastic tissue in Barrett's Esophagus with in vivo probe-based confocal endomicroscopy (DONT BIOPCE). Final results of a prospective international RCT: image guided versus 4 quadrant random biopsies? *Gastroenterology.* 2010;138:S-155.
31. Bajbouj M, Vieth M, Rösch T, Miehlke S, Becker V, Anders M, Pohl H, et al. Probe-based confocal laser endomicroscopy compared with standard four quadrant biopsy for evaluation of neoplasia in Barrett's esophagus. *Endoscopy.* 2010;42:435-40.
32. Meining A, Saur D, Bajbouj M, Becker V, Peltier E, Höfler H, et al. In vivo histopathology for detection of gastrointestinal neoplasia with a portable, confocal miniprobe: an examiner blinded analysis. *Clin Gastroenterol Hepatol.* 2007;5:1261-7.

33. Becker V, Vercauteren T, von Weyhern CH, Prinz C, Schmid RM, Meining A. High-resolution miniprobe-based confocal microscopy in combination with video mosaicing (with video). *Gastrointest Endosc.* 2007;66:1001-7.
34. Pohl H, Rösch T, Vieth M, Koch M, Becker V, Anders M, et al. Miniprobe confocal laser microscopy for the detection of invisible neoplasia in patients with Barrett's oesophagus. *Gut.* 2008;57:1648-53.
35. Wallace MB. Accuracy and inter-observer agreement of experts for probe-based confocal laser endomicroscopy detection of dysplasia in Barrett's Esophagus. *Gastrointest Endosc.* 2009;69:AB351.
36. Dunbar KB, Canto MI. Confocal laser endomicroscopy in Barrett's esophagus and endoscopically inapparent Barrett's neoplasia: a prospective, randomized, double-blind, controlled, crossover trial. *Gastrointest Endosc.* 2010;72:668.
37. Kara M, DaCosta RS, Wilson BC, Marcon NE, Bergman J. Autofluorescence-based detection of early neoplasia in patients with Barrett's esophagus. *Dig Dis.* 2004;22:134-41.
38. Buchner AM, Wallace MB. Future expectations in digestive endoscopy: competition with other novel imaging techniques. *Best Pract Res Clin Gastroenterol.* 2008;22:971-87.
39. Reddymasu SC, Sharma P. Advances in endoscopic imaging of the esophagus. *Gastroenterol Clin North Am.* 2008;37:763-74.
40. Egger K, Werner M, Meining A, Ott R, Allescher HD, Höfler H, et al. Biopsy surveillance is still necessary in patients with Barrett's oesophagus despite new endoscopic imaging techniques. *Gut.* 2003;52:18-23.
41. Niepsuj K, Niepsuj G, Cebula W, ZieleŸnik W, Adamek M, Sielańczyk A, et al. Autofluorescence endoscopy for detection of high-grade dysplasia in short-segment Barrett's esophagus. *Gastrointest Endosc.* 2003;58:715-9.
42. Kara MA, Peters FP, Ten Kate FJ, Van Deventer SJ, Fockens P, Bergman JJ. Endoscopic video autofluorescence imaging may improve the detection of early neoplasia in patients with Barrett's esophagus. *Gastrointest Endosc.* 2005;61:679-85.
43. Borovicka J, Fischer J, Neuweiler J, Netzer P, Gschossmann J, Ehmann T, et al. Autofluorescence endoscopy in surveillance of Barrett's esophagus: a multicenter randomized trial on diagnostic efficacy. *Endoscopy.* 2006;38:867-72.
44. Wilson BC. Detection and treatment of dysplasia in Barrett's esophagus: a pivotal challenge in translating biophotonics from bench to bedside. *J Biomed Opt.* 2007; 12:051401.
45. Georgakoudi I, Jacobson BC, Van Dam J, Backman V, Wallace MB, Müller MG, et al. Fluorescence, reflectance, and light-scattering spectroscopy for evaluating dysplasia in patients with Barrett's esophagus. *Gastroenterology.* 2001;120:1620-9.
46. Wallace MB, Perelman LT, Backman V, Crawford JM, Fitzmaurice M, Seiler M, et al. Endoscopic detection of dysplasia in patients with Barrett's esophagus using light-scattering spectroscopy. *Gastroenterology.* 2000;119: 677-82.
47. Kendall C, Stone N, Shepherd N, Geboes K, Warren B, Bennett R, et al. Raman spectroscopy, a potential tool for the objective identification and classification of neoplasia in Barrett's oesophagus. *J Pathol.* 2003;200:602-9.
48. Wong Kee Song LM. Optical spectroscopy for the detection of dysplasia in Barrett's esophagus. *Clin Gastroenterol Hepatol.* 2005;3:S2-7.
49. Mayinger B, Horner P, Jordan M, Gerlach C, Horbach T, Hohenberger W, et al. Endoscopic fluorescence spectroscopy in the upper GI tract for the detection of GI cancer: initial experience. *Am J Gastroenterol.* 2001;96:2616-21.
50. Bourg-Heckly G, Blais J, Padilla JJ, Bourdon O, Etienne J, Guillemin F, et al. Endoscopic ultraviolet-induced autofluorescence spectroscopy of the esophagus: tissue characterization and potential for early cancer diagnosis. *Endoscopy.* 2000;32:756-65.
51. von Holstein CS, Nilsson AM, Andersson-Engels S, Willén R, Walther B, Svanberg K. Detection of adenocarcinoma in Barrett's oesophagus by means of laser induced fluorescence. *Gut.* 1996;39:711-6.
52. Brand S, Wang TD, Schomacker KT, Poneros JM, Lauwers GY, Compton CC, et al. Detection of high-grade dysplasia in Barrett's esophagus by spectroscopy measurement of 5-aminolevulinic acid-induced protoporphyrin IX fluorescence. *Gastrointest Endosc.* 2002;56:479-87.
53. Ortner MA, Ebert B, Hein E, Zumbusch K, Nolte D, Sukowski U, et al. Time gated fluorescence spectroscopy in Barrett's oesophagus. *Gut.* 2003;52:28-33.

5 Endoscopic Eradication Therapies for Barrett's Neoplasia

Oliver Pech, Gary W Falk

ABSTRACT

The risk of esophageal adenocarcinoma increases with higher grades of dysplasia specifically high-grade intraepithelial neoplasia (HGIN) that warrants endoscopic treatment. Endoscopic treatment techniques include photodynamic therapy (PDT), radiofrequency ablation (RFA), cryoablation, argon plasma coagulation (APC), multipolar electrocoagulation (MPEC), endoscopic resection (ER), and endoscopic submucosal dissection (ESD). The choice of endoscopic treatment technique depends upon the stage and extent of Barrett's neoplasia, the presence of visible lesion, and the availability of expertise and equipment. These modalities are safe and very effective in maintaining complete remission comparable to surgery. In this chapter, we will discuss the different endoscopic treatment strategies for Barrett's neoplasia in detail.

INTRODUCTION

There is a wide armamentarium of endoscopic treatment techniques available for eradication of early Barrett's neoplasia. Some of them have never found wide acceptance, some of them, like photodynamic therapy (PDT), emerged and disappeared, and some became more and more popular in recent years [e.g., endoscopic resection (ER) and radiofrequency ablation (RFA)]. Like most fields in medicine, there is no single treatment method for all different indications such as low-grade and high-grade intraepithelial neoplasia, and early Barrett's cancer. This chapter provides an overview on different endoscopic eradication therapies of early Barrett's neoplasia.

INDICATIONS FOR ENDOSCOPIC TREATMENT

Nondysplastic Barrett's Esophagus

The choice of treatment method in patients with Barrett's esophagus is highly dependent on different stages of the disease. Nondysplastic Barrett's esophagus should not be ablated for several reasons. First, ablative techniques are associated with complications. Therefore, their use is not justified, given the overall cancer risk in patients with Barrett's esophagus is approximately 0.5–0.6% per year.[1,2] Secondly, complete ablation of Barrett's epithelium cannot be guaranteed. Thirdly, there are no data whatsoever that ablation has the potential to further reduce the already small risk of malignant progression. Moreover, recurrence of Barrett's epithelium cannot be excluded even after complete eradication.[3] Therefore, follow-up endoscopies would still be necessary. For these reasons, ablation of nondysplastic Barrett's esophagus should only be performed within the context of prospective clinical trials at the present time.

RFA has been studied for both nondysplastic and dysplastic Barrett's esophaguses. Sharma et al. described their 12-month results on the outcome of circumferential RFA of nondysplastic Barrett's epithelium in 70 patients and achieved complete elimination of intestinal metaplasia without any buried glands in 69% of subjects.[4] Subsequently, long-term follow-up for up to 30 months after additional focal RFA demonstrated complete elimination of metaplasia in 97% of patients.[5] No buried intestinal metaplasia was encountered in any of the biopsy specimens at 12 and 30 months. The preliminary results of 5-year follow-up of 50 treated nondysplastic patients report maintenance of remission of intestinal metaplasia in 92% of these patients.[6] Adverse events, most of which were minor, were encountered in 15.1% after the circumferential ablation phase of the study and 2.6% after the focal ablation phase of the study. Any post-ablation symptoms were resolved within 4 days of the procedure.

Barrett's Esophagus with Neoplastic Lesions

Once any grade of dysplasia is found in a patient with Barrett's esophagus, the pendulum swings from surveillance to endoscopic eradication therapies. In individuals with low-grade intraepithelial neoplasia (LGIN), progression to high-grade intraepithelial neoplasia (HGIN) is observed in up to 85% of cases.[7,8] However, a major concern with LGIN is its difficult histological diagnosis. Frequently, regenerative changes are overdiagnosed as LGIN, and therefore, a second opinion by a GI expert pathologist should always be sought.[8] In a study from the Wiesbaden group, histological slides of 50 patients with the referral diagnosis of LGIN were reviewed by two independent expert pathologists blinded for the primary diagnosis; 50% of LGIN diagnoses were considered incorrect.[9] Overdiagnosis was made in 42% and an underdiagnosis was suggested in 8% (1 HGIN and 3 adenocarcinomas). The Amsterdam group nicely demonstrated that LGIN is often overdiagnosed by nonexpert pathologists.[8] The natural history of LGIN in a large community-based cohort of patients with Barrett's esophagus was investigated after the original histological diagnosis was reviewed by a panel of expert pathologists. After the primary histological slides were reviewed, 85% of the diagnoses of 147 patients with LGIN made by the community-based pathologist were downstaged to nondysplastic Barrett's esophagus or indefinite for dypslasia. The diagnosis of LGIN was considered to be correct in 15% of patients only. Interestingly, for patients with a consensus diagnosis of LGIN, the cumulative risk for progression to HGIN or cancer was 85% after 109 months compared to 4.6% after 107 months for patients downstaged to nondysplastic Barrett's esophagus. These findings highlight the importance of obtaining a second opinion by an expert pathologist in the field of Barrett's esophagus, especially, in case of LGIN, to correctly stratify the risk of progression to higher grades of dysplasia. In case of confirmed LGIN on biopsy, an ER should be performed, if a visible lesion is present, since LGIN is often contiguous to lesions with higher grades of dysplasia. However, in many patients, LGIN cannot be relocalized. In those situations, both, follow-up endoscopies or ablative treatment can be performed. Till date, one study has examined RFA vs. a strategy of continued surveillance in patients with LGIN.[10] This randomized sham control study demonstrated complete resolution of low-grade dysplasia in 91% of the treatment group compared to 23% of the sham group using a combination of the circumferential and focal probes at 1-year follow-up. Progression to HGIN occurred in 4.8% of the treatment group compared to 13.6% of the sham group.

There is a wide agreement that HGIN is an indication for endoscopic treatment, since patients with HGIN harbor an increased risk of the disease progressing to cancer, with yearly rates of up to 19%.[10] A recent systematic review found that endoscopic ablation reduces the rate of cancer progression from 65.8 to 16.76/1000 years.[11] In addition, HGIN is very often located next to cancer lesions, and adenocarcinoma is diagnosed in the resected specimen after ER or surgery in up to 40% of cases.

Mucosal Barrett's adenocarcinoma should also be treated endoscopically. It is well-known that these patients have almost no risk of lymph node metastasis, and cancer is limited to the mucosal layer (T1m1-4). Therefore, endoscopic treatment can be considered as curative in these lesions.[12-14] However, in cases of deep submucosal invasion, lymphatic (L1), or blood vessel infiltration (V1), radical surgical resection should be performed, since there is an increased risk for lymph node metastasis in these cases.[15,16] It is yet not clear, whether cancers limited to the upper submucosal layer (sm1) are eligible for ER. Surgical series suggest that patients with sm1 Barrett's cancer have a very low-risk of lymph node metastasis. However, studies with larger patient numbers reporting on the endoscopic treatment of patients with incipient submucosal cancer are still awaited.[9,10] The Wiesbaden group has recently published a series on ER in these patients. They were able to demonstrate that ER appears to be safe in patients with low-risk submucosal cancer (defined as: T1sm1, G1-2, L0, V0, macroscopic type I or IIa,b). All 21 patients in this series were treated by ER.[15] One patient opted for surgery and one patient died before complete remission could be achieved. The cause of death was not tumor-related. After a mean of 2.9 ER and 5.3 months, 18 out of the remaining 19 patients achieved complete remission. Recurrent or metachronous neoplasia was detected in 5 patients after a mean follow-up of 62 months. Repeat endoscopic treatment was successful in all of these patients. The 5-year overall survival rate was 66%. There was no tumor-related death in this series. These promising results suggest that ER may have a potential in low-risk submucosal Barrett's cancer in a highly experienced center. However, a recently published retrospective analysis of histological samples after esophagectomy from 80 patients with submucosal Barrett's cancer showed that 12.9% of patients with Tsm1

Barrett's cancer had metastatic lymph nodes.[16] Final conclusions cannot be made on this issue currently, and further studies are needed in order to give final recommendations based on a wider evidence.

ABLATIVE TREATMENT METHODS FOR EARLY BARRETT'S NEOPLASIA

All ablative treatment methods have in common that they do not provide a specimen of the neoplastic lesion. Thus, exact histological confirmation of the infiltration, depth, and probable presence of infiltration of lymph vessels (L-status) or blood vessels (V-status) cannot be connected. When treating neoplasia with one of the available ablative treatment modalities, a possible problem will be the underestimation of the neoplastic lesion, and the endoscopist might end up treating a submucosal carcinoma or cancer infiltrating lymph vessels. Unfortunately, there is no pretherapeutic diagnostic method available that enables the endoscopist to accurately predict infiltration and depth of neoplasia. Endoscopic ultrasound (EUS) has been considered as the most accurate diagnostic tool. However, recent studies demonstrate that EUS and even miniprobe EUS cannot accurately differentiate between mucosal and submucosal disease.[17,18] Therefore, all visible and detectable lesions within the Barrett's segment should be treated by ER to provide optimal staging information.

Argon Plasma Coagulation

Argon plasma coagulation (APC) is a noncontact thermal technique using ionized argon gas to deliver a monopolar high frequency current in order to coagulate tissue (Figure 5-1). In the majority of all published studies, APC was used to ablate nondysplastic Barrett's esophagus. However, there are several series that have investigated its use in patients with LGIN and/or HGIN. Attwood et al. treated 29 patients with HGIN at an energy setting of 70 watts.[19] After a median of 2 treatment sessions, complete remission was achieved in 86% (25 of 29 patients). After a mean follow-up of 38 months, recurrence or progression was observed in 4 out of 25 patients (16%). In a further study by Ragunath et al., 26 patients with LGIN (n = 23) and HGIN (n = 3) were randomized to treatment with APC or PDT with photofrin, respectively.[20] The dysplasia eradication rate at 12 months was 67% in the APC arm and 77% in the PDT arm. A mean of 5 APC treatment sessions at 65 watts were performed. PDT was more effective but also more expensive than APC. Complications of APC include strictures and bleedings. Perforations after APC are rarely observed. A major problem of APC seems to be subsquamous Barrett's epithelium (buried Barrett's), found in 5–25% of patients.[19,20] Currently, APC has no role in the primary ablation of Barrett's esophagus but may be considered for touch up of areas after circumferential ER.

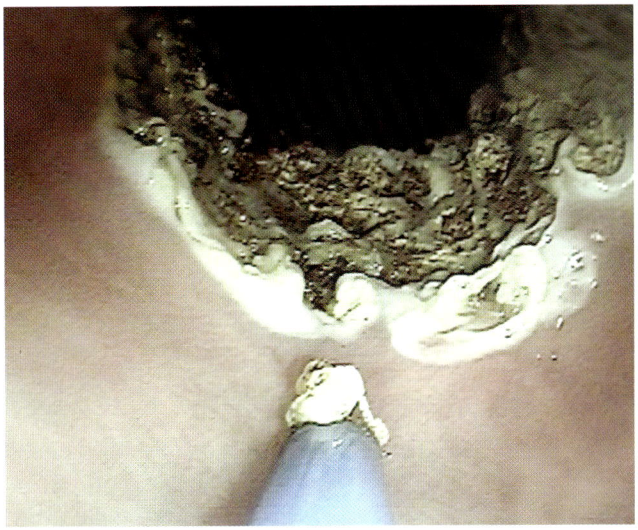

FIGURE 5-1 Ablation of remaining Barrett's epithelium with argon plasma coagulation.

Multipolar Electrocoagulation

Sharma et al. published a prospective randomized trial where they compared APC and multipolar electrocoagulation (MPEC) for ablation of nondysplastic Barrett's esophagus in 35 patients.[21] They described a comparable complete remission rate of Barrett's esophagus in both groups (75 vs. 63%; p = 0.49). The investigators were not able to identify any predictors associated with achieving complete reversal of Barrett's epithelium.

These clinical trials have highlighted the difficulty in obtaining complete endoscopic and histologic ablation with APC and MPEC.[19-21] Studies of these techniques routinely found incomplete macroscopic regression of the Barrett's segment and buried intestinal metaplasia beneath the neosquamous epithelium, which not surprisingly, led to reports of subsquamous cancers developing in patients with previously nondysplastic Barrett's epithelium.[22-24] As such, it appears that techniques, such as MPEC, the heater probe, and APC have all fallen by the wayside. The reasons that these techniques are likely to have no long-term future include difficulty in obtaining uniform ablation, cost, side effects, and persistent endoscopically evident or microscopic columnar epithelium after therapy. The only conceivable place at present for techniques, such as MPEC and APC is for smaller islands and areas of residual Barrett's esophagus after treatment with another more effective modality, e.g., ER.

Cryotherapy

Cryotherapy freezes the gut mucosa to induce cell death. There are two current techniques:

1. Carbon dioxide
2. Liquid nitrogen.

However, very limited data are available till date for either of these methods, and there are no randomized controlled trials. Johnston et al. treated 11 patients with liquid nitrogen with complete endoscopic and histologic reversal in 7 of the 11 patients at 6 months.[25] A case series reported on 26 patients with high-grade dysplasia and Barrett's cancer who were deemed inoperable or refused surgery were treated with liquid nitrogen, of whom 32% were dysplasia free at 12 months of follow-up.[26] The largest experience with liquid nitrogen cyrotherapy is a retrospective study of 60 patients with high-grade dysplasia who completed therapy of the Barrett's segment.[27] At a mean follow-up of 10.5 months, 97% had complete eradication of high-grade dysplasia, 87% had complete eradication of all dysplasia, and 57% had complete eradication of intestinal metaplasia. Buried subsquamous intestinal metaplasia was encountered in 3%. The side effect profile was excellent with no serious adverse events and strictures in 3%.

It appears that cryotherapy has the potential as a simple and relatively inexpensive ablation option. However, a number of concerns remain, including uncertainty regarding optimal dosimetry, technique, limited number of patients studied, short-term follow-up, and lack of comparisons of carbon dioxide vs. liquid nitrogen based techniques. Furthermore, the uneven application inherent in spraying of the cryogen rather than direct balloon based application to isolated segments of the esophagus raises concerns regarding controlled depth of injury.

Photodynamic Therapy

PDT is a process in which a light sensitive drug concentrates in neoplastic tissue. The drug is activated by laser light of an appropriate wavelength directed at the abnormal tissue producing a cytotoxic substance, singlet oxygen, which selectively damages neoplastic tissue. PDT in Barrett's esophagus has involved a variety of different agents, including porfimer sodium, hematoporphyrin derivative and 5-aminolevulinic acid (5-ALA). Each of these compounds is characterized by a different depth of tissue destruction and duration of cutaneous photosensitivity. Only porfimer sodium sodium is available in the US.

PDT has been successfully used to treat early neoplasia in Barrett's esophagus for many years and is one of the best investigated ablation techniques.[28-36] A randomized controlled study evaluated PDT with porfimer sodium compared to a strategy of continued surveillance for patients with high-grade dysplasia.[31] At two years, complete ablation of high-grade dysplasia occurred in 77% of the PDT group compared to 39% of patients in the surveillance group with progression to cancer in 13 and 28%, respectively. Importantly, complete elimination of all intestinal metaplasia and dysplasia occurred in only 52% of the PDT group and 7% of the surveillance group with common complications like strictures occurred in 36% and photosensitivity in 69%. At five years, the probability of complete ablation of high-grade dysplasia after PDT was only 48% and progression to cancer occurred in 15%.[32] However, work from the Mayo Clinic found that high-grade dysplasia patients treated with PDT, with or without concomitant endoscopic mucosal resection, had long-term survival comparable to patients treated with esophagectomy and low-rates of cancer-associated death.[33]

A major concern of PDT in patients with HGIN and cancer is the squamous overgrowth of incompletely treated neoplastic lesions after ablation. However, a recent prospective randomized study was able to show that there was no significant difference in squamous overgrowth between patients treated by PDT or receiving omeprazole alone and more importantly, the highest grade of neoplasia was not found exclusively beneath squamous mucosa in any patient.[37]

However, PDT has several disadvantages leading to a dramatic decrease of its use; PDT with porfimer sodium is expensive and is associated with a high complication rate. Photosensitivity and stricture formation occur in up to 30% of patients and are important drawbacks of this method.[31] Recent studies were able to identify the following risk factors for stricture formation: multiple PDT courses, longer length of Barrett's esophagus, presence of intramucosal carcinoma, ER before PDT, and prior history of esophageal stricture.[38,39] The use of 5-ALA acid as a photosensitizer for PDT is associated with considerably fewer complications and showed promising short- and long-term results.[28,30] Given the advent of other techniques with a more favorable side effect profile, PDT appears to have a limited role today.

Radiofrequency Ablation

Due to several reasons, in recent years, PDT of Barrett's epithelium has been replaced by RFA in most centers. it involves the application of high power radiofrequency energy using bipolar electrodes, thereby, causing rapid heating of the tissue with ablation to a depth of approximately 0.5 mm. A balloon catheter 3 cm in length with circular electrodes delivering the energy designed for circumferential ablation (HALO-360) is used for long segments of Barrett's epithelium. A focal device (HALO-90) that fits over the tip of the endoscope is also available and can be used for ablation of smaller areas.

In an US multicenter registry with 16 centers, the safety and efficacy of RFA in patients with HGIN in Barrett's esophagus was investigated in 142 patients.[40] The median Barrett-length was 6 cm. An ER prior to RFA was permitted in this study. During follow-up, only 1 patient developed a stricture and no buried Barrett's epithelium was found. Complete ablation of HGIN could be confirmed in 90.2% out of 92 patients with at least one follow-up endoscopy. However, the eradication rate of Barrett's epithelium was only 54.3%.

The efficacy of RFA was investigated in a large prospective randomized sham controlled trial in 127 patients with LGIN (n = 63) and HGIN (n = 64). The study was conducted in 19 US centers. Patients were randomized to RFA or sham treatment in a 2:1 fashion. After one year, 74% of patients in the RFA arm achieved complete remission of Barrett's metaplasia compared to none in patients randomized into the sham arm. HGIN was successfully ablated by RFA in 81% (34 out of 42 patients). In contrast, none of the patients in the sham arm had clearance of HGIN. RFA was also able to reduce the rate of neoplasia progression from HGIN to cancer. The results of this study demonstrate that RFA is more effective than proton-pump inhibitors (PPI) alone, but a HGIN eradication rate of 81% after one year was too low to recommend this method alone for treatment of HGIN. The question arises whether the treated lesions were real HGIN or Barrett's cancer incorrectly diagnosed on biopsy samples.

ER of visible neoplastic lesions combined with RFA of the remaining Barrett's esophagus containing HGIN in 23 patients was investigated in two recently published studies from the Amsterdam group.[41,42] RFA without prior ER was performed in 10 patients with flat lesions containing HGIN. Barrett's metaplasia and neoplasia was successfully ablated by RFA in all the 23 patients included in this study. Subsquamous Barrett's esophagus was found in none of the 836 biopsies of the neosquamous mucosa.

RFA seems to provide a high rate of complete Barrett's eradication without residual Barrett's mucosa underneath the newly developed squamous epithelium ("buried glands"). A major advantage of RFA to PDT seems to be the low complication rate. RFA of the remaining non-dysplastic Barrett's epithelium should be performed after successful ER of localizable HGIN and adenocarcinoma. ER of all neoplastic lesions provides a histological specimen that can be evaluated by the pathologist. They can provide important information regarding infiltration, depth, and risk factors for lymphatic metastasis in order to prevent under-treatment. Afterwards, ablation of the nondysplastic Barrett's mucosa can significantly reduce the rate of metachronous neoplasia or recurrences.[43] This strategy was followed in a recently published prospective study. Pouw et al. treated 16 patients with adenocarcinoma and 7 patients with HGIN in the EURO-I study.[44] ER was performed for all visible lesions followed by RFA of the remaining Barrett's segment. Neoplasia and intestinal metaplasia were eradicated in 95 and 88% of patients, respectively, after a median follow-up of 22 months. Recruitment of the EURO-II study with more than 140 patients treated by the same protocol has just ended, and results are eagerly awaited.

Taken together with other data on RFA, the investigators now know and a combination of circumferential and focal probes provides the optimal results, and this technique can be safely combined with endoscopic mucosal resection, preexisting genetic abnormalities resolve, and buried intestinal metaplasia appears to be rare. It is also known that this method does not completely eliminate cancer risk or progression of low-grade dysplasia to high-grade dysplasia. As with other ablative techniques other than endoscopic mucosal resection, RFA does not allow tissue confirmation, leaving a measure of uncertainty for each patient. Only a limited number of patients have been studied till date, and we still do not know about the long durability of this technique.

ENDOSCOPIC RESECTION

ER is a therapeutic option for patients with either high-grade dysplasia or intramucosal carcinoma in the setting of appropriate risk stratification. ER permits accurate histological staging of neoplasia arising in Barrett's epithelium when compared to ER specimens. Negative margins on ER specimens correlate well with the absence of residual disease at the time of surgery, but submucosal involvement is associated both with residual disease at the time of surgery and lymph node metastases. Methods of ER are snare resection with prior submucosal injection, the widely used suck and cut technique, either with a cap or a ligation device, and endoscopic submucosal dissection (ESD).

Until recently, few studies with large patient numbers or long follow-up were available for ER. Excellent long-term results for ER in 100 consecutive patients with low-risk mucosal Barrett's cancer [(lesion diameter <20 mm and macroscopically type I (polypoid), IIa (flat and slightly elevated), or IIb (flat and level), IIc (flat depressed <10 mm); well or moderately differentiated histologic grade; lesions limited to the mucosa proven by histology of the resected specimens; and no invasion of lymph vessels or veins)] have been provided by the Wiesbaden group.[14] Complete remission of adenocarcinoma was achieved in 99% of patients. The calculated 5-year overall survival rate was 98%. Metachronous neoplasias were detected in only 11% after a mean of 36.7 months. There were no tumor-related deaths in this series. A disadvantage of this series was that treatment was performed in a highly selected cohort of patients. All patients were treated for low-risk Barrett's carcinoma. This did not reflect the general population of patients with Barrett's neoplasia. However, it clearly demonstrated the safety and efficacy of ER in an expert center. The results with regard to the complete response rate and recurrence rate were not quite as good in a general patient population with HGIN and mucosal Barrett's cancer, with the majority not fulfilling low-risk criteria (Table 5-1).[14,43] Recently, the so far largest series on endoscopic treatment of high-grade dysplasia (n = 61) and mucosal adenocarcinoma (n = 288) in 349 patients was published by Pech et al.[43] ER was performed in 279 patients, PDT with 5-ALA as a photosensitizer in 55 patients, and both methods were combined in 13 patients. Majority (96.6%) of patients achieved complete remission, but metachronous neoplasia was detected in 21.5% of patients during a follow-up of more than 5 years. Endoscopic retreatment was successful in most of these patients and long-term complete response could be achieved in 94.5%. Long-term survival of patients treated for Barrett's neoplasia in this series did not differ significantly from that of the normal German population, with the same age and gender distribution.

Above results clearly demonstrated that ER is safe and effective in patients with high-grade dysplasia (HGD) and mucosal Barrett's cancer even on long-term follow-up. Major problem of endoscopic treatment are local recurrences or metachronous lesions, although retreatment is successful in almost all patients. The reason for the high rate of recurrence appears to be related to the fact that the residual Barrett's metaplasia seems to have an increased risk of malignant transformation due to genetic abnormalities. Those cannot be influenced by focal ER. Table 5-2 illustrates the risk factors for recurrence that have been identified.[43] An important finding in this study was that ablative therapy of the remaining nondysplastic Barrett's epithelium after ER can significantly reduce recurrence rate. This was also confirmed in a prospective randomized trial by the Wiesbaden group comparing ER of Barrett's cancer followed by ablation of the nondysplastic Barrett's epithelium with APC and follow-up.[45] These data clearly show that ablation of the remaining nondysplastic Barrett's epithelium after successful ER of all detectable

TABLE 5-1 Low-risk Criteria for Early Barrett's Cancer

- Cancer limited to the mucosal layer
- Well or moderate differentiation grade (G1 and G2)
- Size ≤2 cm for macroscopic types I, IIa, IIb
- Size ≤1 cm for macroscopic type IIc
- No lymph vessel infiltration (L0)
- No blood vessel infiltration (V0)
- No ulceration (macroscopic type III)

(All criteria have to be fulfilled)

TABLE 5-2 Risk Factors for Recurrence after Endoscopic Resection of Early Barrett's Neoplasia

Variables	*Relative risk (95% CI)*	*p*
Long-segment Barrett's esophagus	1.9 (1.06–3.3)	0.03
Time until CLR achieved >10 months	0.3 (0.12–0.75)	0.009
Piecemeal resection	2.44 (1.13–4.89)	0.02
Multifocal neoplasia	2.1 (1.16–3.99)	0.01
No ablative therapy of BE after CLR	2.5 (0.26–0.66)	0.0003

BE, Barrett's esophagus; CLR, complete local remission.
From Pech O, Behrens A, May A, Nachbar L, Gossner L, Rabenstein T, et al. Long-term results and risk factor analysis for recurrence after curative endoscopic therapy in 349 patients with high-grade intraepithelial neoplasia and mucosal adenocarcinoma in Barrett's oesophagus. *Gut*. 2008;57:1200-6.

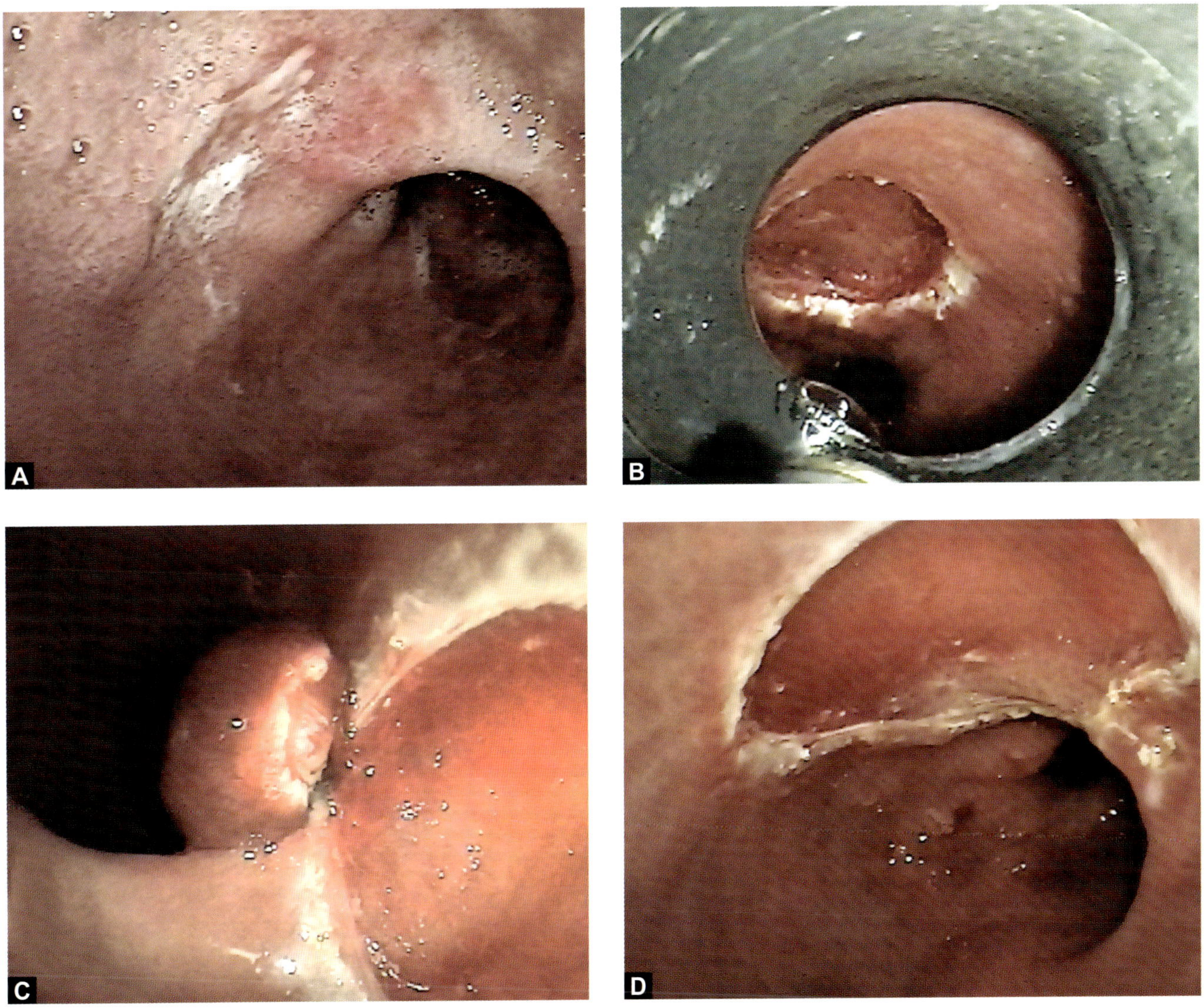

FIGURE 5-2 Endoscopic resection of a mucosal Barrett's cancer with a reusable ligation device.

neoplastic lesions can significantly reduce the rate of metachronous neoplasia and is an important part of the whole treatment concept (Figure 5-2).

Complete Circumferential Endoscopic Resection

A further concept to remove the whole Barrett epithelium in order to reduce the rate of recurrent neoplasia after successful ER is complete circumferential ER. Studies to date suggest that complete ER results in complete remission of intraepithelial neoplasia and Barrett's esophagus in 75–100% of patients. Chennat et al. published the largest US series on circumferential ER till date. They studied 33 patients with HGD and 16 patients with mucosal cancer.[46] Complete elimination of neoplasia and Barrett's epithelium was achieved in all except 1 of the 32 patients who completed treatment. However, esophageal stenosis developed in 37% of patients, all of whom could be managed endoscopically. No other severe complications were observed.

A recently published multicenter study from Europe provides the largest experience with circumferential ER. A total of 169 patients with high-grade dysplasia or early carcinoma in Barrett's esophagus with a segment length <5 cm underwent radical ER of their Barrett's segment. Neoplasia was eliminated in 97.6% of cases, and intestinal metaplasia in 85.2%.[47] After a median of 27 months of follow-up, remission of neoplasia was maintained in

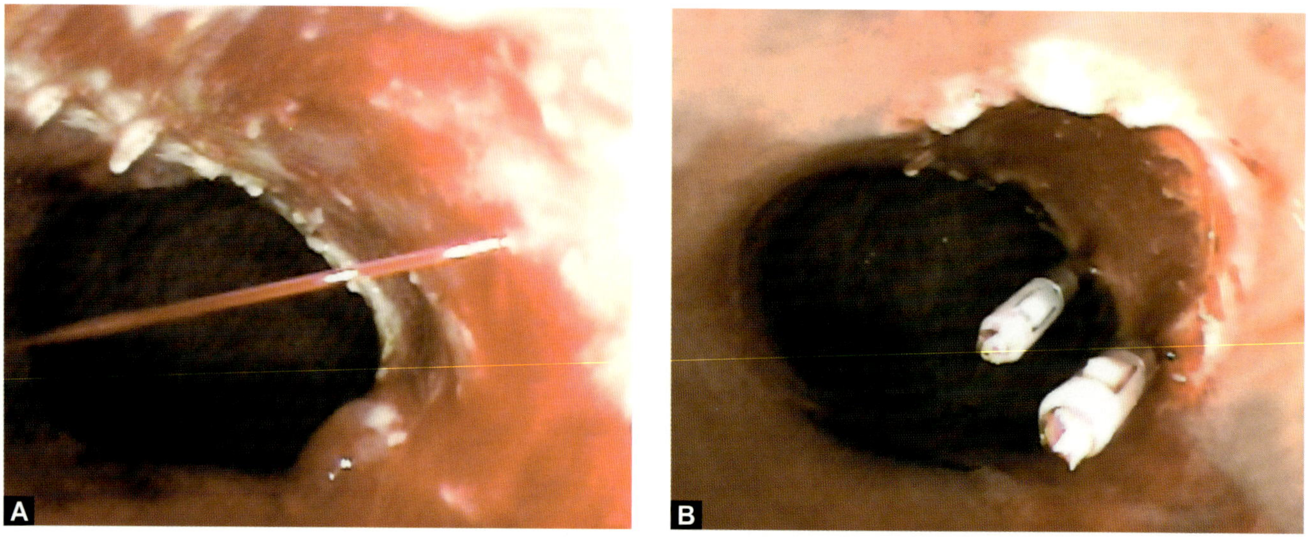

FIGURE 5-3 Complications of endoscopy resection. **A,** Bleeding following endoscopy resection. **B,** Use of clips to control bleeding.

97.5% and remission of intestinal metaplasia in 85%. Metachronous neoplasia was detected in 1.8% of patients. Complications were perforation in 1%, delayed bleeding in 1% (Figure 5-3), and strictures requiring dilation in 50% of the study population. Importantly, the most advanced histologic findings were always encountered at the initial ER session, where the most suspicious lesion was removed first.

Recent work from Australia included 75 patients with HGIN (n = 67) and mucosal Barrett's carcinoma (n = 8) treated by circumferential ER.[48] The complete remission rate of neoplasia was 94 and 11% developed metachronous lesions. The stricture rate was only 8% in this series. Interestingly, ER changed staging in 48% of patients: 17 patients with HGIN were downstaged to LGIN or nondysplastic Barrett's esophagus. More importantly, 8 patients with the biopsy diagnosis of HGIN had mucosal and 5 had submucosal adenocarcinoma in the ER specimen. These results again highlight the importance of ER in all detectable neoplastic lesions rather than simply ablating them.

One of the major advantages of radical ER of neoplastic Barrett's esophagus is the possibility that the whole Barrett's segment can be evaluated by the pathologist in order to detect and stage even endoscopically inapparent neoplasia. One major disadvantage of circumferential ER of the whole Barrett's segment is the high stricture rate associated with this method requiring repeated dilatation. Therefore, a combination of ER of all visible neoplastic lesions followed by ablation of the residual Barrett's epithelium seems to be the best treatment strategy at present (Figure 5-4). The positive effect of tissue acquisitions combined with a low complication rate associated with ablation.[43-45] The risk for recurrence of metachronous neoplasia is attenuated but cannot be fully eliminated by this treatment strategy and long-term follow-up is still necessary.

Endoscopic Submucosal Dissection

There is almost no experience with ESD in patients with early Barrett's neoplasia. A small study by Kakushima et al. reported on ESD in 30 patients with tumors of the esophagogastric junction.[49] Only 4 patients had early Barrett's cancer. The average maximum diameters of the lesions and resected specimens were 22.4 mm and 40.6 mm, respectively. The vertical and lateral margins were free of neoplasia in 97% (29 of 30) patients. Histology revealed lymph vessel invasion in 5 patients and submucosal infiltration of more than 500 μm was detected also in 5 cases. Another series from Japan reported on ESD of superficial adenocarcinoma of the esophagogastric junction.[50] ESD was performed in 25 cancers in 24 patients. The en bloc resection rate was 100% in this series, but only 72% of lesions were judged as curative resection. During a median follow-up of 30.1 months, no recurrences were observed in this cohort.

A Belgium group performed a prospective randomized trial comparing cap ER with ESD in patients with early Barrett's neoplasia. This has so far only been published in an abstract form.[51] Twenty-five patients were included in each group. Piecemeal ER was performed in larger

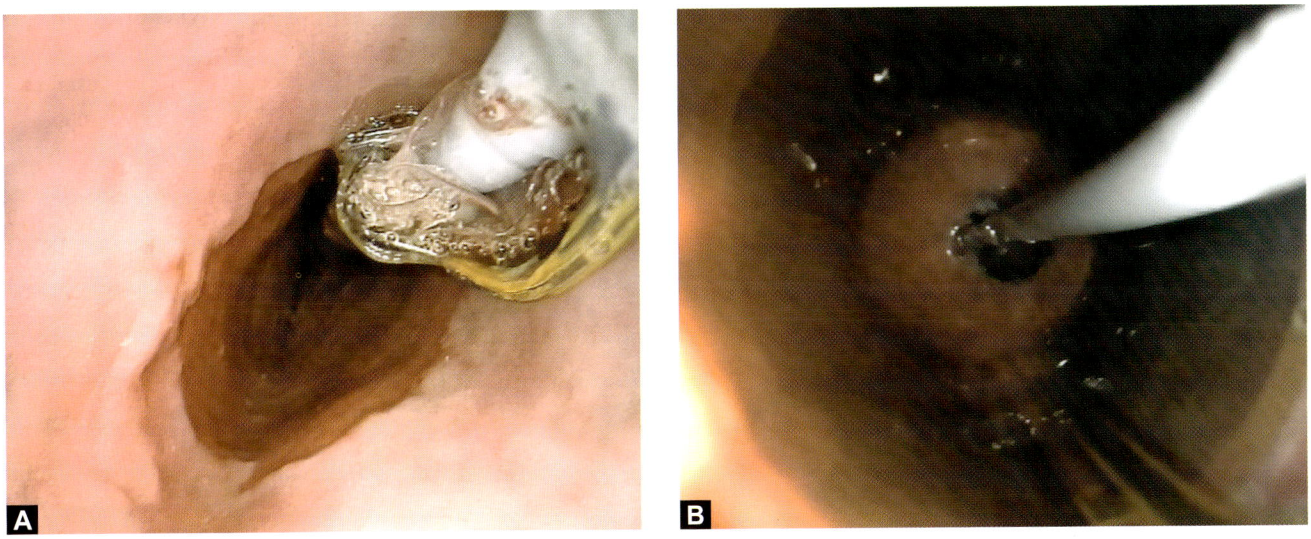

FIGURE 5-4 Radiofrequency ablation of remaining Barrett's epithelium after successful endoscopic resection of mucosal Barrett's cancer.

lesion, and therefore, tumor-free margins (R0) of the resected specimens were only observed in 24%. In contrast, a tumor-free margin was found in 64% in the ESD group. However, complete resection of all neoplasia was achieved in both groups, and no recurrences were observed in both groups after a follow-up of 15 months. Perforations were observed in 2 and 1 patient in the ESD and the ER groups, respectively. Strictures occurred in significantly more patients in the ESD group than in the ER group (44 vs. 20%).

Although ESD is theoretically the ideal treatment technique in patients with early Barrett's neoplasia, data so far do not support its use for Barrett's neoplasia outside prospective studies. Results from Western series are rare, and the results after ESD do not seem to be superior to those obtained with conventional ER. The question arises whether ESD, a demanding and time consuming procedure, with a flat learning curve and a high-complication rate can really improve the excellent results of ER combined with ablation, associated with remission rates of more than 90% already achieved by most centers from Europe and the US.

Comparisons to Surgical Therapy

While there are no randomized controlled trials that have compared endoscopic to surgical approaches for the management of high-grade dysplasia and superficial carcinoma, a number of observational studies now suggest that long-term survival of the two techniques is comparable.[52-54] Studies extending over 5 years are now available on endoscopic mucosal resection, PDT, and a combination of the two demonstrating comparable long-term survival to esophageal surgery for high-grade dysplasia or superficial carcinoma and low-rates of cancer-associated death.[32,43,52] A recent population-based study of patients with early esophageal cancer found comparable long-term survival for patients managed with endoscopic therapy compared to those treated with surgical resection. However, while the 5-year survival is comparable between the two treatment modalities, cancer may develop during follow-up of endoscopically treated patients in approximately up to 12%.[52]

CONCLUSION

Endoscopic treatment of early neoplasia in Barrett's esophagus (HGIN and mucosal adenocarcinoma) has become the method of choice in most countries. Long-term results for endoscopic treatment in a large group of patients are now available. These emerging data suggest that endoscopic eradication therapies are safe and highly effective with long-term complete remission rates of more than 94%. All visible lesions should be treated by ER for histological confirmation of the neoplastic lesion rather than by ablative techniques. After successful ER of all visible and localizable HGIN and mucosal cancer, ablative treatment of the remaining Barrett's epithelium at risk should be performed in order to reduce the rate of recurrent or metachronous neoplasia.

REFERENCES

1. Shaheen NJ, Crosby MA, Bozymski EM, Sandler RS. Is there publication bias in the reporting of cancer risk in Barrett's esophagus? *Gastroenterology.* 2000;119:333-8.
2. Sikkema M, de Jonge PJ, Steyerberg EW, Kuipers EJ. Risk of esophageal adenocarcinoma and mortality in patients with Barrett's esophagus: a systematic review and meta-analysis. *Clin Gastroenterol Hepatol.* 2010;8:235-44.
3. Madisch A, Miehlke S, Bayerdorffer E, Wiedemann B, Antos D, Sievert A, et al. Long-term follow-up after complete ablation of Barrett's esophagus with argon plasma coagulation. *World J Gastroenterol.* 2005;11:1182-6.
4. Sharma VK, Wang KK, Overholt BF, Lightdale CJ, Fennerty MB, Dean PJ, et al. Balloon-based, circumferential, endoscopic radiofrequency ablation of Barrett's esophagus: 1-year follow-up of 100 patients. *Gastrointest Endosc.* 2007;65:185-95.
5. Fleischer DE, Overholt BF, Sharma VK, Reymunde A, Kimmey MB, Chuttani R, et al. Endoscopic ablation of Barrett's esophagus: a multicenter study with 2.5-year follow-up. *Gastrointest Endosc.* 2008;68:867-76.
6. Fleischer DE, Overholt BF, Sharma VK, Reymunde A, Kimmey MB, Chuttani R, et al. Endoscopic radiofrequency ablation of Barrett's esophagus: 5-year durability outcomes from a prospective multicenter trial. *Gastrointest Endosc.* 2010;71:AB117.
7. Reid BJ, Levine DS, Longton G, Blount PL, Rabinovitch PS. Predictors of progression to cancer in Barrett's esophagus: baseline histology and flow cytometry identify low- and high-risk patient subsets. *Am J Gastroenterol.* 2000;95:1669-76.
8. Curvers WL, ten Kate FJ, Krishnadath KK, Visser M, Elzer B, Baak LC, et al. Low-grade dysplasia in Barrett's esophagus: overdiagnosed and underestimated. *Am J Gastroenterol.* 2010;105:1523-30.
9. Pech O, Vieth M, Schmitz D, Gossner L, May A, Seitz G, et al. Conclusions from the histological diagnosis of low-grade intraepithelial neoplasia in Barrett's oesophagus. *Scand J Gastroenterol.* 2007;42:682-8.
10. Shaheen NJ, Sharma P, Overholt BF, Wolfsen HC, Sampliner RE, Wang KK, et al. Radiofrequency ablation in Barrett's esophagus with dysplasia. *N Engl J Med.* 2009; 360:2277-88.
11. Wani S, Puli SR, Shaheen NJ, Westhoff B, Slehria S, Bansal A, et al. Esophageal adenocarcinoma in Barrett's esophagus after endoscopic ablative therapy: a meta-analysis and systematic review. *Am J Gastroenterol.* 2009; 104:502-13.
12. Buskens CJ, Westerterp M, Lagarde SM, Bergman JJ, ten Kate FJ, van Lanschot JJ. Prediction of appropriateness of local endoscopic treatment for high-grade dysplasia and early adenocarcinoma by EUS and histopathologic features. *Gastrointest Endosc.* 2004;60:703-10.
13. Stein HJ, Feith M, Bruecher BL, Naehrig J, Sarbia M, Siewert JR. Early esophageal cancer: pattern of lymphatic spread and prognostic factors for long-term survival after surgical resection. *Ann Surg.* 2005;242:566-73.
14. Ell C, May A, Pech O, Gossner L, Guenter E, Behrens A, et al. Curative endoscopic resection of early esophageal adenocarcinomas (Barrett's cancer). *Gastrointest Endosc.* 2007;65:3-10.
15. Manner H, May A, Pech O, Gossner L, Rabenstein T, Günter E, et al. Early Barrett's carcinoma with "low-risk" submucosal invasion: long-term results of endoscopic resection with a curative intent. *Am J Gastroenterol.* 2008; 103:2589-97.
16. Badreddine RJ, Prasad GA, Lewis JT, Lutzke LS, Borkenhagen LS, Dunagan KT, et al. Depth of submucosal invasion does not predict lymph node metastasis and survival of patients with esophageal carcinoma. *Clin Gastroenterol Hepatol.* 2010;8:248-53.
17. Pech O, Günter E, Dusemund F, Ell C. Value of high-frequency miniprobes and conventional radial endoscopic ultrasound in the staging of early Barrett's carcinoma. *Endoscopy.* 2010;42:98-103.
18. Pech O, Günter E, Dusemund F, Origer J, Lorenz D, Ell C. Accuracy of endoscopic ultrasound in preoperative staging of esophageal cancer: results from a referral center for early esophageal cancer. *Endoscopy.* 2010;42:456-61.
19. Attwood SE, Lewis CJ, Caplin S, Hemming K, Armstrong G. Argon beam plasma coagulation as therapy for high-grade dysplasia in Barrett's esophagus. *Clin Gastroenterol Hepatol.* 2003;1:258-63.
20. Ragunath K, Krasner N, Raman VS, Haqqani MT, Phillips CJ, Cheung I. Endoscopic ablation of dysplastic Barrett's oesophagus comparing argon plasma coagulation and photodynamic therapy: a randomized prospective trial assessing efficacy and cost-effectiveness. *Scand J Gastroenterol.* 2005;40:750-8.
21. Sharma P, Wani S, Weston AP, Bansal A, Hall M, Mathur S, et al. A randomised controlled trial of ablation of Barrett's oesophagus with multipolar electrocoagulation versus argon plasma coagulation in combination with acid suppression: long term results. *Gut.* 2006;55:1233-9.
22. Van Laethem JL, Peny MO, Salmon I, Cremer M, Devière J. Intramucosal adenocarcinoma arising under squamous re-epithelialisation of Barrett's oesophagus. *Gut.* 2000;46: 574-7.
23. Shand A, Dallal H, Palmer K, Ghosh S, MacIntyre M. Adenocarcinoma arising in columnar lined oesophagus following treatment with argon plasma coagulation. *Gut.* 2001;48:580-1.
24. Mino-Kenudson M, Ban S, Ohana M, Puricelli W, Deshpande V, Shimizu M, et al. Buried dysplasia and early adenocarcinoma arising in Barrett esophagus after porfimer-photodynamic therapy. *Am J Surg Pathol.* 2007; 31:403-9.

25. Johnston MH, Eastone JA, Horwhat JD, Cartledge J, Mathews JS, Foggy JR. Cryoablation of Barrett's esophagus: a pilot study. *Gastrointest Endosc.* 2005;62:842-8.
26. Dumot JA, Vargo JJ 2nd, Falk GW, Frey L, Lopez R, Rice TW. An open-label, prospective trial of cryospray ablation for Barrett's esophagus high-grade dysplasia and early esophageal cancer in high-risk patients. *Gastrointest Endosc.* 2009;70:635-44.
27. Shaheen NJ, Greenwald BD, Peery AF, Dumot JA, Nishioka NS, Wolfsen HC, et al. Safety and efficacy of endoscopic spray cryotherapy for Barrett's esophagus with high-grade dysplasia. *Gastrointest Endosc.* 2010;71:680-5.
28. Gossner L, Stolte M, Sroka R, Rick K, May A, Hahn EG, et al. Photodynamic ablation of high-grade dysplasia and early cancer in Barrett's esophagus by means of 5-aminolevulinic acid. *Gastroenterology.* 1998;114:448-55.
29. Overholt BF, Panjehpour M, Haydek JM. Photodynamic therapy for Barrett´s esophagus: follow-up in 100 patients. *Gastrointest Endosc.* 1999;49:1-7.
30. Pech O, Gossner L, May A, Rabenstein T, Vieth M, Stolte M, et al. Long-term results of photodynamic therapy with 5-aminolevulinic acid for superficial Barrett's cancer and high-grade intraepithelial neoplasia. *Gastrointest Endosc.* 2005;62:24-30.
31. Overholt BF, Lightdale CJ, Wang KK, Canto MI, Burdick S, Haggitt RC, et al. Photodynamic therapy with porfimer sodium for ablation of high-grade dysplasia in Barrett's esophagus: international, partially blinded, randomized phase III trial. *Gastrointest Endosc.* 2005;62:488-98.
32. Overholt BF, Wang KK, Burdick JS, Lightdale CJ, Kimmey M, Nava HR, et al. Five-year efficacy and safety of photodynamic therapy with Photofrin in Barrett's high-grade dysplasia. *Gastrointest Endosc.* 2007;66:460-8.
33. Prasad GA, Wang KK, Buttar NS, Wongkeesong LM, Krishnadath KK, Nichols FC 3rd, et al. Long-term survival following endoscopic and surgical treatment of high-grade dysplasia in Barrett's esophagus. *Gastroenterology.* 2007;132:1226-33.
34. Krishnadath KK, Wang KK, Taniguchi K, Sebo TJ, Buttar NS, Anderson MA, et al. Persistent genetic abnormalities in Barrett's esophagus after photodynamic therapy. *Gastroenterology.* 2000;119:624-30.
35. Hage M, Siersema PD, Vissers KJ, Steyerberg EW, Haringsma J, Kuipers EJ, et al. Molecular evaluation of ablative therapy of Barrett's oesophagus. *J Pathol.* 2005;205:57-64.
36. Hage M, Siersema PD, Vissers KJ, Dinjens WN, Steyerberg EW, Haringsma J, et al. Genomic analysis of Barrett's esophagus after ablative therapy: persistence of genetic alterations at tumor suppressor loci. *Int J Cancer.* 2006; 118:155-60.
37. Bronner MP, Overholt BF, Taylor SL, Haggitt RC, Wang KK, Burdick JS. Squamous overgrowth is not a safety concern for photodynamic therapy for Barrett's esophagus with high-grade dysplasia. *Gastroenterology.* 2009;136:56-64.
38. Yachimski P, Puricelli WP, Nishioka NS. Patient predictors of esophageal stricture development after photodynamic therapy. *Clin Gastroenterol Hepatol.* 2008;6:302-8.
39. Prasad GA, Wang KK, Buttar NS, Wongkeesong LM, Lutzke LS, Borkenhagen LS. Predictors of stricture formation after photodynamic therapy for high-grade dysplasia in Barrett's esophagus. *Gastrointest Endosc.* 2007;65:60-6.
40. Ganz RA, Overholt BF, Sharma VK, Fleischer DE, Shaheen NJ, Lightdale CJ, et al. Circumferential ablation of Barrett's esophagus that contains high-grade dysplasia: a U.S. Multicenter Registry. *Gastrointest Endosc.* 2008;68:35-40.
41. Gondrie JJ, Pouw RE, Sondermeijer C, Peters FP, Curvers WL, Rosmolen WD, et al. Effective treatment of early Barret's neoplasia with stepwise circumferential and focal ablation using the HALO system. *Endoscopy.* 2008;40:370-9.
42. Gondrie JJ, Pouw RE, Sondermeijer C, Peters FP, Curvers WL, Rosmolen WD, et al. Stepwise circumferential and focal ablation of Barrett's esophagus with high-grade dysplasia: results of the first prospective series in 11 patients. *Endoscopy.* 2008;40:359-69.
43. Pech O, Behrens A, May A, Nachbar L, Gossner L, Rabenstein T, et al. Long-term results and risk factor analysis for recurrence after curative endoscopic therapy in 349 patients with high-grade intraepithelial neoplasia and mucosal adenocarcinoma in Barrett's oesophagus. *Gut.* 2008;57:1200-6.
44. Pouw RE, Wirths K, Eisendrath P, Sondermeijer CM, Ten Kate FJ, Fockens P, et al. Efficacy of radiofrequency ablation combined with endoscopic resection for Barrett's esophagus with early neoplasia. *Clin Gastroenterol Hepatol.* 2010;8:23-9.
45. Manner H, Rabenstein T, Braun K, May A, Pech O, Pohl J, et al. What should we do with the remainder of the Barrett's segment after endoscopic resection of early Barrett's cancer? Intermediate results of the first prospective-randomized trial on the APC ablation of residual Barrett's mucosa with concomitant esomeprazole therapy versus surveillance without ablation after ER of Early Barrett's Cancer. *Gastrointest Endosc.* 2010;71:AB175.
46. Chennat J, Konda VJ, Ross AS, de Tejada AH, Noffsinger A, Hart J, et al. Complete Barrett's Eradication Endoscopic Mucosal Resection (CBE-EMR): An Effective Treatment Modality for High Grade Dysplasia (HGD) and Intra-mucosal Carcinoma (IMC) - An American Single Center Experience. *Am J Gastroenterol.* 2009;104:2684-92.
47. Pouw RE, Seewald S, Gondrie JJ, Deprez PH, Piessevaux H, Pohl H, et al. Stepwise radical endoscopic resection for eradication of Barrett's oesophagus with early neoplasia in a cohort of 169 patients. *Gut.* 2010;59:1169-77.
48. Moss A, Bourke MJ, Hourigan LF, Gupta S, Williams SJ, Tran K, et al. Endoscopic resection for Barrett's high-grade dysplasia and early esophageal adenocarcinoma: an essential staging procedure with long-term therapeutic benefit. *Am J Gastroenterol.* 2010;105:1276-83.

49. Kakushima N, Yahagi N, Fujishiro M, Kodashima S, Nakamura M, Omata M. Efficacy and safety of endoscopic submucosal dissection for tumors of the esophagogastric junction. *Endoscopy.* 2006;38:170-4.
50. Yoshinaga S, Gotoda T, Kusano C, Oda I, Nakamura K, Takayanagi R. Clinical impact of endoscopic submucosal dissection for superficial adenocarcinoma located at the esophagogastric junction. *Gastrointest Endosc.* 2008;67:202-9.
51. Deprez PH, Piessevaux H, Aouattah T, Yeung RC, Sempoux C, Mourin AJ. ESD in Barrett's Esophagus High Grade Dysplasia and Mucosal Cancer: Prospective Comparison with CAP Mucosectomy. *Gastrointest Endosc.* 2010;71:AB126.
52. Prasad GA, Wu TT, Wigle DA, Buttar NS, Wongkeesong LM, Dunagan KT, et al. Endoscopic and surgical treatment of mucosal (T1a) esophageal adenocarcinoma in Barrett's esophagus. *Gastroenterology.* 2009;137:815-23.
53. Das A, Singh V, Fleischer DE, Sharma VK. A comparison of endoscopic treatment and surgery in early esophageal cancer: an analysis of surveillance epidemiology and end results data. *Am J Gastroenterol.* 2008;103:1340-5.
54. Schembre DB, Huang JL, Lin OS, Cantone N, Low DE. Treatment of Barrett's esophagus with early neoplasia: a comparison of endoscopic therapy and esophagectomy. *Gastrointest Endosc.* 2008;67:595-601.

6 Detection of Premalignant and Malignant Gastric Lesions

Philip WY Chiu, Joseph JY Sung

ABSTRACT

Globally, gastric cancer is the second most common cause of cancer-related deaths. It is associated with a poor survival rate, which makes early diagnosis of gastric cancer essential. Gastric intestinal metaplasia (IM) has been recognized as a premalignant lesion for gastric cancer. The presence of IM, gastric atrophy, and early gastric cancer, which are curable, is often missed on routine endoscopy. Recent imaging techniques like chromoendoscopy, narrow band imaging (NBI), magnifying endoscopy, endocytoscopy, and confocal imaging have been successful in the diagnosis of IM and early gastric cancer. These imaging techniques are discussed in depth in this chapter.

INTRODUCTION

Stomach cancer is the second leading cause of cancer deaths in Asia and worldwide.[1,2] Carcinoma of the stomach is notoriously difficult to treat with a wide variation in the incidence and prognosis. A comparative study on stomach cancer incidence and survival across four continents, including Latin America, North America, Europe, and Japan showed that there was a significant difference in survival and prognosis.[3] The survival for advanced carcinoma of stomach after treatment amounts to 20% at 5 years.[4,5] One of the reasons for such poor survival is that these cancers are diagnosed at an advanced stage. Everett et al. however, showed that worldwide early gastric cancer can have excellent 5-year survival of more than 90%.[6] Hamashima et al. reviewed the currently used four methods of gastric cancer screening; photofluorography, endoscopy, serum pepsinogen testing, and *H. pylori* antibody testing.[7] In the absence of prospective randomized trials, most evidences were established through case-controlled study and showed that photofluorography reduced gastric cancer mortality by 40–60%. While no prospective study was conducted to evaluate the efficacy of endoscopic screening for gastric cancer, a cohort study on endoscopic screening was performed in Linqu County, China.[8] Out of 4,394 residents being screened with endoscopy, 85 gastric cancers were detected, of which 29 cases were at early stage. However, there was no impact on mortality for patients screened for gastric cancers when compared to those detected without screening. Another study from Japan showed a sensitivity of 84%. Although not recommended as a standard method of screening by Japanese guidelines, the authors foresee the potential of endoscopic screening as an alternative to photofluorography. With advancement in the technology of endoscopy, the detection of premalignant and malignant gastric lesions is greatly enhanced. This chapter reviews the current endoscopic approaches and new advances in the recognition of premalignant and malignant neoplastic lesions.

PREMALIGNANT AND MALIGNANT GASTRIC LESIONS

Gastric intestinal metaplasia (IM) has been considered as a premalignant condition. Correa et al. proposed a hypothetical relationship between chronic gastritis, atrophy, IM, dysplasia, and carcinoma known as Correa cascade.[9] In a multistep model for gastric carcinogenesis, atrophic gastritis with IM develop through dysplasia into adenocarcinoma.[10,11] *H. pylori* serves an important role in this process of chronic inflammation and malignant changes. IM is defined as replacement of the mucous cells that line the normal gastric mucosa with an epithelium

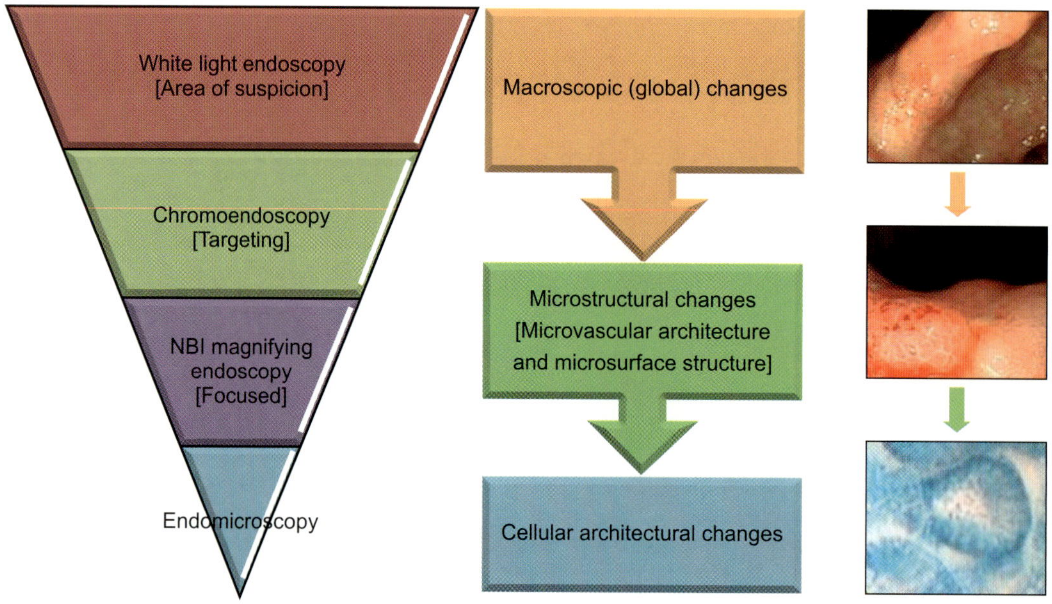

FIGURE 6-1 The endoscopic scheme to recognize premalignant and malignant gastric lesions.

similar to that of small intestine. The histological features of gastric IM include the presence of absorptive brush border, goblet cells, and immature intermediate cells with production of sialo- and sulfomucins. Gastric IM can be classified into 3 types; type I has brush border and no sialomucins, type II comprises of no brush border and rare sulfomucins, while type III has brush border, cellular disarray, and abundant sulfomucins. Type III gastric IM is considered as a high risk premalignant condition, while type I is considered as having no risk of malignancy. The recognition of gastric IM upon endoscopy, however, posed significant interobserver variation.[12,13] Moreover, as gastric mucosa is distributed over a wide area, random biopsy may not be able to obtain a representative sample. The risk of neoplastic change correlates with the pattern of distribution of gastric IM, and the risk is highest among patients with diffuse involvement over the entire gastric mucosa.[14] The distinction between gastric IM, dysplasia, and early gastric cancer posed significant difficulty among endoscopists under ordinary white light endoscopy (WLE), as gross appearance of these lesions shared similar features.[15] The development of endoscopic techniques, application of new technologies, and standardization of features to recognize these lesions are important to distinguish atrophic gastritis, gastric IM, and dysplasia, which are distinct clinical entities with different implications and treatments. Our focus will be on the endoscopic recognition for gastric IM and dysplasia.

Endoscopic Recognition of Premalignant and Malignant Gastric Lesions: From Macroscopic to Microscopic Features

The recognition of gastric pathologies by endoscopy is through the appreciation of gross appearances and color changes in the lumen. These changes in the macroscopic view would be enhanced by improvement in endoscopic technologies. Figure 6-1 outlines our usual practice in recognizing premalignant and malignant gastric lesions. We first start with the observation of an abnormal or suspicious area using WLE. The suspicious area would be further examined using either chromoendoscopy or narrow band imaging (NBI) coupled with magnifying endoscopy to detect microstructural features. By observing macroscopic and microscopic features, differentiation between benign and malignant gastric lesions can be made. The description of early gastric cancer will be refined according to the Paris classification.[16] The Paris classification unified the endoscopic description of early neoplasia of the gastrointestinal (GI) tract. Type 0 is assigned to superficial gastric cancers to distinguish from those lesions classified by Borrmann classification for gastric cancer in 1926.[17] Morphologically, type 0 early gastric cancer can be classified into; type 0-I: polypoid, type 0-II: non-polypoid and non-excavated, and type 0-III: non-polypoid with a frank ulcer. Type 0-II can be further classified into; type 0-IIa: elevated, type 0-IIb: flat, and

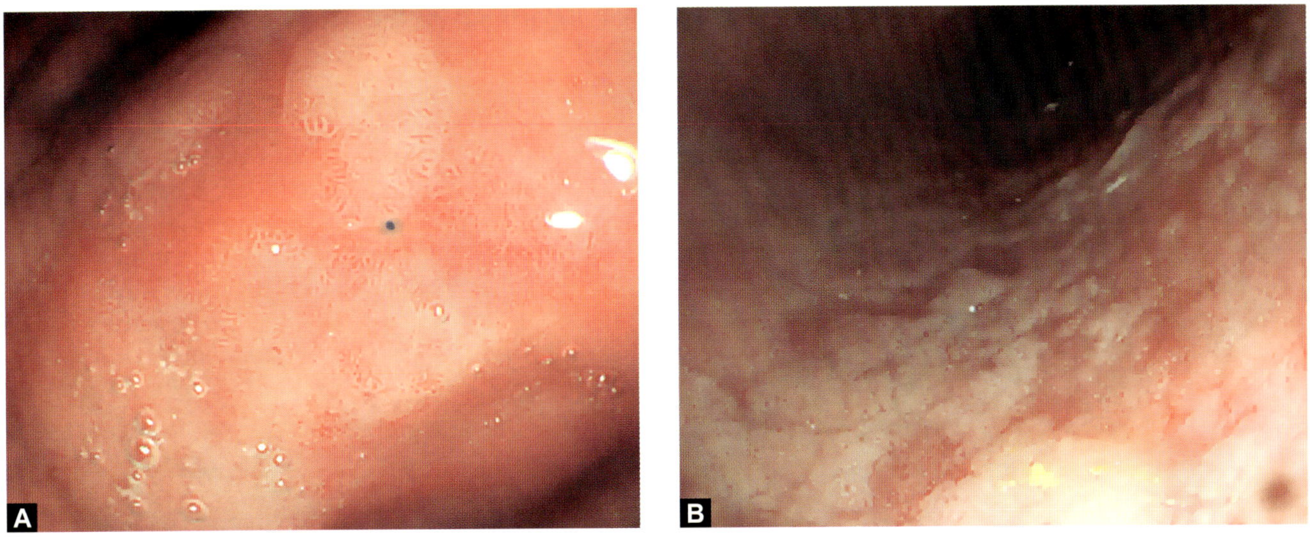

FIGURE 6-2 Endoscopic appearance of gastric intestinal metaplasia upon ordinary white light endoscopy.

type 0-IIc: depressed. If the superficial neoplasic lesion has elements of elevation and depression, the classification can be a combination of IIa and IIc, depending on which proportion dominates. This classification facilitated communication between endoscopists on the description of the lesion and subsequent management of early gastric cancer.

Conventional Endoscopic Detection of Premalignant and Malignant Gastric Lesions Using White Light Endoscopy and Chromoendoscopy

In the past, differentiation between atrophic gastritis, gastric IM, and dysplasia upon WLE was extremely difficult.[18,19] Ordinary WLE examination is an analogue to gross histopathology. There is a significant limitation in achieving accurate diagnosis based on gross appearance alone. Belair et al. conducted a study to investigate the accuracy of endoscopy for diagnosis of gastritis.[20] There was a poor correlation between endoscopic features and ultimate histological diagnosis. The receiver operator characteristics curve correlating the global endoscopic impression of the diagnosis to histopathology showed an area under curve of 0.65 only. More often, premalignant lesions were diagnosed by surprise upon histopathology.[20,21] The appearance of gastric IM was often described as reddish patch of abnormal mucosa upon WLE (Figure 6-2). These appearances mimic other types of gastritis, including chronic active gastritis, atrophic gastritis, and eosinophilic gastritis.[18] For dysplasia and early gastric cancer, ordinary WLE also show features, such as slight mucosal elevation, depression, and irregularity with reddish discoloration (Figure 6-3).

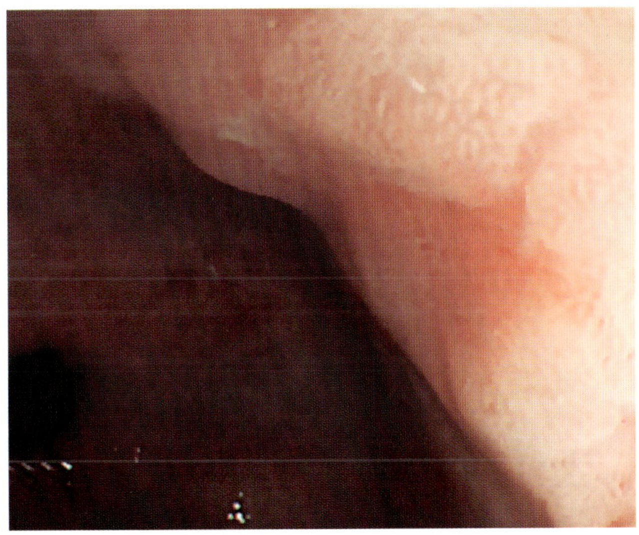

FIGURE 6-3 Endoscopic appearance of type 0-IIa early gastric cancer.

The development of chromoendoscopy aimed to augment the contrast between normal and abnormal gastric epithelium by using safe and effective chemical agents. The various agents used for chromoendoscopy can be classified into vital or absorptive stains, reactive stains, and contrasting agents.[22] Indigo carmine is a contrasting dye, which is not absorbed by the mucosal cells. It acts by pooling between crevices and ridges to improve the contrasting effect. Under WLE, the color difference between normal and abnormal epithelium varies from white, pink, or red. Indigo carmine pooled between the grooves adds a contrasting blue color to augment the color difference. The dose of indigo carmine used varies from 0.2–05%, and is applied through a dye-spraying catheter. The technique of evenly spreading out the indigo carmine dye through the whole area includes spraying generally, collapse, and re-expand the stomach with suction. Figures 6-4 and 6-5 demonstrate the difference between WLE and indigo carmine chromoendoscopy in identifying an early gastric cancer at antrum. Numerous studies reported the effectiveness of indigo carmine dye in improving the diagnosis and recognition of precancerous gastric lesions and early gastric cancers.[23-26]

Methylene blue is a vital dye which is absorbed by dysplastic cells and active epithelial cells within the IM. The authors usually use 1% methylene blue and spray it to the area of suspicion through the catheter. The suspected precancerous or cancerous area is examined by magnifying endoscopy to recognize the mucosal pit pattern. Dinis-Ribeiro et al. employed methylene blue enhanced magnifying endoscopy for examination of gastric IM and dysplasia in 141 patients.[27] The images

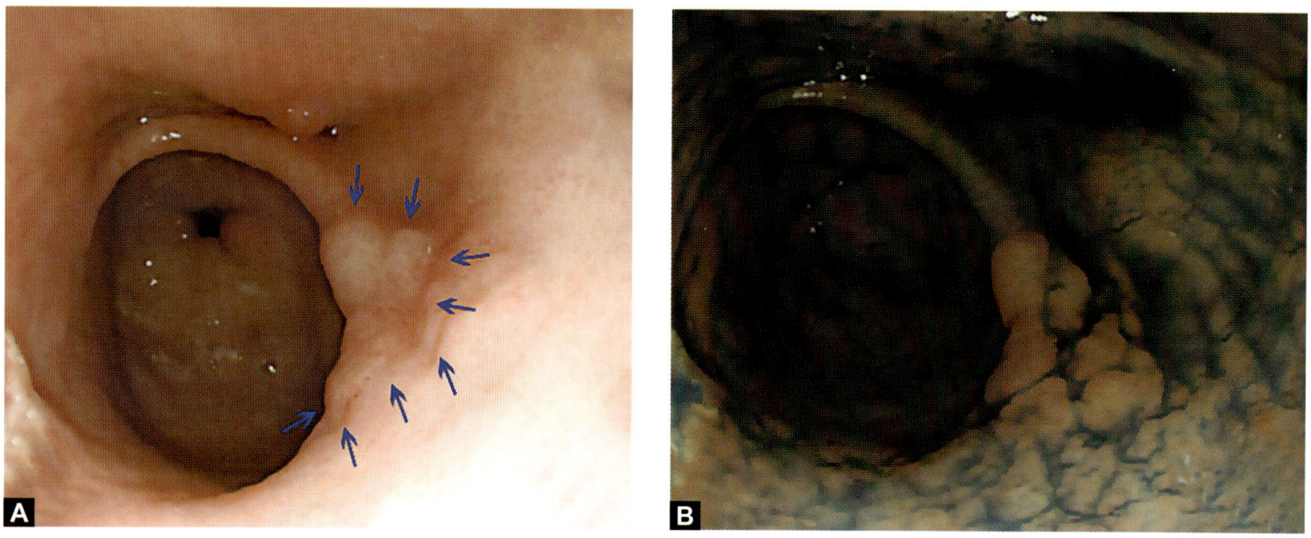

FIGURE 6-4 Early gastric cancer located at posterior antrum. **A,** Type 0-IIa early gastric cancer under WLE (blue arrows). **B,** After indigo carmine chromoendoscopy.

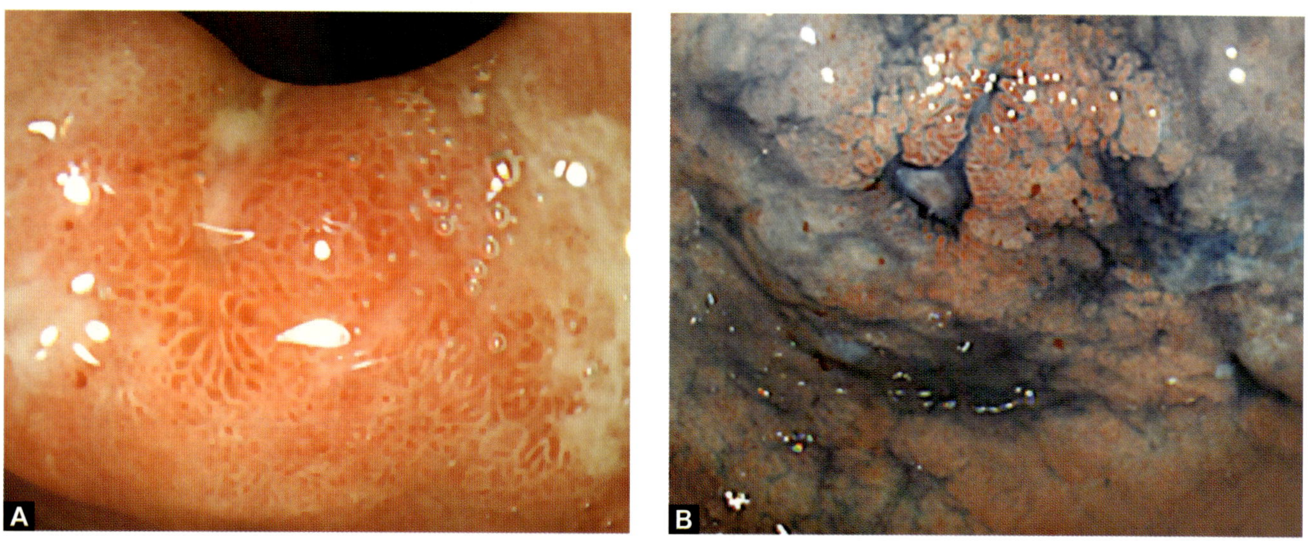

FIGURE 6-5 A case of early gastric cancer located at angular incisura. **A,** Detection of a type 0-IIc + IIa early gastric cancer, under WLE. **B,** The appearance of the early gastric cancer after indigo carmine dye spray chromoendoscopy.

were grouped into three; group 1 of non-metaplastic and nondysplastic lesions, group 2 of metaplastic mucosa, and group 3 of dysplastic mucosa. From these images, appearances of the stained pits can be further classified into various patterns. For metaplastic mucosa, the pits were irregular, round and tubular, villi, or small. For dysplastic mucosa, the pits loses clear pattern with depression or slight elevation. With the recognition of these features, the sensitivity and specificity to diagnose IM was 76.4 and 86.6%, respectively, while the sensitivity and specificity to diagnose dysplasia was 97.4 and 81.1%, respectively. This classification was externally validated in a multicenter prospective study.[28] It resulted in excellent reproducibility and correlation, with 99% specificity for diagnosis of dysplasia.

NOVEL DEVELOPMENTS IN ENDOSCOPIC TECHNOLOGY TO ENHANCE DETECTION: NARROW BAND IMAGING AND MAGNIFYING ENDOSCOPY

Although most agents used for chromoendoscopy are inert to human body, the preparation and spraying process significantly prolong the examination time. Moreover, dye-enhanced magnifying endoscopy recognizes early gastric cancers through changes in the architecture without appreciation of the vascular alternations. Technological advances can now attain virtual or optical chromoendoscopy without the necessity of spraying contrast. NBI is a novel endoscopic technique, which narrows the bandwidth of the ordinary white light into a focused combination.[29] In NBI mode, the optical filter allows the light to pass at 400–430 and 525–555 nm. This limits the depth of penetration of the emitted light and suppresses the background signals from reflections of deep structures, while enhancing the light signals from superficial mucosa. In combination with a magnifying endoscope, the images are magnified 80 times on a 14-inch TV monitor which allows the observation of fine mucosal details including the vascular and pit patterns. A short and soft transparent cap of 2 mm in length is attached at the distal end to allow fixation of the endoscope to the mucosa. This facilitates fine observation upon magnification at a fixed distance and prevents excessive movement (Figure 6-6). The combined use of NBI and magnifying endoscopy improved the diagnostic power of the endoscopist to detect premalignant and malignant gastric neoplasia. Before the performance of magnifying endoscopy, a clear view on the gastric mucosa is essential to improve the diagnostic accuracy. In Japan, patients

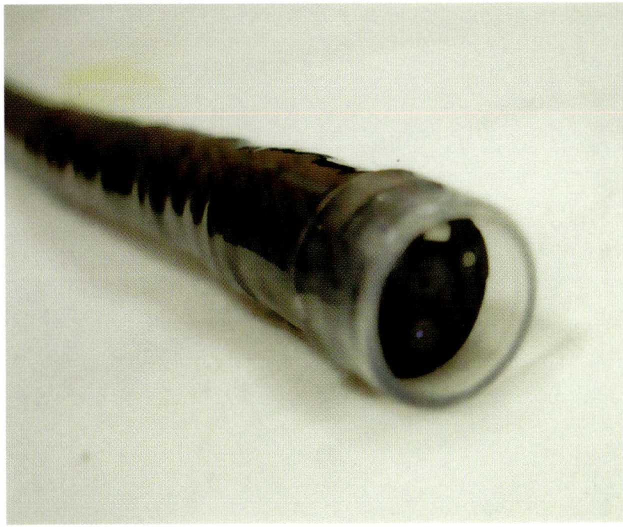

FIGURE 6-6 The setup for magnifying endoscopy with a distal short transparent cap.

were given a mixture of pronase, sodium bicarbonate, and dimethylpolysiloxane, 30 minutes before the procedure.[30] Pronase may not be available in all parts of the world, so Yao et al. suggested an alternative of giving 100 mL of water mixed with 2 mL of acetylcysteine and 0.5 mL (40 mg/mL) of activated dimethicone to clear up the mucus and bile from the stomach.[30] It is our routine practice to give intravenous sedation during this procedure, as a prolonged procedure is expected for surveillance and close observation to identify early gastric cancers.

Capelle et al. examined the use of NBI without magnification against WLE for recognition of gastric IM and dysplasia.[31] The investigators defined endoscopic suspicion of IM upon NBI as bluish whitish areas with irregular mucosal pattern and dysplasia as complete loss of architectural and mucosal patterns. Of all the IM cases detected, WLE and NBI were able to detect IM in 69%, while NBI alone detected IM in 30%. For the detection of dysplasia, 89% of these were detected by both WLE and NBI, while NBI recognized an addition of 11%. The investigators concluded that NBI achieved more accurate results in surveillance of patients with IM and dysplasia when compared to WLE. Figure 6-7 shows the endoscopic appearance of gastric IM upon NBI without magnification. Figure 6-8 compares the appearance of normal gastric mucosa under magnifying endoscopy with NBI-assisted magnifying endoscopy.

Uedo et al. reported the light blue crest (LBC) sign as a diagnostic criteria for gastric IM upon NBI-assisted magnifying endoscopy (Figure 6-9).[32] In an initial investigational study, LBC sign was observed in the gastric mucosa

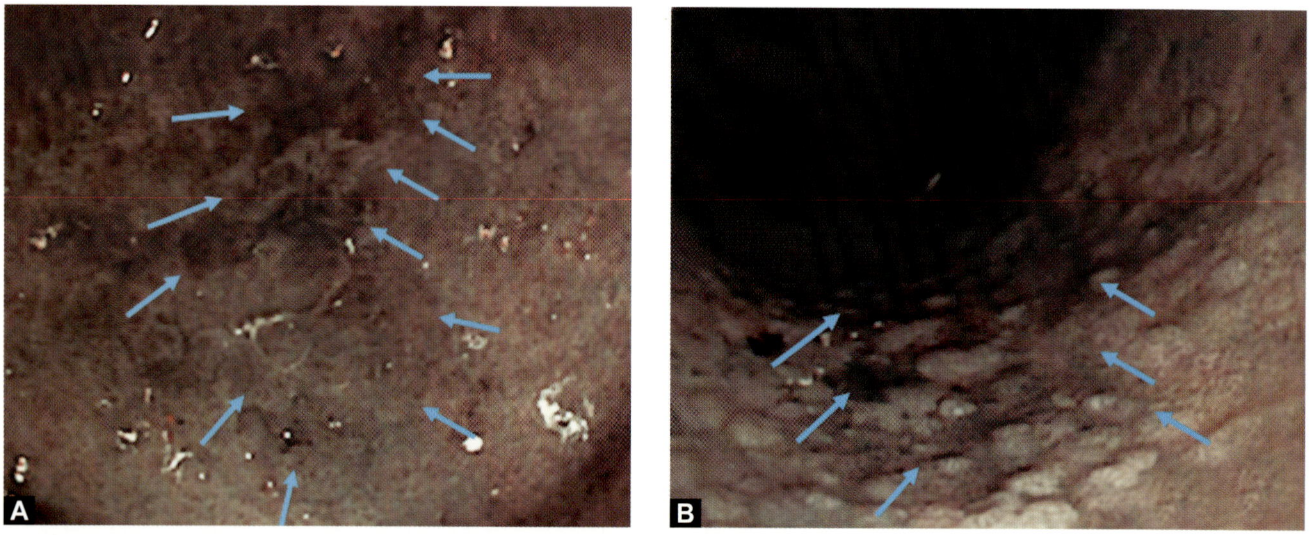

FIGURE 6-7 Endoscopic appearance of gastric IM upon NBI (blue arrows).

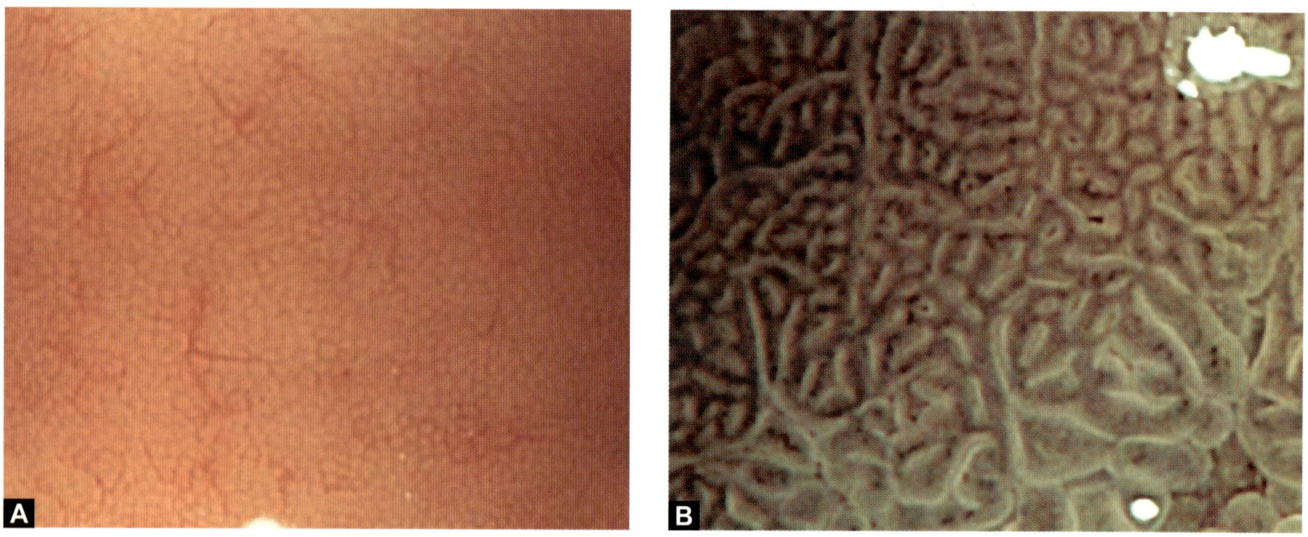

FIGURE 6-8 Appearance of normal mucosa of gastric body. **A,** Under magnifying endoscopy. **B,** Under NBI-assisted magnifying endoscopy.

of 25 patients. The accuracy of LBC sign in diagnosing IM was 91% when compared to histopathology. The LBC sign was observed in 400–430 nm reflection images and not in 525–555 nm. This implies that the LBC sign is a dense reflection of shorter wavelength light. The investigators further validated the diagnostic accuracy of LBC sign in recognizing gastric IM. One hundred and twenty-four biopsies were obtained from LBC sign mucosa and 95 from non-LBC mucosa. The LBC sign showed a sensitivity of 89% and specificity of 91% in diagnosing gastric IM.

The diagnosis of dysplasia and early intramucosal gastric cancer upon NBI magnifying endoscopy depends on microstructural changes, including microvascular architecture (MV) and microsurface structures (MS) (the "VS classifications").[33,34] Yao et al. reported the application of the VS system to define various characteristics of early gastric cancers observed through NBI magnifying endoscopy.

Microvascular Pattern

It comprises of changes in the subepithelial capillary network (SECN), connecting venules, and microvessels. The microvessels could be either capillary, connecting

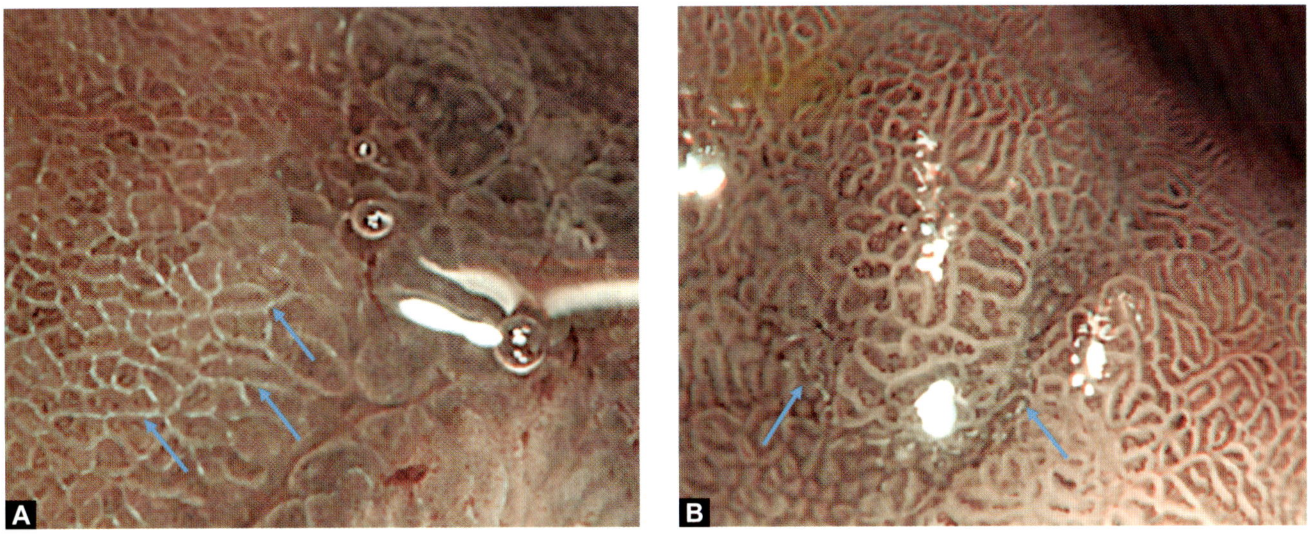

FIGURE 6-9 NBI-assisted magnifying endoscopy for gastric IM which shows light blue crest sign (blue arrows).

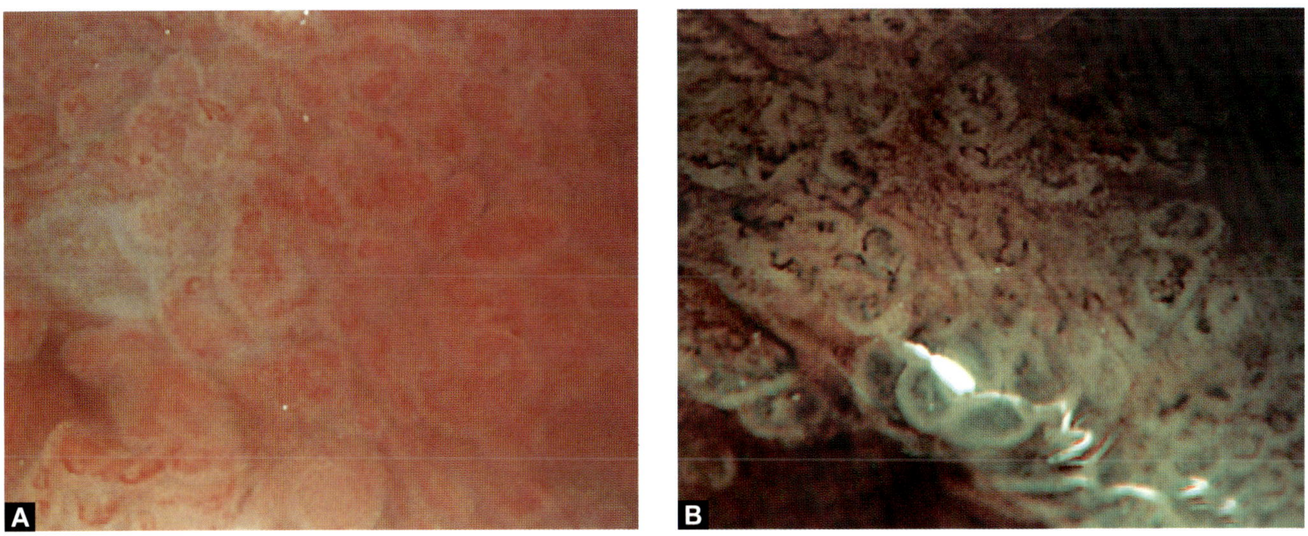

FIGURE 6-10 The abnormal microvascular architecture. **A,** Under magnifying endoscopy. **B,** NBI-assisted magnifying endoscopy.

venules, or neovascularization. The types of pattern observed can be classified as:

1. *Regular MV:* The mucosal SECN are in uniform shape with a close- or an open loop. They are consistent in sizes and arrangements.
2. *Irregular MV:* The vessels vary in shape, sizes and arrangements. They are torturous, branched, with or without network. The SECN is dilated and increased in size (Figures 6-10 and 6-11).
3. *Absent MV:* The SECN is obscured by the presence of a whitish matter named white opaque substance (WOS).[34]

Microsurface Pattern

The change in the structural arrangements and patterns of the gastric pits is another main feature to observe for differentiation between gastritis, IM, dysplasia, and early gastric cancer. Moreover, the presence of WOS could be another feature to delineate adenoma from carcinoma when SECN is obscured (Figure 6-12).[35] The surface pattern can be classified as:

1. *Regular MS:* These lesions have regular arrangements of the pits with uniform shape of round, oval, tubular, linear, or papillary structures. The pits are regular in sizes.

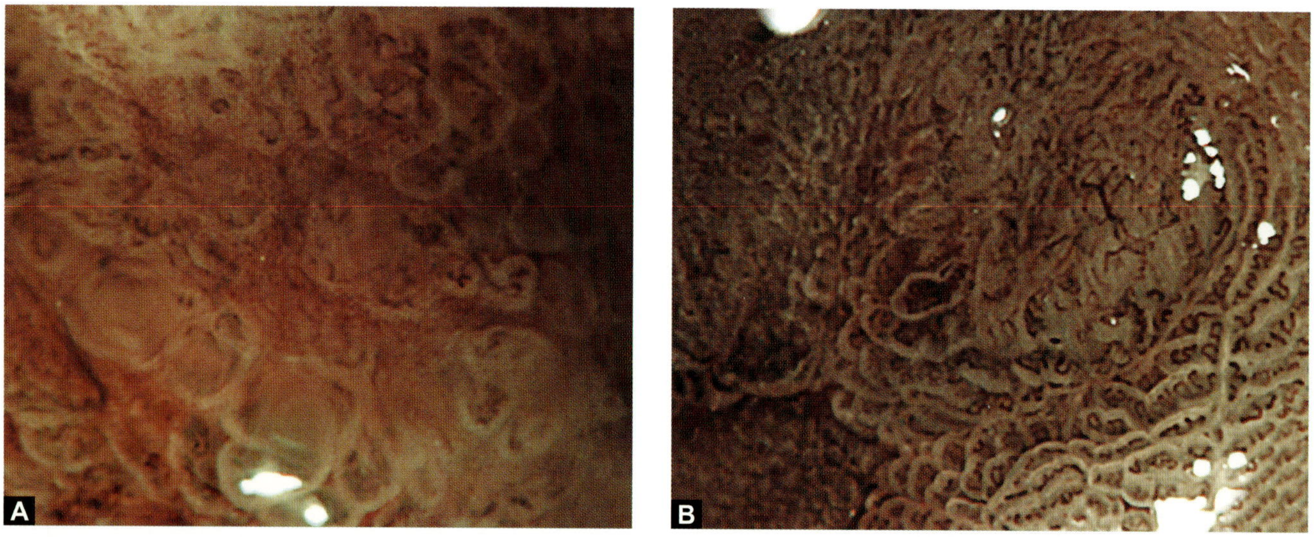

FIGURE 6-11 Abnormal vascular pattern observed in early gastric cancer with dilated, torturous SECN. **A,** With NBI. **B,** Without NBI.

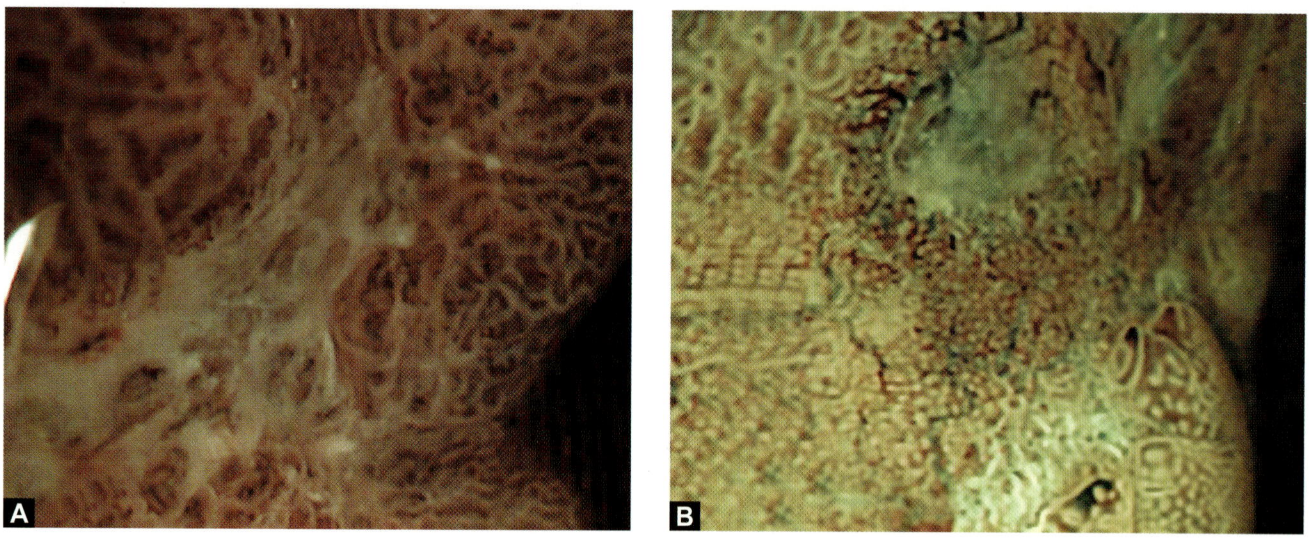

FIGURE 6-12 Whitish opaque substance upon NBI-assisted magnifying endoscopy.

2. *Irregular MS:* The arrangements of pits show irregularity in sizes and distribution. The width varies between different pits, and the pattern is disorganized. Also there is a loss of the crypt opening within the pits (Figures 6-13 and 6-14).
3. *Absent MS:* No epithelial structure can be identified (Figure 6-15).

With the application of this MV and MS classification on 100 cases of early gastric cancer, Yao et al. showed that 97% of these cancers showed features of either irregular MV or MS pattern.[33] A clear demarcation line can be observed between normal epithelium and malignant area. Yoshida et al. reported the use of non-structural microsurface changes in predicting the depth of invasion for early gastric cancer.[35] The non-structural pattern could be interpreted as similar to absent MS (Figure 6-15). When the MS pattern became non-structural without identifiable epithelial structures, the risk of submucosal invasion became significant. Among all the 11 cases of adenoma and 29 of the 31 cases of mucosal gastric cancer, the non-structural pattern was not identified. However, 9 of the 11 submucosal gastric cancers showed non-structural pattern. Indeed the MV and MS features do not only enlighten the differentiation between benign

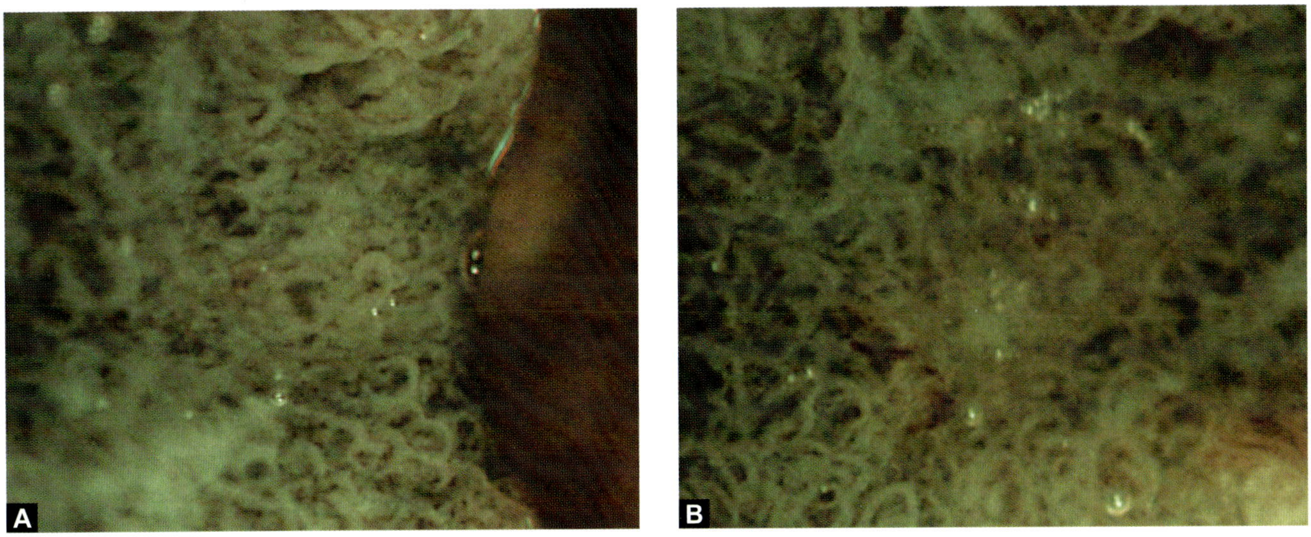

FIGURE 6-13 Abnormal microsurface structure.

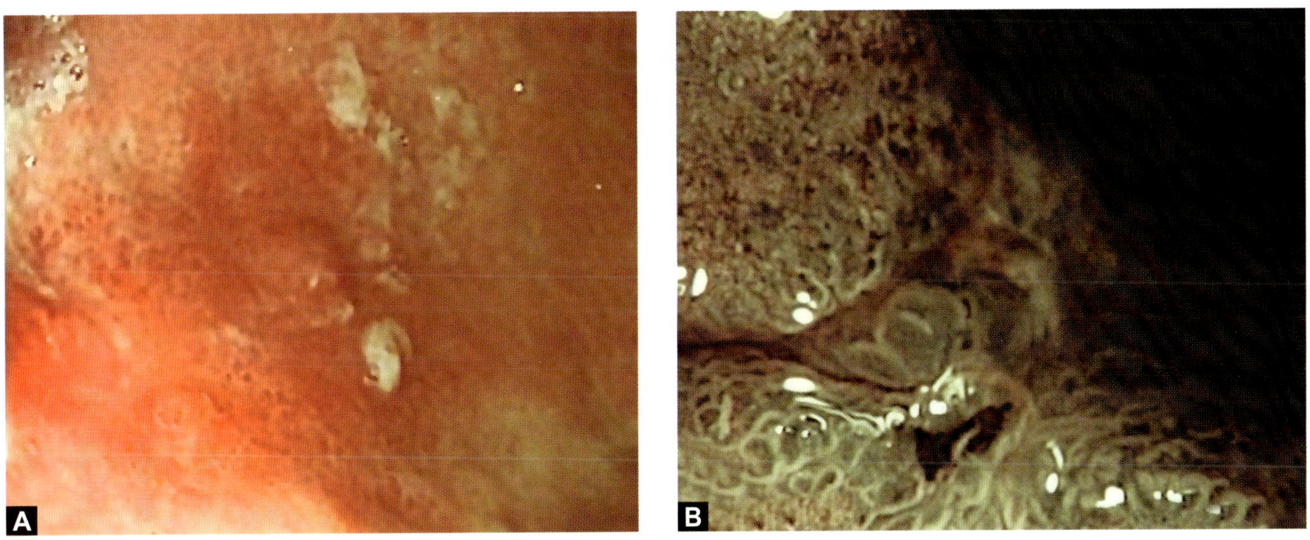

FIGURE 6-14 Type 0-IIc + IIa early gastric cancer located at greater curvature of body. **A,** Under white light endoscopy. **B,** Narrow band imaging magnifying endoscopy showed features of irregular microsurface and microvascular pattern.

and malignant lesions, they could also be applied to predict the depth of invasion. Further correlation study is necessary to confirm this application.

ENDOMICROSCOPY FOR DIAGNOSIS OF PREMALIGNANT AND MALIGNANT GASTRIC LESIONS

Although the developments in endoscopy has enhanced the recognition of macro- and microstructural changes within the mucosa to predict various pathologies, biopsy is still necessary for confirmation of the pathology. Current novel technologies can allow endoscopists to directly examine the cellular architectures, thus achieving an optical biopsy and histopathology. Endocytoscope is a catheter type of contact endoscope with high magnification to allow observation of living cells, and it can be passed through the therapeutic channel (>3.7 mm) of a double channel endoscope. The prototype endocytoscope had a magnification of 450 and 1,125 times on a 14-inch monitor (Figure 6-16A).[36] After washing with water and mucolytics to remove the mucus, gastric mucosa is sprayed

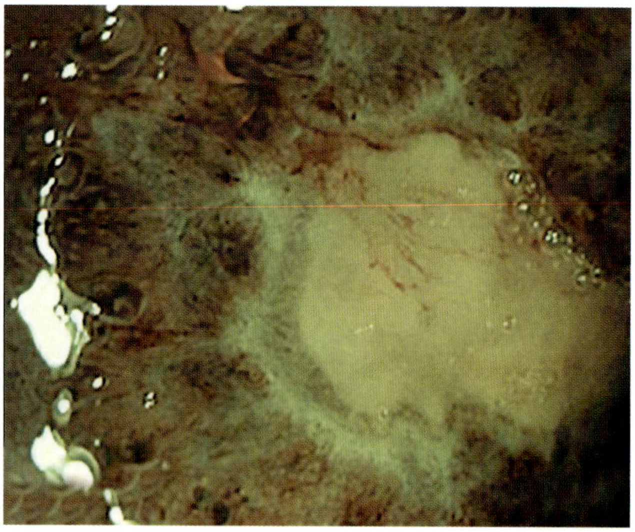

FIGURE 6-15 Absent microsurface pattern or non-structural pattern, which represent early gastric cancer with submucosal invasion.

with 0.5% methylene blue. After 5 minutes, the stained area is observed by the endocytoscope (Figure 6-16B). The investigators conducted a prospective study on the differentiation of gastric IM using endocytoscopy in 20 patients. Hundred areas within the stomach suspicious of IM were examined and the diagnosis was confirmed upon histology. Eighty-eight biopsies showed features of IM, while 14 were diagnosed as chronic gastritis. The image quality upon endocytoscopy was significantly better for areas of IM as compared to those of gastritis ($p < 0.05$; OR 21.7; 95% CI 4.5–105.9). Multiple stepwise logistic regression confirmed that the observation of goblet cell predicted the presence of IM ($p < 0.05$). The application of endocytoscopy in stomach will need further validation, especially when the image quality could be hindered by the presence of mucus, variation in staining, and movement of the gastric wall.[37] Confocal endomicroscopy is another technology to allow observation of gastric epithelial cells at a magnification of 1,000 times. From *in vitro* studies, it was found that confocal laser scanning microscopy differentiated between normal and gastric cancer cells; and achieved good image quality when compared to formal histopathology.[38,39] The development of technology allowed the development of confocal endomicroscopy, which could be catheter-based or build into a conventional endoscope. Prior to examination by confocal endomicroscope, intravenous injection of fluorescein is necessary to enhance fluorescence observation of cellular architecture and morphology. Kakeji et al. compared 27 images of normal mucosa to 27 images of gastric cancers using confocal endomicroscopy.[40] The mean size of the nucleus was significantly larger in gastric cancer when compared to normal mucosal cells. The accuracy of diagnosing gastric cancer was 96.3% for endoscopist and 94.4% for pathologist. The investigators are currently conducting a prospective study on the diagnosis of gastric IM using catheter-based confocal endomicroscopy. Figure 6-17 shows the recognition of gastric IM upon confocal endomicroscopy with the presence of goblet cells (blue arrow).

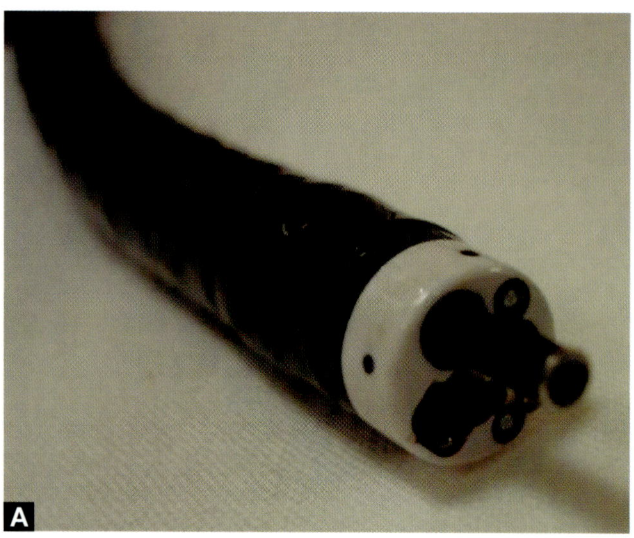

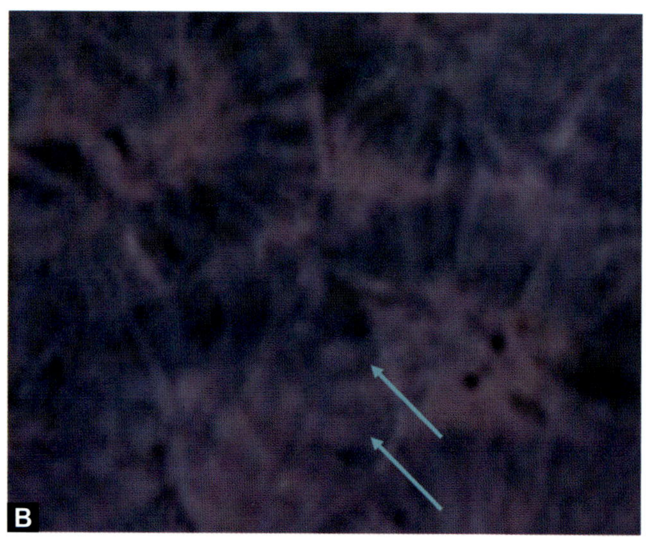

FIGURE 6-16 Endocytoscopy for observation of gastric IM. **A,** The prototype endocytoscope. **B,** Endocytoscopy (x450) with the presence of goblet cells (blue arrows).

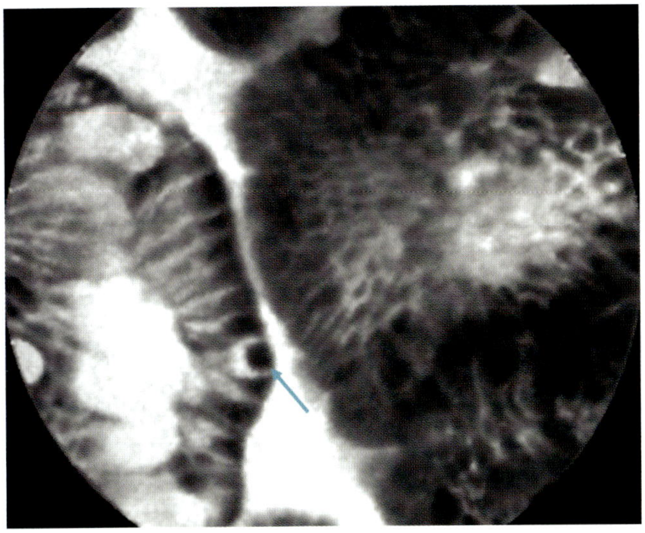

FIGURE 6-17 Confocal endomicroscopy image for identification of gastric IM with the presence of goblet cells (blue arrow).

CONCLUSION

Carcinoma of stomach develops from atrophic gastritis, IM, and dysplasia. Endoscopic detection and differentiation between IM, dysplasia, and early gastric cancer is extremely important in the management. Macroscopic changes in gastric mucosa should be carefully appreciated to recognize the area of suspicion for premalignant and malignant lesions. Targeted examination by NBI magnifying endoscopy can differentiate between IM, dysplasia, and early gastric cancer with observation of MV and MS patterns. Further research should focus on validation of these features differentiating between premalignant and malignant lesions, the prediction of depth of invasion for early gastric cancers, and the development of endomicroscopy.

REFERENCES

1. International Association of Cancer Registry (IACR): GLOBOCAN 2002.
2. Hundahl SA, Menck HR, Mansour EG, Winchester DP. The National Cancer Data Base report on gastric carcinoma. *Cancer*. 1997;80:2333-41.
3. Verdecchia A, Mariotto A, Gatta G, Bustamante-Teixeira MT, Ajiki W. Comparison of stomach cancer incidence and survival in four continents. *Eur J Cancer*. 2003;39:1603-9.
4. Bonenkamp JJ, Hermans J, Sasako M, van de Velde CJ, Welvaart K, Songun I, et al. Extended lymph-node dissection for gastric cancer. *N Engl J Med*. 1999;340: 908-14.
5. Cuschieri A, Fayers P, Fielding J, Carven J, Bancewicz J, Joypaul V, et al. Postoperative morbidity and mortality after D1 and D2 resections for gastric cancer: preliminary results of the MRC randomized controlled surgical trial. *Lancet*.1996;347:995-9.
6. Everett SM, Axon AT. Early gastric cancer in Europe. *Gut*. 1997;41:142-50.
7. Hamashima C, Shibuya D, Yamazaki H, Inoue K, Fukao A, Saito H, et al. The Japanese guidelines for gastric cancer screening. *Jpn J Clin Oncol*. 2008;38:259-67.
8. Riecken B, Pfeiffer R, Ma JL, Jin ML, Li JY, Liu WD, et al. No impact of repeated endoscopic screens on gastric cancer mortality in a prospectively followed Chinese population at high risk. *Prev Med*. 2002;34:22-8.
9. Correa P. Chronic gastritis as a cancer precursor. *Scand J Gastroenterol Suppl*. 1984;104:131-6.
10. Correa P. Human gastric carcinogenesis: a multistep and multifactorial process - First American Cancer Society Award Lecture on Cancer Epidemiology and Prevention. *Cancer Res*. 1992;52:6735-40.
11. Genta RM, Rugge M. Review article: pre-neoplastic states of the gastric mucosa - a practical approach for the perplexed clinician. *Aliment Pharmacol Ther*. 2001;15:43-50.
12. Laine L, Cohen H, Sloane R, Marin-Sorensen M, Weinstein WM. Interobserver agreement and predictive value of endoscopic findings for *H. pylori* and gastritis in normal volunteers. *Gastrointest Endosc*. 1995;42:420-3.
13. Redeen S, Petersson F, Jonsson KA, Borch K. Relationship of gastroscopic features to histological findings in gastritis and *Helicobacter pylori* infection in a general population sample. *Endoscopy*. 2003;35:946-50.
14. Cassaro M, Rugge M, Gutierrez O, Leandro G, Graham DY, Genta RM. Topographic patterns of intestinal metaplasia and gastric cancer. *Am J Gastroenterol*. 2000;95:1431-8.
15. Taghavi SA, Membari ME, Eshraghian A, Dehghani SM, Hamidpour L, Khademalhoseini F. Comparison of chromoendoscopy and conventional endoscopy in the detection of premalignant gastric lesions. *Can J Gastroenterol*. 2009; 23:105-8.
16. Participants in the Paris Workshop. The Paris endoscopic classification of superficial neoplastic lesions: esophagus, stomach and colon. *Gastrointest Endosc*. 2003;58:S3-43.
17. Borrmann R, Geschwulste des Magens und Duodenums. In: Henke F, Lubarch O, editors. Handbuch der speziellem pathologischen anatomie und histology. Berlin: Springer Verlag; 1926.
18. Lin BR, Shun CT, Wang TH, Lin JT. Endoscopic diagnosis of intestinal metaplasia of stomach - accuracy judged by histology. *Hepatogastroenterology*. 1999;46:162-6.
19. Carpenter HA, Talley NJ. Gastroscopy is incomplete without biopsy: clinical relevance of distinguishing gastropathy from gastritis. *Gastroenterology*. 1995;108:917-24.
20. Belair PA, Metz DC, Faigel DO, Furth EE. Receiver operator characteristic analysis of endoscopy as a test for gastritis. *Dig Dis Sci*. 1997;42:2227-33.

21. Fennerty MB. Gastric intestinal metaplasia on routine endoscopic biopsy. *Gastroenterology*. 2003;125:586-90.
22. Canto MI. Staining in gastrointestinal endoscopy: the basics. *Endoscopy*. 1999;31:479-86.
23. Ida K, Hashimoto Y, Takeda S, Murakami K, Kawai K. Endoscopic diagnosis of gastric cancer with dye scattering. *Am J Gastroenterol*. 1975;63:316-20.
24. Demirci S, Gohchi A. A comparative study for fiberoptic and video endoscopic determination of the extent in minimal changes of gastric mucosa using indigo dye spraying. *Surg Endosc*. 1990;4:80-2.
25. Okabayashi T, Gotoda T, Kondo H, Ono H, Oda I, Fujishiro M, et al. Usefulness of indigo carmine chromoendoscopy and endoscopic clipping for accurate preoperative assessment of proximal gastric cancer. *Endoscopy*. 2000;32:S62.
26. Sakai Y, Eto R, Kasanuki J, Kondo F, Kato K, Arai M, et al. Chromoendoscopy with indigo carmine dye added to acetic acid in the diagnosis of gastric neoplasia: a prospective comparative study. *Gastrointest Endosc*. 2008;68:635-41.
27. Dinis-Ribeiro M, da Costa-Pereira A, Lopes C, Lara-Santos L, Guilherme M, Moreira-Dias L, et al. Magnification chromoendoscopy for the diagnosis of gastric intestinal metaplasia and dysplasia. *Gastroinest Endosc*. 2003;57: 498-504.
28. Areia M, Amaro P, Dinis-Ribeiro M, Cipriano MA, Marinho C, Costa-Pereira A, et al. External validation of a classification for methylene blue magnification chromoendoscopy in premalignant gastric lesions. *Gastrointest Endosc*. 2008;67:1011-8.
29. Gono K, Obi T, Yamaguchi M, Ohyama N, Machida H, Sano Y, et al. Appearance of enhanced tissue features in narrow-band endoscopic imaging. *J Biomed Opt*. 2004;9:568-77.
30. Yao K, Anagnostopoulos GK, Ragunath K. Magnifying endoscopy for diagnosing and delineating early gastric cancer. *Endoscopy*. 2009;41:462-7.
31. Capelle LG, Haringsma J, de Vries AC, Steyerberg EW, Biermann K, van Dekken H, et al. Narrow band imaging for the detection of gastric intestinal metaplasia and dysplasia during surveillance endoscopy. *Dig Dis Sci*. 2010;55: 3442-8.
32. Uedo N, Ishihara R, lishi H, Yamamoto S, Yamada T, Imanaka K, et al. A new method of diagnosing gastric intestinal metaplasia: narrow band imaging with magnifying endoscopy. *Endoscopy*. 2006;38:819-24.
33. Yao K, Iwashita A, Matsui T. A new diagnostic VS classification system produced by magnification endoscopy plus narrow band imaging in the stomach: microvascular architecture and microsurface structure. New Challenges in gastrointestinal endoscopy. Springer; 2008.
34. Yao K, Iwashita A, Tanabe H, Nishimata N, Nagahama T, Maki S, et al. White opaque substance within superficial elevated gastric neoplasia as visualized by magnification endoscopy with narrow-band imaging: a new optical sign for differentiating between adenoma and carcinoma. *Gastrointest Endosc*. 2008;68:574-80.
35. Yoshida T, Kawachi H, Sasajima K, Shiokawa A, Kudo SE. The clinical meaning of a nonstructural pattern in early gastric cancer on magnifying endoscopy. *Gastrointest Endosc*. 2005;62:48-54.
36. ASGE Technology Committee, Kwon RS, Wong Kee Song LM, Adler DG, Conway JD, Diehl DL, et al. Endocytoscopy. *Gastrointest Endosc*. 2009;70:610-2.
37. Eberl T, Jechart G, Probst A, Golczyk M, Bittinger M, Scheubel R, et al. Can an endocytoscope system (ECS) predict histology in neoplastic lesions? *Endoscopy*. 2007; 39:497-501.
38. Inoue H, Cho JY, Satodate H, Sakashita M, Hidaka E, Fukami S, et al. Development of virtual histology and virtual biopsy using laser-scanning confocal microscopy. *Scand J Gastroenterol Suppl*. 2003;237:37-9.
39. Chiu PW, Inoue H, Satodate H, Kazawa T, Yoshida T, Sakashita M, et al. Validation of the quality of histological images obtained of fresh and formalin fixed specimens of esophageal and gastric mucosa by laser scanning confocal microscopy. *Endoscopy*. 2006;38:236-40.
40. Kakeji Y, Yamaguchi S, Yoshida D, Tanoue K, Ueda M, Masunari A, et al. Development and assessment of morphologic criteria for diagnosing gastric cancer using confocal endomicroscopy: an ex vivo and in vivo study. *Endoscopy*. 2006;38:886-90.

7 Endoscopic Management of Early Gastric Cancer

Brigitte Schumacher, Horst Neuhaus

ABSTRACT

The diagnosis of early stomach cancer has become very important since the development of new endoscopic local resection techniques. Advantages of these procedures compared to surgery are maintenance of organ, low morbidity, and improved quality of life. Patients need to be selected for local therapy by assessment of high- and low-risk criteria with regard to depth of infiltration and risk of lymph node metastasis. Several endoscopic techniques have been advocated for mucosal resection. Endoscopic resection (ER) by snare or cap for lesions up to 2 cm in size is the most common procedure; lesions larger than 2 cm should be resected by endoscopic submucosal dissection (ESD), as high risk of recurrence by piecemeal technique has been reported. In Japan, ESD is the standard procedure for therapy of early gastric cancer (EGC). It is still unclear whether these data are transferable to Europe. The procedure is time-consuming, and shows a higher risk of complications and a high learning curve. Possibly, further refinements of endoscopes and technical equipments may simplify the procedure, and ESD will become the first option for the treatment of EGC.

INTRODUCTION

Few years ago, early gastric cancer (EGC) was routinely treated by (subtotal) gastrectomy; today, in many cases, a minimally invasive endoscopic therapy can be performed. The fundamental of the establishment of endoscopic procedures is the fact that mucosal carcinoma is rarely associated with lymph node metastasis. Thus, complete curative endoscopic resection (ER) is possible, while preserving the organ. Endoscopic mucosal resection (EMR) has been widely accepted as a useful standard technique for neoplasms confined to the superficial layers of the gastrointestinal (GI) tract.[1] EMR is potentially curative for treatment of early neoplasias, provided that the histopathology of the resected specimen indicates no tumor infiltration of the submucosal layer. The risk of lymph node metastasis is very low in mucosal cancer but increases in case of submucosal involvement depending on the depth of invasion and the anatomical location. Despite its efficacy, the EMR procedure is associated with a high rate of local recurrence, especially when lesions larger than 20 mm are resected in a piecemeal manner.[2] Various EMR techniques have been proven effective for resection of mucosal lesions with a very low morbidity rate.[1,2] All of them are limited in resection size, and large lesions have to be removed in several fragments. In addition, the targeted area cannot be precisely controlled by the endoscopist, which might cause incomplete resection of even small lesions and also unnecessary resection of nonneoplastic mucosa. Endoscopic submucosal dissection (ESD) may overcome these limitations and allows precise insulation of targeted mucosal lesions, with subsequent resection in an en bloc fashion.[3] This method was originally developed for resection of large neoplastic gastric lesions. A variety of prospective and retrospective trials from Japan showed that ESD achieves higher rates of en bloc resection and curative resection of early gastric lesions than EMR.[4-7] These advantages can explain lower rates of residual tumors or recurrences. However, ESD is more time-consuming than EMR, and is correlated with a higher rate of complications, such as perforation or bleeding. The endoscopist's experience affects the outcome of ESD.[6] It is difficult to overcome the flat learning curve in Western countries because of the low rate of detection of EGC.

INDICATIONS FOR ENDOSCOPIC RESECTION

EGC is defined as a mucosal or submucosal invasive cancer (T1 cancer) irrespective of the presence of lymph node metastasis. ER should be done only in patients having no risk of nodal metastasis and that can be resected in a single fragment. Criteria for node-negative cancer have been defined in a large database of more than 5,000 patients with EGC who underwent gastrectomy with lymph node dissection.[8] Considering the risks of gastrectomy and the decreasing quality of life, it is logical to offer local treatment for these patients.

Prior to any therapy, an accurate staging by means of modern endoscopic equipment is essential. After macroscopic characterization according to the Paris-classification (type 0-Ip and Is, IIa-c, III), particularly the lateral tumor extension, the infiltration depth and enlarged local lymph nodes must be described. In addition to this, the potential risk of lymph node metastasis must be evaluated. According to the guidelines of the Japanese Gastric Cancer Association,[9] ER is indicated in well-differentiated elevated lesions less than 2 cm in size and small (<1 cm) flat/depressed well differentiated lesions (type IIb/c) without ulceration.

A large retrospective Japanese study detected a very low risk of lymph node metastasis in mucosal gastric cancer (2.7%) and an elevated risk in case of infiltration of the submucosal layer (18.7%).[8] Therefore, criteria for ER were extended to:

- Differentiated mucosal EGC pT1a, P0, V0, <3 cm of size, with or without ulceration
- Differentiated mucosal EGC pT1a, P0, V0, of any size, without ulceration
- Differentiated submucosal EGC pT1b (sm1, <500 µm infiltration depth), P0, V0, <3 cm of size
- Undifferentiated mucosal EGC pT1a, P0, V0, <2 cm of size.

DIAGNOSIS OF EARLY CANCER

Diagnosis and staging is performed by means of high-resolution endoscopes, chromoendoscopy, and endoscopic ultrasound. In selected cases, zoom endoscopy or confocal laser microscopy are applied. Several studies of magnification endoscopy in patients with premalignant gastric lesions or early cancer have found an excellent correlation with histological diagnosis.[10-14] The addition of magnification to chromoendoscopy improves visualization of the stemming surface and allows a better distinction between the neoplastic lesion and nonneoplastic tissue. Recently developed magnification endoscopy with narrow band imaging (NBI) may offer a better description of the extent of EGCs and can be used to improve the safety margin and cure rate when EMR or ESD are performed.[15-18] NBI is based on the fact that the depth of light penetration depends on its wavelength. The longer the wavelength, the deeper is the penetration. The most important wavelengths are 412 and 540 nm. The result of selective reflection of the NBI light (shortened wavelength) is an improving image of the superficial layers in the GI tract. For application of ESD, an accurate diagnosis of gastric lesions is important before the endoscopic procedure can start.

TECHNIQUES

A variety of different ER procedures are distinguished:

Piecemeal Resection

- *Snare resection without injection*
- *Lift-and-cut technique:* Submucosal injection of saline solution to lift the lesion from the muscularis propria layer (positive "lifting-sign")
- *Band-and-snare technique:* After ligation of the lesion, the created "pseudopolyp" is resected. Using this technique, the gastroscope is fitted with a ligation device. The lesion is ligated with prior submucosal injection and then snared by a standard polypectomy snare
- *Suck-and-cut technique:* A transparent cap is used for endoscopic mucosal resection using a cap-fitted endoscope (EMRC) (Figure 7-1).

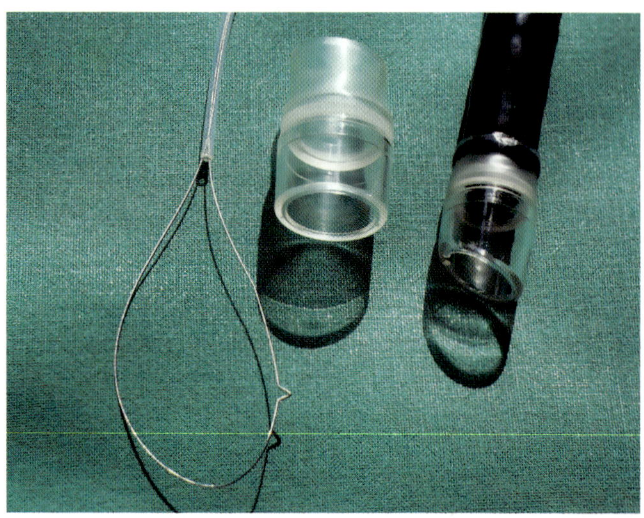

FIGURE 7-1 Endoscopic mucosal resection using a cap-fitted endoscope: different plastic caps with snare.

This technique requires a specialized small transparent cap at the tip of the endoscope. Different sizes of caps are available according to the diameter of the gastroscope and the size of the lesion. After sucking the lesion into the cap, a prelooped snare into the rim of the cap is pushed down onto the base of the aspirated lesion; and after closure of the snare, the lesion is strangulated. By using endocut mode, the lesion can be removed. The cap allows a safety aspiration of the resected specimen.

En Bloc Resection

ESD enables en bloc resection of larger mucosal lesions. It is characterized by three steps (Figure 7-2):

- Injecting fluid into the submucosa to elevate the lesion
- Cutting the surrounding mucosa of the lesion
- Dissecting the submucosa beneath the lesion.

Particularly, in ESD, the technical progress is impressive. Apart from variable knives (Needle knife, Insulated tip knife, Hook knife, Flex knife, Triangle tip knife, and Dual knife), new multifunctional instruments have been developed that appear to facilitate the endoscopic procedure (R-scope Olympus, water jet hybrid knife, ERBE).

Conventional Endoscopic Submucosal Dissection (Different Needle Knives)

ESD using several knives has been developed to prepare one piece resection (Figure 7-3). A transparent hood

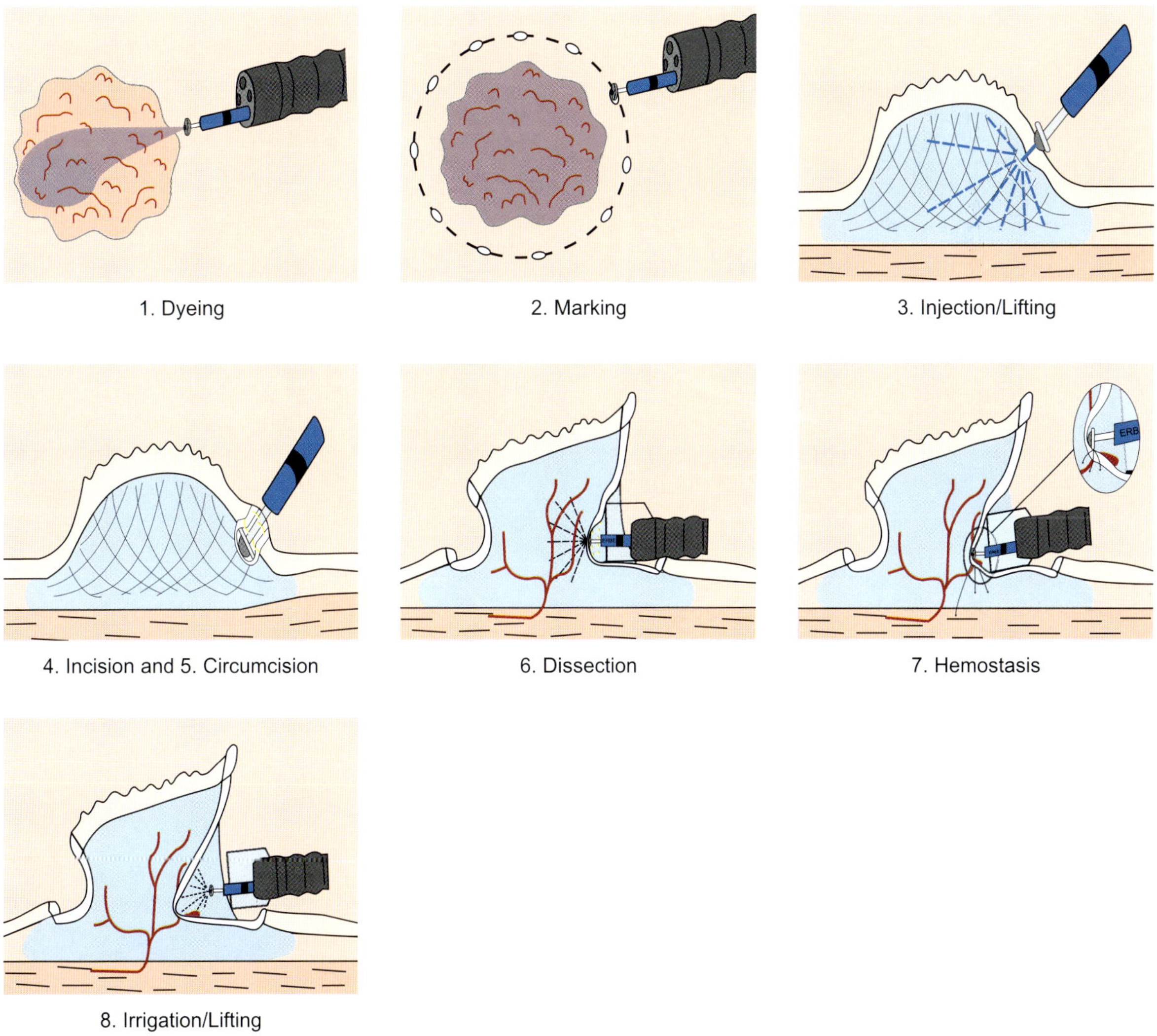

FIGURE 7-2 Schematic diagram of endoscopic submucosal dissection: En bloc resection.

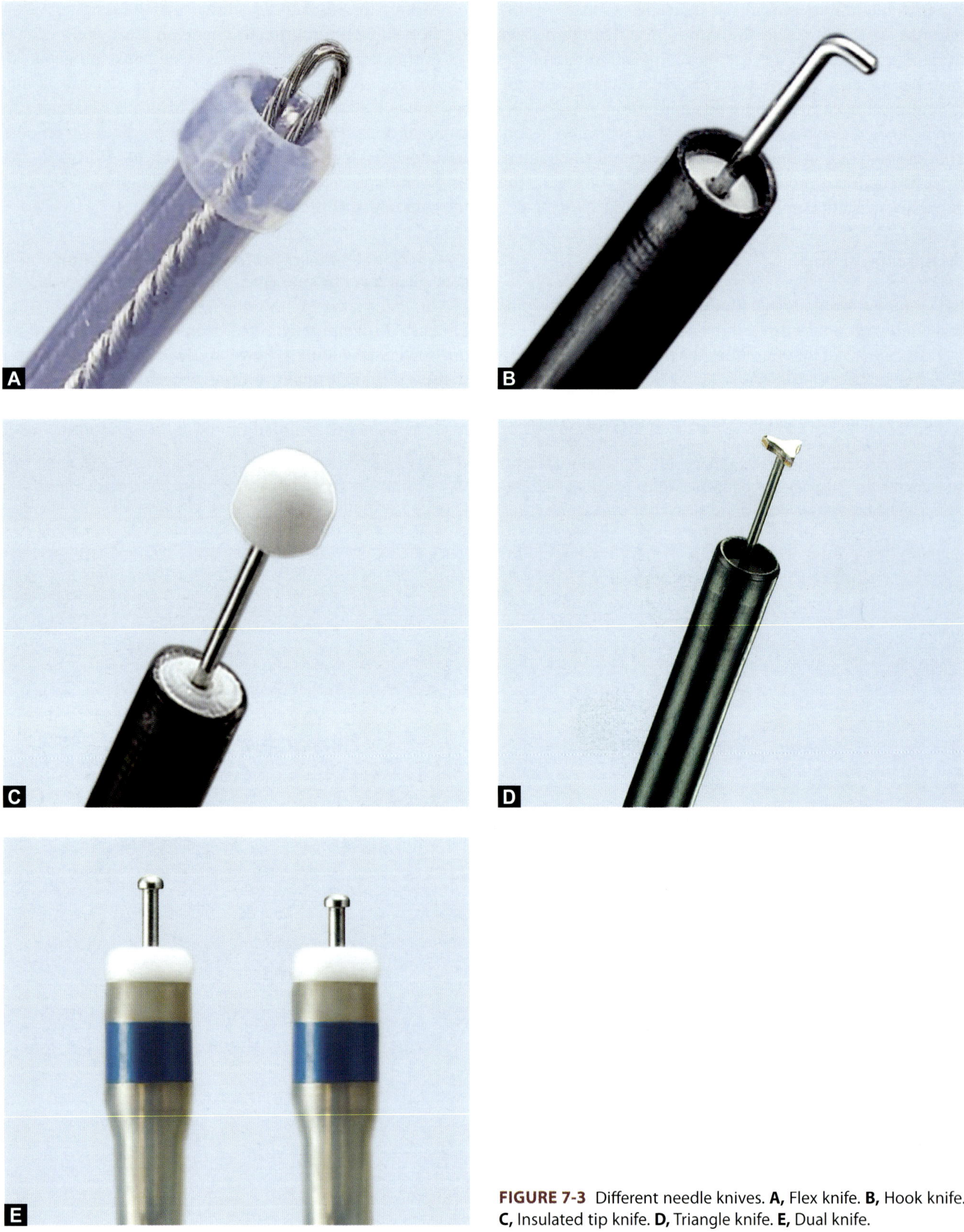

FIGURE 7-3 Different needle knives. **A,** Flex knife. **B,** Hook knife. **C,** Insulated tip knife. **D,** Triangle knife. **E,** Dual knife.

attached to the endoscope tip is used to safely assist precise control of a needle knife tip while incising the mucosa for better visualization of the submucosal tissue. Combined with submucosal thickening by locally injected saline solution or sodium hyaluronate, the transparent hood enables safe dissection of the submucosal layer with a needle knife. Effective control of bleeding can be done by using a hemostatic forceps.

R-scope

To simplify the ESD with time and to decrease complications, new endoscopes were developed. One of them, R-scope, is a 2-channel instrument, one for lifting the lesion and another for dissection with different knives. Both channels can be moved independent from each other (Figure 7-4). This scope was tested in two small series.[19,20] The European authors concluded that the use of R-scope was technically difficult, dependent on lesion location, time-consuming, and combined with a high-risk of perforation.

Water Jet Hybrid Knife

This knife is a new device developed by a German company and is a combination of high pressure water jet and high frequency technology performing in one instrument (Figure 7-5). This device allows submucosal injection or

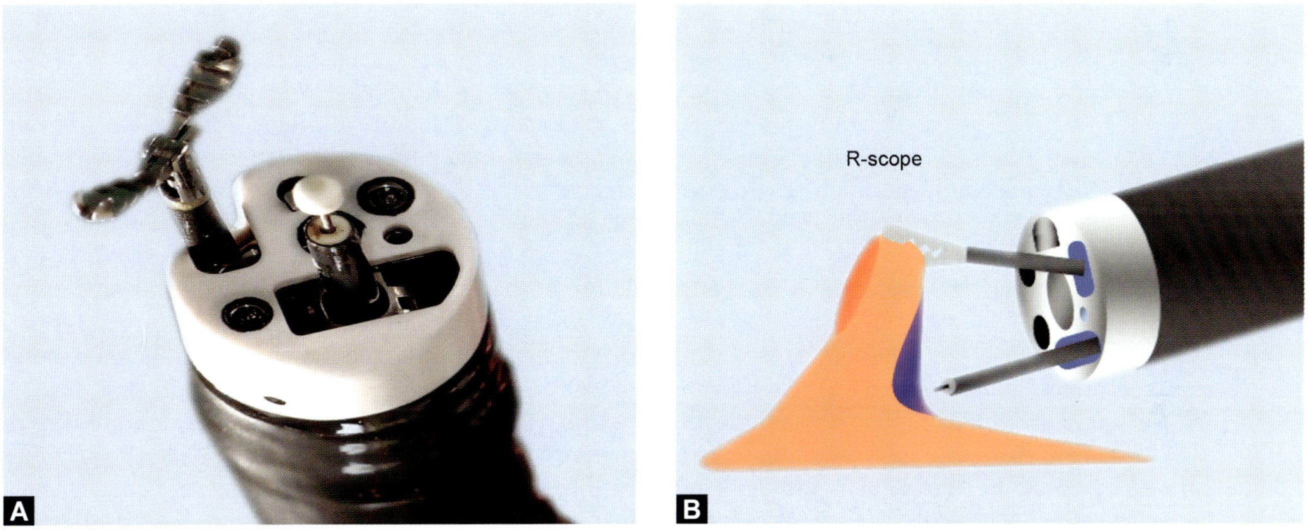

FIGURE 7-4 R-scope. **A,** Prototype from Olympus. **B,** ESD with R-scope.

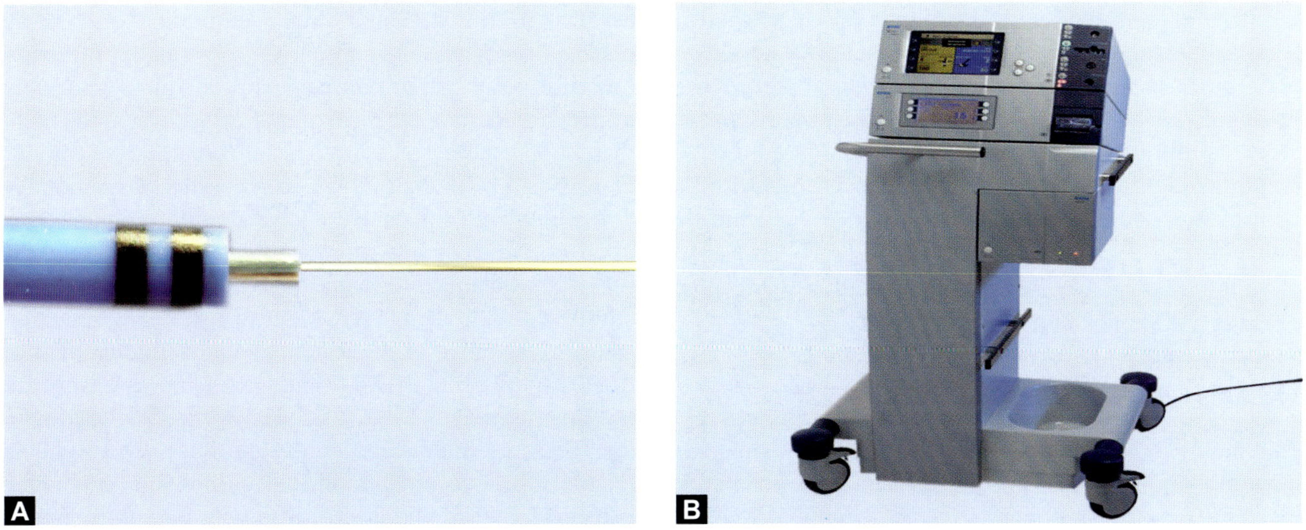

FIGURE 7-5 Hybrid knife is a combination of water jet and radiofrequency technology (ERBE).

flushing with a preselected pressure through an axial water jet channel. Dye-spraying, needle submucosal injection and lifting, flushing of the targeted lesion, dissection, and coagulation can be performed by the same device without need for changing the instrument (Figure 7-6). The instrument has an outer diameter of 2.1 mm and can be used with any standard endoscope.[21,22]

This technique was first evaluated in a pig model (EASIE), followed by a randomized study comparing EMR with ESD of esophageal lesion in a porcine model.[23,24] The use of the new water jet dissector in combination with the hybrid knife seems to accelerate the ESD procedure and may increase its safety and efficacy according to the experimental trials.[24]

In the described study, 13 lesions were randomized to EMR and 12 to ESD of early gastric neoplasia with water jet hybrid knife (ESDH). ESDH achieved complete resection, significantly more frequently than EMR (10/12 vs. 6/13). All ESDH resections were performed as a single piece, whereas a mean of 2.5 resections were needed for EMR. The procedural duration was longer for ESDH than for EMR (28.2 vs. 12.2 min). There was no perforation in either group.[24]

PATHOLOGY

All resected specimens, independent of the removing technique, are immediately flattened and fixed to the periphery on the cork by using thin needles (Figure 7-7A). All marking dots should be included in the resected lesion. One piece resection enables precise and complete histological staging (Figure 7-7B). The treatment is judged as curative resection, if the lesion is resected en bloc with negative margins and fulfills the criteria of node-negative neoplasm. In case of piecemeal resection as well as node-negative neoplasm, a defined endoscopic follow-up should be performed to detect residual neoplasm or local recurrences. Additional surgery should strongly be recommended in case of deeper submucosal infiltration or recurrences, which could not be resected endoscopically due to scars.

COMPLICATIONS AND THEIR MANAGEMENT AFTER ENDOSCOPIC SUBMUCOSAL DISSECTION

The main complications of ESD in the stomach are bleeding and perforation. To prevent postprocedural bleeding, hemostasis of appearing vessels after removing the specimen is essential. Hemostasis is performed by hemostatic forceps, hot biopsy forceps, or endoclips in severe bleedings. According to the perforation data recently published, it was suggested that small perforation can be successfully closed by using endoclips combined with a conservative treatment of the patient by fasting, antibiotics, and careful surveillance.[25,26] ESD should be performed in hospitalized patients, and in most of the cases under sedation with propofol and midazolam. After ESD, eating is started after 24 h of fasting, if there are no complications. Proton pump inhibitors (PPIs) are administered to relieve pain, prevent postoperative bleeding, and promote ulcer healing. Ulcers after ESD heal within 6–8 weeks. In the first year, endoscopic surveillance should be performed every 3 months to detect local recurrence early.

RESULTS

A retrospective Japanese multicenter study revealed significantly higher rates of en bloc resection and curative resection of EGC by use of ESD in comparison with EMR (93 vs. 56%; 74 vs. 61%, respectively). However, there were significantly more perforations in the ESD group (3.6 vs. 1.2%). Tumor-free survival after 3 years was 98% in the ESD group and 93% in the EMR group.[3]

Another large study found out that en bloc resection of EGC with tumor-free margins was possible in 87% (1,019/1,167 patients) in the ESD group and only 42% in the EMR group.[4] The advantage of ESD was even higher with increasing diameter of the lesion. As a consequence of these results, ESD established a gold-standard for patients with EGC in Japan. On the other hand, it is important to consider that ESD is time-consuming and associated with a higher rate of complications. These disadvantages must be compared with a higher mortality and morbidity rate of the surgical procedures (mortality of EGC patients after gastrectomy with lymph node dissection was 0.2–0.5% in a specialized Japanese clinic).[5] However, the results of these studies are not completely consistent and none have allowed definite conclusions about the efficacy and safety of these two approaches. A recently published meta-analysis with 15 nonrandomized studies identified high en bloc and curative resection rates, irrespective of the lesion size and independent of the organ by using ESD. Local recurrence was lower with ESD compared to EMR.[27] Clinical long-term follow-up after ESD for expanded criteria lesions has not been widely studied. Three recently published studies showed en bloc resection rates of about 93%, complete resection rates of 88%, and curative resection rates of 91%. Complications

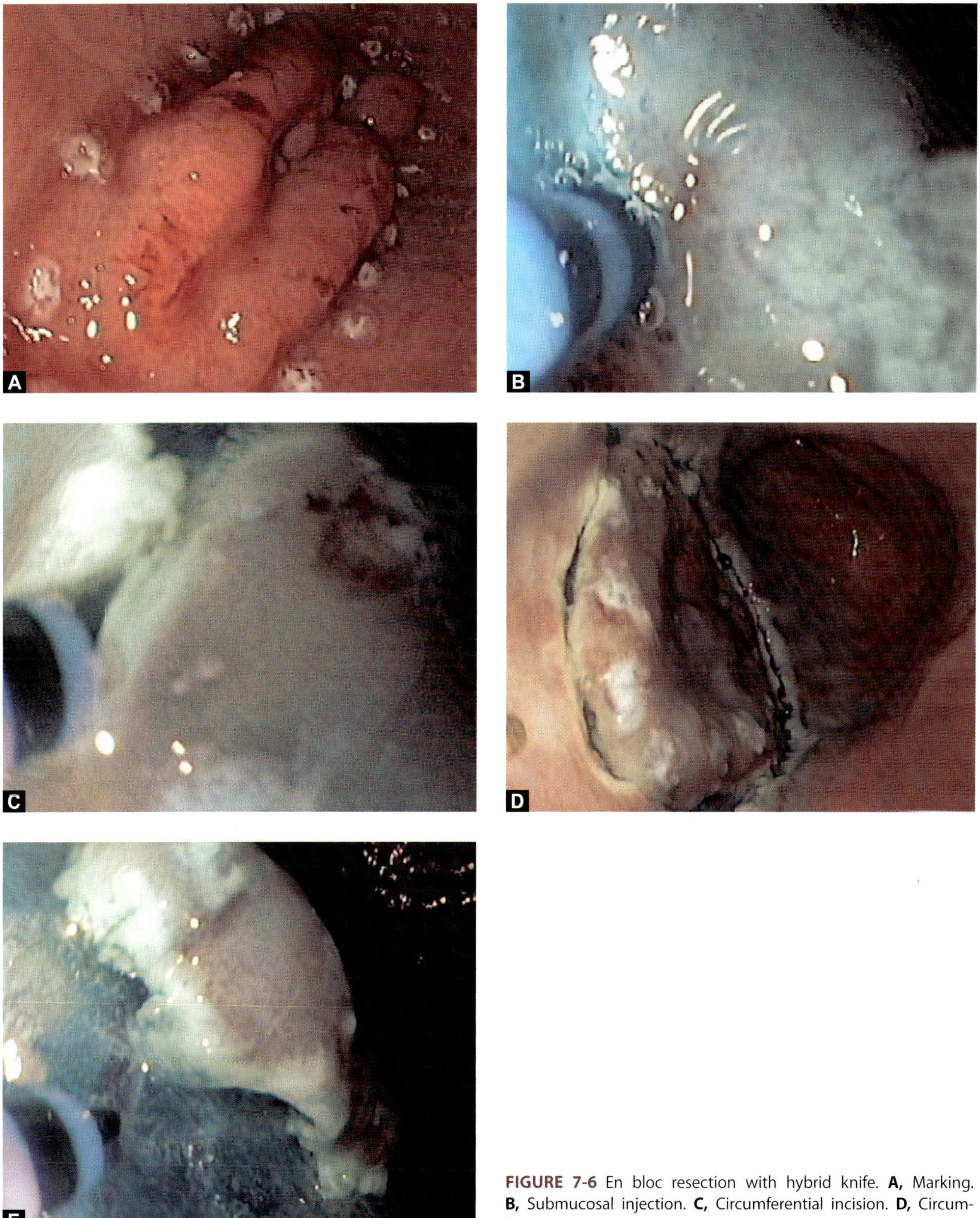

FIGURE 7-6 En bloc resection with hybrid knife. **A,** Marking. **B,** Submucosal injection. **C,** Circumferential incision. **D,** Circumferential incision completed. **E,** Submucosal dissection.

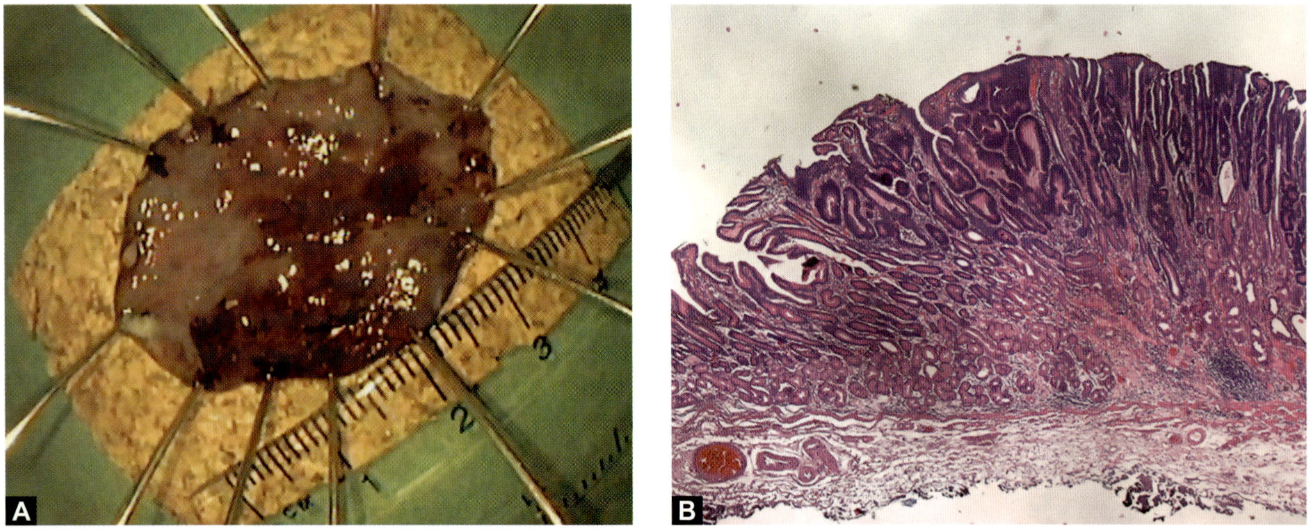

FIGURE 7-7 En bloc resection of gastric lesion. **A,** Specimen flattend and fixed on the cork. **B,** Histology showed adenoma with focal adenocarcinoma.

like bleeding and perforation were reported with 5 and 6.6%, respectively. The 5-year overall survival rate ranged between 96.9 and 100%. Recurrences or metachronous lesion occurred in 2.4–4.5% after a follow-up of 6–16 months.[28-30] The procedural duration of ESD is significantly longer compared to the EMR procedure. Recent clinical data indicated that the procedure can be performed effectively and safely after the experience of 40 cases, with a significant shortening of the procedural time during the learning curve.[31] However, even with increasing experience, ESD is more time consuming than EMR, which seems to be acceptable in view of its higher effectiveness. New techniques like the water jet system and the use of a hybrid knife should accelerate ESD and may increase its safety and efficacy because of time saving changes between lifting and cutting by use of the same device.[21,23] Our study group could demonstrate that this technique achieved complete resection of esophageal lesions more frequently with less number of specimens than EMR in a randomized controlled trial in pigs under general anesthesia.[24] Water jet assisted ESD is still more time-consuming than EMR, but is potentially shorter than conventional ESD, because there is no need for exchange of accessories.

First ESD results of Western endoscopists indicated lower success rates concerning en bloc resection, but revealed that even submucosal tumors can be treated endoscopically.[32] Rösch et al. reported on attempted en bloc resections of upper GI tumors in 37 patients.[32] Complete en bloc resection was achieved in 25% of 24 mucosal lesions and 36% of 14 submucosal tumors. Complications occurred in 16% of the cases. Neuhaus et al. evaluated ESD of early gastric neoplasia, which was performed by use of R-scope in several European centers.[19] They achieved complete en bloc resection in 6 out of 10 cases in this feasibility study. Four patients underwent surgery because of perforation and/or incomplete resection or submucosal tumor infiltration. These results indicate lower rates of complete resection and a higher morbidity compared to most of trials from Asia. They also demonstrated an unfavorable outcome at the beginning of the learning curve even after training in an experimental setting. Probst et al. performed ESD in 71 epithelial or submucosal lesions in the upper and lower GI tract.[33] The results demonstrated a learning curve resulting in a decreasing procedural duration and an increasing rate of complete en bloc resection over time.

The data of the first prospective Western study evaluating the ESDH of early gastric neoplasia in human were presented by Schumacher et al.[34] Thirty-three patients were included with histologically confirmed gastric neoplasia according to the Japanese guidelines. En bloc resection of the targeted area could be achieved in 30 cases and histology confirmed complete resection in 27/33 patients. The vertical margins were free of neoplasia in all cases, which could not be confirmed for the horizontal margins in 6 patients. Follow-up was done after 10 weeks, 5, 9, and 12 months. ESD showed complete remission in 94–96%. Recurrent neoplasia was found in 3 cases. One was managed endoscopically, 2 underwent surgery. Complications like 3 perforations and 2 severe bleedings were managed endoscopically. Furthermore, complications decreased with growing experience of the investigator. Recently, a large retrospective Korean study on ESD (1,000 cases of EGC) revealed a perforation rate of only 1.2%.[35] Only 0.2% of all patients had to be transferred for surgery because of complications.

CONCLUSION

Numerous convincing reports from Asian centers have confirmed that ESD achieves complete en bloc resection of early gastric neoplasia more frequently than EMR, which is needed to avoid gastrectomy as a potential alternative with excellent results. In addition, ESD is associated with a lower recurrence rate. Therefore, the clinical relevance is considered to be high from a Western point of view too. The main problem is to overcome the flat learning curve in view of the low number of detected cases of early gastric lesions in Western countries. A better acceptance of ESD requires improvement of the technique to allow an easier, faster, and safer approach. There is a strong demand for structured training courses and limitations of human cases in selected centers, which participate in prospective trials. A close collaboration between Western and Asian centers is recommended for improvement of the ESD technique and its clinical application.

REFERENCES

1. Larghi A, Waxman I. State of the art on endoscopic mucosal resection and endoscopic submucosal dissection. *Gastrointest Endosc Clin N Am.* 2007;17:441-69.
2. Soetikno R, Kaltenbach T, Yeh R, Gotoda T. Endoscopic mucosal resection for early cancers of the upper gastrointestinal tract. *J Clin Oncol.* 2005;23:4490-8.
3. Ono H, Kondo H, Gotoda T, Shirao K, Yamaguchi H, Saito D, et al. Endoscopic mucosal resection for treatment of early gastric cancer. *Gut.* 2001;48:225-9.
4. Oka S, Tanaka S, Kaneko I, Mouri R, Hirata M, Kawamura T, et al. Advantage of endoscopic submucosal dissection compared with EMR for early gastric cancer. *Gastrointest Endosc.* 2006;64:877-83.
5. Oda I, Saito D, Tada M, Lishi H, Tanabe S, Oyama T, et al. A multicenter retrospective study of endoscopic resection for early gastric cancer. *Gastric Cancer.* 2006;9:262-70.
6. Fujishiro M. Perspective of the practical indications of endoscopic submucosal dissection of gastrointestinal neoplasms. *World J Gastroenterol.* 2008;14:4289-95.
7. Yamamoto H, Yahagi N, Oyama T, Gotoda T, Dio T, Hirasaki S, et al. Usefulness and safety of 0.4% sodium hyaluronate solution as a submucosal fluid "cushion" in endoscopic resection for gastric neoplasms: a prospective multicenter trial. *Gastrointest Endosc.* 2008;67:830-9.
8. Gotoda T, Yanagisawa A, Sasako M, Ono H, Nakanishi Y, Shimoda T, et al. Incidence of lymph node metastasis from early gastric cancer: estimation with a large number of cases at two large centers. *Gastric Cancer.* 2000;3:219-25.
9. Japanese Gastric Cancer Association. JGCA gastric cancer treatment guideline. 2nd ed. Japan: JGCA; 2004.
10. Nakagawa S, Kato M, Shimizu Y, Nakagawa M, Yamamoto J, Luis PA, et al. Relationship between histopathologic gastritis and mucosal microvascularity: observations with magnifying endoscopy. *Gastrointest Endosc.* 2003;58:71-5.
11. Tajiri H, Doi T, Endo H, Nishina T, Terao T, Hyodo I, et al. Routine endoscopy using a magnifying endoscope for gastric diagnosis. *Endoscopy.* 2002;34:772-7.
12. Yagi K, Nakamura A, Sekine A. Comparison between magnifying endoscopy and histological, culture and urease test findings from the gastric mucosa of the corpus. *Endoscopy.* 2002;34:376-81.
13. Kim S, Harum K, Ito M, Tanaka S, Yoshihara M, Chayama K. Magnifying gastroendoscopy for diagnosis of histologic gastritis in the gastric antrum. *Dig Liver Dis.* 2004;36:286-91.
14. Guelrud M, Herrera I, Essenfeld H, Castro J, Antonioli DA. Intestinal metaplasia of the gastric cardia: a prospective study with enhanced magnification endoscopy. *Am J Gastroenterol.* 2002;97:584-9.
15. Sumiyama K, Kaise M, Nakayoshi T, Kato M, Mashiko T, Uchiyama Y, et al. Combined use of a magnifying endoscope with a narrow band imaging system and a narrow band imaging system and a multibending endoscope for en bloc EMR of early stage gastric cancer. *Gastrointest Endosc.* 2004;60:79-84.
16. Nakayoshi T, Tajiri H, Matsuda K, Kaise M, Ikagami M, Sasaki H. Magnifying endoscopy combined with narrow band imaging system for early gastric cancer: correlation of vascular pattern with histopathology (including video). *Endoscopy.* 2004;36:1080-4.
17. Uedo N, Ishihara R, Lishi H, Yamamoto S, Yamamoto S, Yamada T, et al. A new method of diagnosing gastric intestinal metaplasia: narrow-band imaging with magnifying endoscopy. *Endoscopy.* 2006;38:819-24.
18. Yoshida T, Inoue H, Usui S, Satodate H, Fukami N, Kudo SE. Narrow-band imaging system with magnifying endoscopy for superficial esophageal lesions. *Gastrointest Endosc.* 2004;59:288-95.
19. Neuhaus H, Costamagna G, Deviere J, Fockens P, Ponchon T, Rosch T, et al. Endoscopic submucosal resection (ESD) of early neoplastic gastric lesions using a new double channel endoscope (the "R-scope"). *Endoscopy.* 2006;38:1016-23.
20. Yonezawa J, Kaise M, Sumiyama K, Goda K, Arakawa H, Tajiri H. A novel double-channel therapeutic endoscope (R-scope) facilitates endoscopic submucosal dissection of superficial gastric neoplasms. *Endoscopy.* 2006;38:1011-5.
21. Kähler GF, Sold MS, Post S, Fisher K, Enderle MD. Selective tissue elevation by pressure injection (STEP) facilitates endoscopic mucosal resection (EMR). *Surg Technol Int.* 2007;16:107-12.

22. Kaehler GFBA, Sold MS, Fischer K, Post S, Enderle M. Selective fluid cushion in the submucosa layer by water-jet: advantage for endoscopic mucosal resection. *Eur Surg Res.* 2007;39:93-7.
23. Schumacher B, Neuhaus H, Enderle MD. Experimental use of new device for mucosectomy. *Acta Endoscopica.* 2007;37:673-8.
24. Neuhaus H, Wirths K, Schenk M, Enderle MD, Schumacher B. Randomized controlled study of endoscopic mucosal resection (EMR) versus endoscopic submucosal dissection with a water-jet hybrid-knife (ESDH) of esophageal lesions in a porcine model. *Gastrointest Endosc.* 2009;70:112-20.
25. Minami S, Gotada T, Ono H, Oda I, Hamanaka H. Complete endoscopic closure of gastric perforation induced by endoscopic resection of early gastric cancer using endoclips can prevent surgery (with video). *Gastrointest Endosc.* 2006; 63:596-601.
26. Fujishiro M, Yahagi N, Kakushima N, Kodashima S, Muraki Y, Ono S, et al. Successful non surgical management of perforation complicating endoscopic submucosal dissection of gastrointestinal epithelial neoplasms. *Endoscopy.* 2006;38:1001-6.
27. Cao Y, Ciao C, Tan A, Gao Y, Mo Z, Gao F. Meta-analysis of endoscopic submucosal dissection versus endoscopic mucosal resection for tumors of the gastrointestinal tract. *Endoscopy.* 2009;41:751-7.
28. Yamaguchi N, Isomoto H, Fukuda E, Ikeda K, Nishiyama H, Akiyama M, et al. Clinical outcomes of endoscopic submucosal dissection for early gastric cancer by indication criteria. *Digestion.* 2009;80:173-81.
29. Isomoto H, Shikuwa, Yamaguchi N, Fukuda E, Ikeda K, Nishiyama H, et al. Endoscopic submucosal dissection for early gastric cancer: a large-scale feasibility study. *Gut.* 2009;58:331-6.
30. Goto O, Fujishiro M, Kodashima S, Ono S, Omata M. Outcomes of endoscopic submucosal dissection for early gastric cancer with special reference to validation for curability criteria. *Endoscopy.* 2009;41:118-22.
31. Choi IJ, Kim CG, Chang HJ, Kim SG, Kook MC, Bae JM. The learning curve for EMR with circumferential mucosal incision in treating intramucosal gastric neoplasm. *Gastrointest Endosc.* 2005;62:860-5.
32. Rösch T, Sarbia M, Schumacher B, Deinert K, Frimberger E, Toermer T, et al. Attempted endoscopic en bloc resection of mucosal and submucosal tumors using insulated-tip knives: a pilot series. *Endoscopy.* 2004;36:788-801.
33. Probst A, Golger D, Arnholdt H, Messmann H. Endoscopic submucosal dissection of early gastric cancers, flat adenomas, and submucosal tumors in the gastrointestinal tract. *Clin Gastroenterol Hepatol.* 2009;7:149-55.
34. Schumacher B, Mayershofer R, Charon JP, Seelhoff A, Vieth M, Neuhaus H. Endoscopic submucosal resection of early gastric neoplasia with a water-jet hybrid-knife (ESDH) a prospective western study in 31 patients. *Gastrointest Endosc.* 2010;71:AB124.
35. Chung IK, Lee JH, Lee SH, Kim SJ, Cho JY, Cho WY, et al. Therapeutic outcomes in 1000 cases of endoscopic submucosal dissection for early gastric neoplasms: Korean ESD Study. Group multicenter study. *Gastrointest Endosc.* 2009;69:1228-35.

8 Imaging for Small Bowel Neoplasms: Capsule Endoscopy and Deep Enteroscopy

Lauren B Gerson

ABSTRACT

Small bowel neoplasms are uncommon tumors of the gastrointestinal (GI) tract. Most of these tumors present late because of the vague presentation and lack of appropriate diagnostic tools. Video capsule endoscopy (VCE) and deep enteroscopy have improved the diagnostic yield of small bowel pathology. They have been successfully used for varied presentations like obscure GI bleed in the surveillance of Peutz-Jeghers syndrome (PJS). VCE and deep enteroscopy have supplemented valuable details to the array of existing imaging techniques like small bowel follow-through (SBFT), computed tomography enteroscopy (CTE), and magnetic resonance enterography (MRE). These tools have both diagnostic and therapeutic potential. VCE has the advantage of imaging the entire small bowel, while deep enteroscopy is useful for obtaining biopsies and other therapeutic potential as well. In this chapter, we will discuss in detail regarding VCE and deep enteroscopy, their advantages, yield, and complications.

SMALL INTESTINAL NEOPLASMS

Background and Epidemiology

Despite the fact that the small intestine accounts for approximately 75% of the length and 90% of the mucosal surface of the alimentary tract, neoplastic disorders involving the small intestine account for approximately 2% of all gastrointestinal (GI) cancers.[1] The age-adjusted yearly incidence of small bowel cancers has been estimated to range between 0.7 and 1.6 cases per 100,000 population.[2,3] While the small intestine can be affected by both malignant and benign tumors, it is often not possible to differentiate between the two entities based on patient's symptoms, which can include overt or occult GI bleeding, abdominal pain, weight loss, and/or intermittent obstruction or intussusception.[4]

Given the vague symptoms of patients with small bowel neoplasms, and prior to the introduction of capsule endoscopy and other advanced imaging techniques for the small bowel, the average delay in the diagnosis of small tumors was approximately 6–8 months, and was associated with a 50% rate of metastases at presentation for patients with malignant tumors.[5,6] More data are needed to determine whether the advent of advanced imaging techniques has shortened the time for diagnosis of small bowel neoplasms, decreased the need for other imaging modalities, and improved the overall prognosis for patients with small bowel neoplasms. In a series of patients diagnosed with tumors by video capsule endoscopy (VCE), each patient underwent a mean of 2–4 examinations before the diagnostic VCE.[7,8]

Presentation, Tumor Types, and Location

The average age of diagnosis for small bowel neoplasms has been estimated to be approximately 60 years,[9] with a proximal slight male prominence for malignant tumors.[10,11] According to the data from the Surveillance, Epidemiology, and End Results (SEER) registry from 1973–2004, neuroendocrine tumors comprised approximately 36.5% of small bowel neoplasms; adenocarcinomas were detected in 31% of patients, sarcomas and gastrointestinal stromal tumors (GISTs) in 10%, lymphomas 19%, and miscellaneous tumor types in 4%.[12] Data from SEER demonstrated that the incidence of sarcomas has remained unchanged from 1973–2004, while neuroendocrine tumors, adenocarcinomas, and

TABLE 8-1 Location of Benign and Malignant Tumors in Selected Series

Series	*Tumors/VCE total*	*Adeno-carcinoma*	*Carcinoid*	*Lymphoma*	*GIST/other*	*Benign*
Schwartz[7]**	**87 all by VCE**	**18 (21%)**	**17 (20%)**	**5 (7%)**	**29 (33%)**	**17 (20%)**
Duodenum		2 (2%)	0 (0%)	1 (1%)	3 (3%)	0 (0%)
Jejunum		11 (13%)	7 (8%)	4 (5%)	14 (16%)	11 (13%)
Ileum		2 (2%)	8 (9%)	0 (0%)	8 (9%)	0 (0%)
Gabos[13] 1975–1989	**818/1244 (66%) No VCE**	**521 (42%)**	**334 (27%)**	**224 (18%)**	**140 (11%)**	*
Duodenum		287 (55%)	13 (4%)	47 (21%)	27 (19%)	
Jejunum		156 (30%)	30 (9%)	65 (29%)	66 (47%)	
Ileum		83 (16%)	291 (87%)	112 (50%)	53 (38%)	
Cobrin[21] 2001-2004	**50/562 (9%)**	**8 (16%)**	**10 (20%)**	**5 (10%)**	**4 (8%)**	**14 (28%)**
Duodenum		2 (22%)	0 (0%)	0 (0%)	0 (0%)	2 (14%)
Jejunum		2 (22%)	2 (20%)	5 (100%)	3 (75%)	8 (57%)
Ileum		3 (33%)	5 (50%)	0 (0%)	1 (25%)	4 (29%)
Multifocal		2 (22%)	3 (30%)	0 (0%)	0 (0%)	0 (0%)
Urbain[30] 2001-2004	**11/443 (2.5%)**	**4 (36%)**	**1 (9%)**	**3 (27%)**	**3 (27%)**	*
Duodenum		0 (0%)	0 (0%)	0 (0%)	0 (0%)	
Jejunum		3 (75%)	0 (0%)	0 (0%)	2 (67%)	
Ileum		1 (25%)	0 (0%)	0 (0%)	1 (33%)	
Multifocal		0 (0%)	1 (100%)	3 (100%)	0 (0%)	
SUMMARY	**966**	**552 (57%)**	**362 (37%)**	**237 (25%)**	**176 (18%)**	
Duodenum		291 (53%)	13 (4%)	48 (20%)	30 (17%)	
Jejunum		172 (31%)	39 (11%)	74 (31%)	85 (48%)	
Ileum		88 (16%)	304 (84%)	112 (47%)	63 (36%)	

*Not reported; **Location not specified for all lesions.
VCE, video capsule endoscopy; GIST, gastrointestinal stromal tumor.

lymphomas have increased approximately two-fold during the time period.

In a population-based study from Canada of 1,244 cases of small bowel cancers, 818 (66%) had data regarding tumor location. Adenocarcinoma was the most common subtype in 42% of patients with cancers, followed by carcinoid in 27%, lymphoma in 18%, and sarcoma in 11% of the patients.[13] Most of the adenocarcinomas were proximal in location, compared to carcinoids that were located in the ileum. A comparison of locations of benign and malignant tumors in selected series is listed in table 8-1.

Involvement of the small intestine from metastases is more frequent than primary involvement. Metastases from breast, lung, and melanoma to the small bowel occurs via hematogenous route, whereas direct invasion or intraperitoneal spread occurs from colon, ovarian, uterine, and gastric cancers.[14]

VIDEO CAPSULE ENDOSCOPY

Background

Capsule endoscopy can be performed using the Given M2A video capsule system (initially FDA-approved for evaluation of small bowel disorders in 2001) or the Olympus Endocapsule released in 2007. The current capsules measure 11 × 26 mm and contain light-emitting diodes (LEDs), a lens, white LEDs for illumination, silver oxide batteries, and a ultra-high frequency band radio telemetry transmitter.[15] The camera for the Given capsule is a complementary metal oxide semiconductor chip

TABLE 8-2 Comparison of Capsule Endoscopy Systems

Manufacturer	*Capsule name*	*Dimension*	*Weight*	*Frames per second*	*Battery life*	*Field of view*
Given	PillCam SB/SB2	11 × 26 mm	3.4 gm	2 fps	8 hours	140°/156°
Olympus	Endocapsule	11 × 26 mm	3.8 gm	2 fps	8 hours	145°
IntroMedic	MiroCam	11 × 24 mm	3.4 gm	3 fps	11 hours	150°

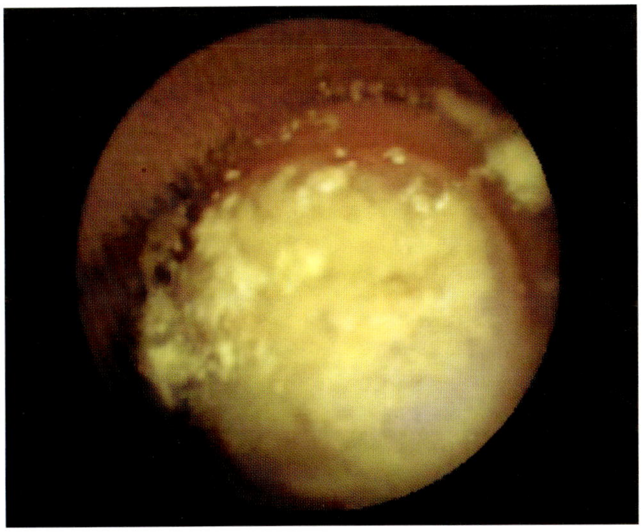

FIGURE 8-1 GIST on VCE study (*Courtesy of Dr Kenneth Binmoeller, CPMC; with permission*).

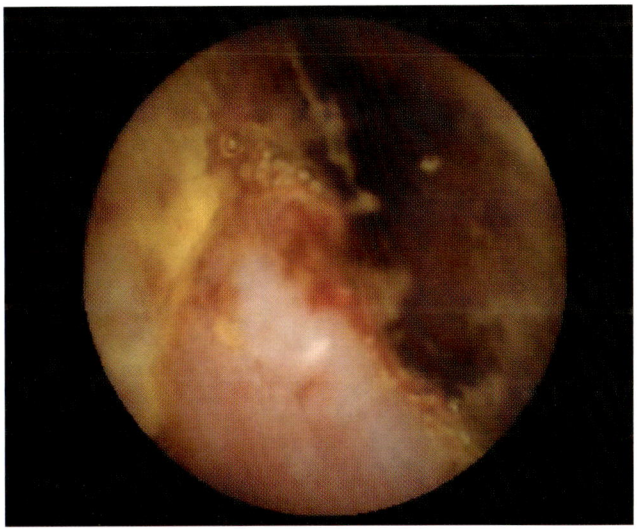

FIGURE 8-2 VCE study demonstrating adenocarcinoma (*Courtesy of Given Imaging, Inc.; with permission*).

while the Olympus capsule uses a charge-coupled device. Two comparative studies did not demonstrate significant differences regarding diagnostic yield between the two capsule systems in patients with obscure GI bleeding.[16,17] The Korean-produced capsule, known as the MiroCam, differs from the two other capsules via a transmission system that utilizes the human body as a conductive medium to transmit the capsule signal to electrodes. The electrical transmission system results in a longer capsule operating time with higher rates of cecal entry.[18] The MiroCam is currently under study for FDA approval in the US, and a comparison of the three capsule systems, is shown in table 8-2.

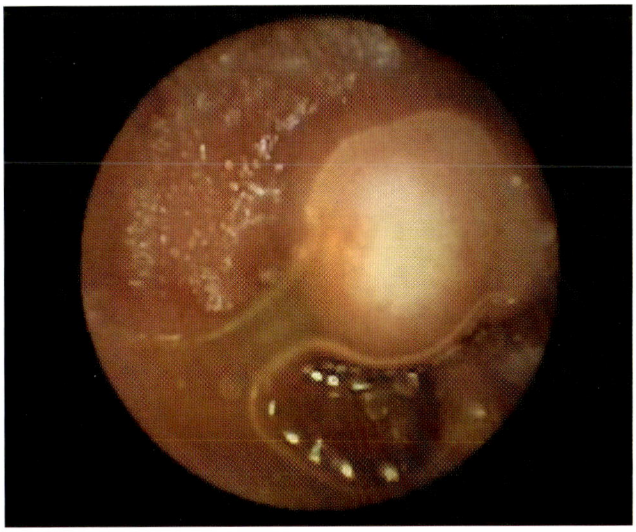

FIGURE 8-3 Carcinoid tumor capsule study (*Courtesy of Given Imaging, Inc.; with permission*).

Appearance of Neoplasms on Video Capsule Endoscopy

Lesions that are suggestive of tumors on VCE can include nonneoplastic lesions including inflammatory polyps and lymphangiectasias; benign neoplasms, including adenomas, GIST (Figure 8-1), lipoma, lymphangioma, hemangioma, hamartoma, and malignant lesions, including adenocarcinoma (Figure 8-2), carcinoid (Figure 8-3), lymphoma, melanoma, and mestastatic lesions from other cancers.

TABLE 8-3 Proposed Classification of Mass Lesions on Video Capsule Endoscopy

Tumor probability	*Major*					*Minor*		
	Bleeding	*Mucosal disruption*	*Irregular surface*	*Polypoid appearance*	*Color*	*Delayed passage*	*White villi*	*Invagination*
High	++	++	++	++	++	++	++	++
Intermediate	±	+	+	+	+			
Low	–	–	–	±	–	–	–	

Source: Mergener K, Ponchon T, Gralnek I, Pennazio M, Gay G, Selby W, et al. Literature review and recommendations for clinical application of small-bowel capsule endoscopy, based on a panel discussion by international experts. Consensus statements for small-bowel capsule endoscopy, 2006/2007. *Endoscopy*. 2007;39:895-909.

Even for the most experienced capsule endoscopy readers, it can be difficult to distinguish bulges from neoplasms on VCE and most often not possible to distinguish benign from malignant tumors. Bulges are more likely to appear as round smooth large base protrusions into the lumen without changes in the surrounding villi.[19] Careful viewing of the video stream can demonstrate that bulges and adjacent loops of bowel move with peristalsis, while neoplasms do not move with the video stream. Additional clues to neoplastic disorders include surface ulcerations or central umbilication that may accompany a submucosal lesion, stretched or thinned mucosa in the area of a tumor, or a multilobulated bulge. Bridging folds that come up to a bulge, but do not cross, it may also signify a submucosal process.[20]

A polypoid appearance is most commonly observed (70–80%)[8,21] followed by ulcerative or stenosed lesions in 20–30% of patients. In a large multicenter study involving 29 centers from 10 European countries, 124 (2.4%) of 5,129 patients undergoing VCE were found to have small bowel tumors (112 primary and 12 metastatic).[22] The most common indication for VCE was obscure GI bleeding in 108 (87%) patients. The frequency of tumors found on VCE ranged from 0.8% (3/400) to 9.3% (7/75) for the 29 centers. The endoscopic appearance of the tumors included a mass or polyp in 94 (76%) cases, ulcerations in 10 (8%) patients, fresh blood in 8 (6.5%), stenoses in 8 (6.5%), and cobblestoned mucosa in 4 (3%). The lesions were single in 111 (90%) and multiple in 13 (11%) cases. In this European study, GIST was the most common subtype in 32%, followed by adenocarcinoma in 21%, and carcinoid in 16%. Metastatic melanoma was the most common subtype in 66% of metastatic cases. The tumors were most commonly found in the jejunum (70%), followed by ileum (22%), and duodenum (7%).

In another small study of 27 patients with known GI lymphoma undergoing VCE in Germany, 7 patients with primary intestinal lymphomas had findings on VCE that included ulcerations (4), nodes (4), villous atrophy (3), and plaques/white villi in 1 patient.[23] The capsule failed to reach the cecum in 2/7 (29%) patients with intestinal lymphoma, in 5/20 (25%) patients with gastric lymphoma, and in 4/30 (13%) control patients with obscure bleeding. In patients with small bowel lymphoma, signs included villous atrophy with or without erythema, edema of the bowel wall with ulcerations, or polypoid nodules. In 5/20 (25%) patients with gastric lymphoma, additional signs of lymphoma in the small bowel were found on VCE examination, which altered the course of therapy.

Another retrospective study from Italy found 13 of 380 (3.4%) patients with small bowel neoplasms on VCE. Findings on VCE included jejunal polyps in 6 (46%), ulcerated strictures in 3 (23%), submucosal nodule in 1 patient, and active bleeding in 1 patient; an ileal stricture with multiple aphthoid ulcers in a patient was found to have ileal carcinoid, complicated by capsule retention.[24]

Based on potential features of mass lesions on VCE, a proposed scoring system was published as part of the International Conference on Capsule Endoscopy (ICCE) in 2006 (Table 8-3).[25] Features considered to be associated with a high probability of a tumor included presence of bleeding, mucosal disruption, irregular surface, polypoid appearance, color change, delayed small bowel passage, white villi, and invagination. However, a formal score has not yet been developed, and this classification system has not been validated to date in any clinical studies.

Capsule Retention in Patients with Small Bowel Neoplasms

According to the consensus statement from the 2005 ICCE, capsule retention is defined as the presence of the capsule endoscope in the digestive tract for a minimum of two weeks or as the capsule remaining in the bowel lumen unless directed medical, endoscopic, or surgical intervention is instituted.[26] Capsule-associated small bowel obstruction has been defined as the development of an acute small bowel obstruction occurring within 24 hours after ingestion of the capsule.[27]

While retention of the capsule endoscope has not been reported in healthy volunteers, the frequency of retention ranges from 0 to 25% in patients with neoplasms,[8,21,22] 4 to 13% in established Crohn's disease, and up to 21% in patients with suspected small bowel obstruction.[19] In a multicenter study by Rondonotti and colleagues,[22] the VCE study was not complete to the cecum in 38 (30.6%) patients; capsule retention at the site of the tumor occurred in 12 (9.7%). Five of the 12 patients had undergone prior small bowel imaging with small bowel series or enteroclysis with normal testing. Capsule retention was more common in patients with stenoses, but occurred equally among tumor subtypes.

The majority of patients with neoplastic capsule retention have been reported to remain asymptomatic,[28] with the retention leading to the necessary subsequent surgical resection. However, acute symptomatic small bowel obstruction due to capsule impaction at sites of stricture and/or neoplasm remains possible, and subsequent perforation has been reported.[29] Deep enteroscopy has been reported as a nonsurgical mean to remove impacted video capsule endoscopes.[27] In a large series of 904 capsule examinations from the Netherlands, retention was reported in 8 patients (5 of which were diagnosed with malignant neoplasms) and caused symptomatic acute small bowel obstruction in 6 patients. Double balloon enteroscopy (DBE) was successful in the removal of all impacted capsules.

Impact on Diagnosis and Therapy

In a small series of 11 tumors from Belgium,[30] VCE was determined to have an influence on therapy in 10/11 patients, although in 3/10 patients, VCE confirmed findings detected on other diagnostic procedures. Therefore, the actual impact on diagnosis was considered to be 64% (7/11 patients) and impact on subsequent therapy occurred in 55% (6/11 patients) of the cases. There is currently a paucity of data regarding the role of VCE and impact on the prognosis of patients with small bowel neoplasms.

Capsule Endoscopy Miss Rates

A pilot randomized controlled trial by Appleyard in 2000, compared diagnostic yields for VCE to push enteroscopy (PE) for the detection of beads sewn into the canine small intestines.[31] Although the overall VCE yield was significantly higher compared to PE (64% compared to 37%), the miss rate for VCE was approximately 36% overall. Because of the tumbling of the capsule and angulation of the duodenum, prior studies have only demonstrated limited sensitivity for detection of pathology in this area. In a clinical assessment of 125 studies, the ampulla was only visualized in 10% of cases.[32]

Other Limitations of Capsule Endoscopy

The approximate location of neoplastic lesions in the small bowel can be estimated by the time of transit of the VCE from the duodenum to the cecum.[33] In one study, the route of subsequent DBE was predicted more accurately when cutoff value for the selection was half of the small bowel transit time in the complete VCE examination.[34] However, the estimation of location will not be accurate, if the capsule does not reach the cecum during the 8-hour recording period, or if the transit is delayed because of the presence of an obstructing lesion. The localization system[35] for the Given capsule system is based on the capsule-emitted signal received by the eight sensors that are placed on the chest and abdomen during the examination. The result is a dynamic display of the course of the capsule as it transits through the small intestine, with the location of the VCE denoted by quadrants. A small Korean study demonstrated good accuracy between VCE localization and subsequent findings on laparoscopy.[36]

The Given "patency capsule" was developed to determine potential clearance of a standard capsule endoscope in patients with suspected stenosis. The capsule is composed of a lactose body that dissolves within 40 hours after ingestion, and contains a radiofrequency identification tag so that it can be identified using a hand-held radiofrequency detector placed on the abdominal wall.[37] In a clinical study of 22 patients with suspected intestinal stenosis, computed tomographic enterography (CTE), or small bowel follow-through (SBFT) examinations were conducted first, followed by the patency capsule in all patients. At 30 hours post-ingestion, the patency capsule was detected in 17 (77%) patients. In patients with capsule retention at the site of stenosis, the abnormality had been suspected on CTE or SBFT examination. In 3 patients, the patency capsule induced a symptomatic intestinal occlusion, which required emergency surgery in 2 patients. The investigators did not detect an increased incremental yield from the patency capsule in this small study of patients with suspected intestinal stenosis.[38]

Usage of Capsule Endoscopy for Hereditary Polyposis Syndromes

The usage of VCE has been proposed for surveillance in patients with inherited polyposis syndromes, including Peutz-Jeghers syndrome (PJS) and familial adenomatous polyposis (FAP), both of which are associated with an increased risk for malignancy. VCE has been shown to be superior to SBFT for the detection of polyps in PJS with the detection ratio of 4:1 when compared to barium studies.[39] Other studies have confirmed the superiority of VCE to barium contrast studies for patients with both PJS and FAP[40] and superiority of VCE compared to PE in FAP patients for detection of jejunal polyps.[41] Despite the superiority of VCE in the detection of numbers of polyps, the usage of MRE has been shown to be more accurate for localization of polyps and size determination.[42,43] While VCE is recommended every 2–3 years in patients with PJS and for surveillance in FAP, particularly in patients with duodenal polyps, the impact of VCE on patient outcomes has not been well studied. In particular, more data is needed regarding the usage of VCE and subsequent deep enteroscopy to remove polyps on reduction of small bowel neoplasms and other outcomes including GI bleeding and small bowel obstruction.

DEEP ENTEROSCOPY

Background

Deep enteroscopy can be defined as the usage of an enteroscope to examine small intestine distal to the ligament of Treitz or proximal to the terminal ileum. Commercially available options for deep enteroscopy include DBE, single balloon enteroscopy (SBE), and spiral enteroscopy. The concept of DBE was introduced by Dr Hinori Yamamoto in 2001,[44] and was subsequently introduced commercially into the US by Fujinon Corporation in 2004. The development of DBE was based on the concept that stretching of the small intestinal wall prevents further endoscopic advancement, and that the usage of a balloon would grip the intestinal wall and prevent subsequent loop formation.[44] The diagnostic enteroscope (EN450P5) has a 200 cm working length, an endoscope diameter of 8.5 mm, and an accessory channel of 2.2 mm. The therapeutic enteroscope (EN450T5) has a diameter of 9.4 mm and an accessory channel of 2.8 mm. Technical details regarding performance of the DBE and SBE examinations are available in a recent publication.[45]

SBE system was developed in 2006 and was introduced into the commercial market on May 19, 2007.[46] The objectives behind development of the SBE were to reduce the learning curve for balloon-assisted enteroscopy, avoid the difficulty of attaching the enteroscope balloon to the distal tip of the scope encountered in DBE, and eliminate the requirement of inflating and deflating two balloons in multiple steps with the current DBE insertion technique. A prospective multicenter trial comparing SBE to DBE examinations using the Fujinon DBE system demonstrated that while instrument preparation was faster with SBE compared to DBE, complete enteroscopy (defined as reaching an India ink tattoo placed during an examination from the opposite approach) was performed in 33/50 (66%) DBE patients compared to 11/50 (22%) patients in the SBE arm, with higher associated diagnostic and therapeutic yields for DBE.[47]

Spiral enteroscopy, introduced in 2007, uses a special overtube, the Discovery Small Bowel (DSB), with raised helices at the distal end.[48] Clockwise rotation of the DSB pleats the small bowel onto the overtube. The current DSB with an outer diameter of 16 mm and length of 130 cm can be used with the Fijinon EN450T5 enteroscope and the Olympus SIF-Q180 enteroscopes. A retrospective trial comparing spiral enteroscopy to single balloon enteroscopy did not show a difference in diagnostic yield (60% for SBE vs. 43% for spiral enteroscopy; $p = 0.12$) or procedure times. The mean depth of insertion distal to the ligament of Treitz was estimated to be higher for spiral enteroscopy (mean 301 vs. 222 cm; $p < 0.001$).[49]

Deep Enteroscopy for Evaluation of Small Bowel Neoplasms

For patients with small bowel neoplasms, deep enteroscopy offers the potential advantages compared to usage of VCE including biopsy, treatment of bleeding lesions, and other therapeutic maneuvers including stricture dilation and stent placement. Lesions located within the proximal 2/3rd of the small bowel transit time on capsule endoscopy are thought to be amenable to deep enteroscopy performed via the anterograde approach. DBE has been reported to be diagnostic in a small percentage of patients with normal capsule examinations, particularly in the situation of ongoing acute obscure hemorrhage.[50]

Majority of outcomes in the literature on deep enteroscopy pertain to DBE, since publications on SBE and spiral enteroscopy remain limited. A summary of

TABLE 8-4 Comparisons of Western vs. Eastern Double Balloon Enteroscopy Studies

	Patients (% bleeding)	*Diagnostic yield*	*Ulcers*	*Neoplasm**	*Vascular lesions**
Eastern					
Yamamoto[64]	66 (37%)	65%	33%	15%	11%
Manabe[70]	31 (100%)	74%	35%	29%	6%
Matsumoto[71]	28 (100%)	43%	21%	4%	7%
Akahoshi[72]	20 (19%)	25%	10%	10%	5%
Zhong[73]	191 (50%)	81%	25%	19%	17%
Sun[74]	152 (80%)	72%	20%	30%	23%
Lin[61]	90 (80%)	76%	12%	26%	39%
Chen[53]	75 (89%)	60%	9%	23%	15%
Li[75]	51 (100%)	67%	12%	33%	18%
Totals (Mean ± SD)	*704 (73 ± 30%)*	*63% ± 18%*	*20% ± 10%*	*21% ± 10%*	*16% ± 11%*
Western					
May[76]	90 (36%)	80%	27%	25%	37%
Ell[77]	64 (44%)	72%	16%	13%	34%
Di Caro[78]	33 (37%)	88%	21%	6%	58%
Mehdizadeh[66]	130 (55%)	57%	12%	6%	37%
Hadithi[79]	35 (100%)	60%	6%	3%	51%
Heine[80]	168 (61%)	87%	2%	5%	36%
Monkemuller[81]	29 (41%)	66%	10%	7%	48%
Gross[82]	101 (50%)	80%	12%	22%	48%
Lahat[83]	59 (48%)	67%	12%	21%	18%
Totals (Mean ± SD)	*709 (52 ± 20%)*	*73% ± 11%*	*13% ± 8%*	*12% ± 9%*	*41% ± 12%*

*p value = 0.05 for tumors (more common in Eastern DBE). p value <0.05 for vascular lesions in Western DBE series. All other p values were not significant.

the published DBE literature has demonstrated similar diagnostic yields to capsule endoscopy. In these published studies, the overall mean diagnostic yield was 67% with a treatment success rate of 64%.[51] A recent meta-analysis comparing capsule endoscopy to DBE from 11 studies demonstrated similar diagnostic yields of both modalities for vascular lesions, inflammatory disorders, and small bowel neoplastic lesions.[52]

There remain important differences between deep enteroscopy examinations performed in patients from Eastern countries compared to Western series. Table 8-4 compares the findings of ulcerative disorders, neoplasms, and vascular lesions in approximately 700 patients from both regions. Neoplasms were more common in patients from Eastern countries ($p = 0.05$) while vascular lesions were more likely to be found in Western patients ($p < 0.05$). The reasons for these differences remain unclear. These studies have also demonstrated that approximately 1/3rd of patients in Eastern countries with neoplasms would have pathology located in the distal small bowel,[53] while patients in the West tend to have pathology located within the reach of the anterograde approach.[54]

Findings in Series of Patients Undergoing Deep Enteroscopy

In a large Japanese series of 1,035 DBE cases, the most common indication for the procedure was obscure GI bleeding in 61 (42%) patients, while suspected presence of a tumor was the indication for DBE in 144 (14%) patients with small bowel neoplasm.[55] Malignant lymphoma was found in 31 (21.5%) and GIST in 27 (19%) cases. As in the prior VCE series, carcinoma was more likely to be found in the upper small bowel (4 in duodenum and upper jejunum, 1 in lower jejunum, and 2 in lower ileum) Biopsies were performed for malignant lymphoma in all 31 subjects, in 22/27 GIST tumors and 12/14 patients with carcinoma. The biopsy was confirmative, however, only in 9 (41%) of GIST cases, the rest of which were confirmed via histology after surgery. Of note, there were 14 (5%) complications, including small-bowel perforation in 2 cases with malignant lymphoma and 2 cases of pancreatitis in patients with PJS.

A smaller case series from Portugal analyzed 96 DBE performed in 78 patients from 2005–2008, which included 9 (12%) patients with small bowel tumors.[56] Five patients had prior abnormal VCE studies and the other 4 had abnormal radiographic examinations. Adenocarcinoma was diagnosed in 33% of the cases, GIST in 33%, lymphoma in 22%, and carcinoid in 11% of the tumors. At a mean follow-up time of 15 months, two patients died of their disease.

In a study assessing the safety of DBE in elderly patients over the age of 75 in Pennsylvania,[57] angioectasias remained the most common finding, and were more common in patients over the age of 75 compared to patients aged less than 75 years (39 vs. 23%; $p = 0.01$). Neoplasms were the second most common finding, and their prevalence did not differ between age cohorts.

To date, there is no information regarding whether DBE changes the outcome of patients diagnosed with small bowel neoplasms. Prior studies have demonstrated that early performance of VCE (within 2 weeks of an overt bleeding episode) is associated with a higher diagnostic yield (91 vs. 34%; $p < 0.05$), including polyps and neoplasms.[58] A retrospective study from the Netherlands examining the role of direct DBE without initial VCE showed a higher prevalence of angiodysplastic lesions that were treated endoscopically, but patients with normal DBE also had high spontaneous cessation rates of bleeding.[59] Further studies regarding early usage of deep enteroscopy and outcomes of patients with small bowel neoplasms is warranted.

Lesions Detected on Deep Enteroscopy Missed by Video Capsule Endoscopy Examination

In a patient with ongoing overt bleeding and a negative capsule examination, further diagnostic studies can be considered, including deep enteroscopy, repeat capsule endoscopy, radiographic examinations, or intraoperative enteroscopy. Repeat VCE studies have been shown to be associated with a higher diagnostic yield, particularly in patients with ongoing overt hemorrhage and drop in hemoglobin levels.[60] Performance of a CTE or MRE examination is another option that might detect the presence of submucosal tumors or vascular lesions that would not be visualized on endoscopic examination (Figure 8-4).[61] Empiric deep enteroscopy is also an option for patients with ongoing bleeding and normal VCE examination. In a retrospective multicenter study of 183 patients undergoing DBE, a small bowel neoplasms was identified in 18 patients. Fifteen of the 18 patients had prior VCE studies showing a mass lesion in 5 patients, fresh blood without an underlying lesion in 7 patients, and nonspecific erythema in 3 patients. Four cases of primary adenocarcinoma were missed by VCE.[50]

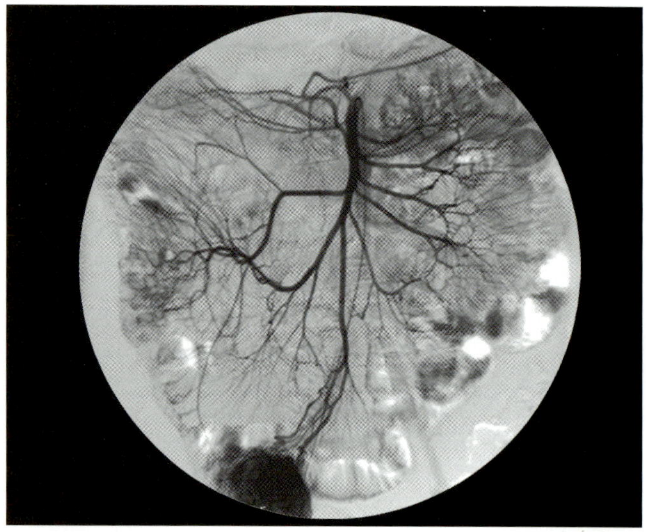

FIGURE 8-4 After retrograde deep enteroscopy demonstrating fresh blood in the ileum, a superior mesenteric angiogram was performed demonstrating a well-circumscribed hypervascular mass lesion in the right lower quadrant. Subsequent CT scan demonstrated a hypervascular mass arising from the distal ileum consistent with a submucosal lesion, most likely a GIST or leiomyoma. The patient underwent resection of the involved segment of ileum revealing a GIST.

Complications Associated with Deep Enteroscopy

Complications that appear to be increased in association with deep enteroscopy have included small bowel perforation and pancreatitis. Studies using DBE have reported perforation rates ranging between 0.3 and 3.4%.[62,63] Perforation risks have been reported to be increased in patients with inflammatory bowel disease,[64] malignancy,[65] and altered anatomy, including ileoanal anastomoses.[66] The presence of small bowel malignancy can be associated with weakening of the intestinal wall, which can be enhanced in patients undergoing chemotherapy. In the original DBE series from Yamamoto published in 2004,[64] for example, a patient with lymphoma undergoing chemotherapy sustained small bowel perforation in areas of necrosis. In an elderly patient with a suspected abdominal tumor, introduction of SBE into the jejunum before the areas of neoplasm was reached, caused small bowel perforation; histology from resected bowel demonstrated metastatic carcinoma from unknown primary with perforation at the site of ulcerations.[65]

In a large retrospective study of DBE complications from 9 US centers, complications were reported in 20 (0.9%) of 2,478 DBE examinations.[67] Perforations occurred in 11 (0.4%) examinations including 3 (0.2%) anterograde examinations and 8 (1.2%) retrograde DBEs. Patients with inflammatory bowel disease or altered surgical anatomy (including ileoanal anastomosis and Roux-en-Y anatomy) were more likely to experience complications, reported in 1/59 (1.6%) anterograde examinations, 5/60 (8%) retrograde DBEs, and 1/5 (20%) peristomal examinations. One anterograde DBE was complicated by an asymptomatic pneumoperitoneum after biopsy of a metastatic breast cancer presenting as a fungating jejunal mass. Two retrograde DBE examinations were notable for perforations occurring after snare polypectomy of ileal carcinoid lesions, which included mesenteric involvement in one patient. On the basis of these available data, deep enteroscopy should be performed with caution in patients with altered surgical anatomy and small bowel malignancy. Further studies are needed to define which patients with small bowel tumors are at greatest risk for endoscopic complications.

Increased risk of small bowel perforation has also been reported after therapeutic interventions, including post-argon plasma coagulation for angiodysplastic lesions, post-stricture dilation,[62] and postpolypectomy of large (>3 cm) polyps in patients with hereditary polyposis syndromes.[63]

Data regarding perforations associated with SBE and spiral enteroscopy are limited, but also suggest a higher rate of perforation in patients with inflammatory bowel disease or malignancy. In a series of 78 patients undergoing SBE, a mucosal tear was observed in one patient with Crohn's disease when the tip of the enteroscope pressed against a longitudinal ulcer scar during insertion of the overtube.[68] In another series of 37 SBE procedures, a perforation occurred in a case of ulcerative colitis postoperatively and was believed to be due to the sliding tube being caught in the mucosa of the ileal pouch when the sliding tube was inserted along the enteroscope.[69] Another case report of SBE reported perforation associated with jejunal ulcerations from metastatic adenocarcinoma of unknown primary; the perforation occurred during insertion of the enteroscope before detection of the lesions that were subsequently found on laparotomy.[65]

On the basis of the experience described earlier, perforation associated with deep enteroscopy is increased compared with standard endoscopic procedures. Traction and distention in association with deep enteroscopy of a weakened intestinal wall may occur in patients with altered surgical anatomy, ulcerative, or neoplastic disorders.

The incidence of pancreatitis is increased in association with deep enteroscopy for unclear reasons. Pancreatitis occurred in 7 (0.3%) patients in the Mensink study; 6 occurred in diagnostic DBE cases.[62] The location of pancreatitis occurred in the body or tail in 4 patients, the head of the pancreas in 1 patient, and the entire pancreas in 2 patients. The incidence of pancreatitis did not seem to increase with the use of the therapeutic DBE enteroscope. Pancreatitis was reported in 6 (0.2%) cases in the multicenter US study; one case occurred in a patient undergoing retrograde DBE examination.[67] None of the procedures involved therapeutic interventions in the area of the ampulla.

The mechanism for post-DBE pancreatitis remains unclear. Potential explanations might include pancreatic duct obstruction by direct compression of the papilla with the inflated balloon, an increase in duodenal intraluminal pressure caused by the overtube and gastrointestinal shortening technique, reflux of duodenal contents into the pancreatic duct due to intraluminal hypertension caused by the inflated balloon, or injury or ischemia due to stretching and shortening of the proximal small bowel. The incidence of post-DBE pancreatitis has not been increased in patients found to have small bowel malignancies.

CONCLUSION

Small bowel neoplasms are unlikely causes of obscure GI hemorrhage, particularly in Western countries. Capsule endoscopy provides opportunity for complete small bowel visualization and has an increased diagnostic yield for all pathology, including small bowel tumors and polyps compared to other imaging studies. Weakness associated with VCE includes visualization of the duodenum where pathology could be missed. In patients with polyposis syndromes, PE or a side-viewing enteroscope should be used to visualize the periampullary region.

Deep enteroscopy allows for tissue biopsy and polypectomy in patients with familial polyposis syndromes. The diagnostic yield is comparable to VCE. Because of an increased risk of complications, DBE should occur after a positive VCE. However, further data are required regarding early usage of direct deep enteroscopy and diagnostic yield. CTE or MRE can be useful to diagnose submucosal pathology in patients with normal VCE examinations and ongoing anemia/bleeding. Tumor type determines location in the small bowel. Adenocarcinomas are more likely to be located in the proximal small bowel, while carcinoids are more likely to be ileal in location. Lymphomas can be located throughout the small bowel, while GISTs are more common in the jejunum and/or ileum. Further studies regarding usage of VCE and/or deep enteroscopy and tumor outcomes are needed.

Small bowel perforation is increased in patients undergoing deep enteroscopy with small bowel malignancy, particularly with associated bowel wall weakness.

REFERENCES

1. DiSario JA, Burt RW, Vargas H, McWhorter WP. Small bowel cancer: epidemiological and clinical characteristics from a population-based registry. *Am J Gastroenterol.* 1994;89:699-701.
2. Barclay TH, Schapira DV. Malignant tumors of the small intestine. *Cancer.* 1983;51:878-81.
3. Jemal A, Murray T, Ward E, Samuels A, Tiwari RC, Ghafoor A, et al. Cancer statistics, 2005. *CA Cancer J Clin.* 2005;55:10-30.
4. Sjoblom SM. Clinical presentation and prognosis of gastrointestinal carcinoid tumours. *Scand J Gastroenterol.* 1988;23:779-87.
5. Ciresi DL, Scholten DJ. The continuing clinical dilemma of primary tumors of the small intestine. *Am Surg.* 1995; 61:698-702.
6. Maglinte DD, O'Connor K, Bessette J, Chernish SM, Kelvin FM. The role of the physician in the late diagnosis of primary malignant tumors of the small intestine. *Am J Gastroenterol.* 1991;86:304-8.
7. Schwartz GD, Barkin JS. Small-bowel tumors detected by wireless capsule endoscopy. *Dig Dis Sci.* 2007;52:1026-30.
8. Bailey AA, Debinski HS, Appleyard MN, Remedios ML, Hooper JE, Walsh AJ, et al. Diagnosis and outcome of small bowel tumors found by capsule endoscopy: a three-center Australian experience. *Am J Gastroenterol.* 2006;101:2237-43.
9. Silberman H, Crichlow RW, Caplan HS. Neoplasms of the small bowel. *Ann Surg.* 1974;180:157-61.
10. Sethi G, Hardin CA. Primary malignant tumors of the small bowel. *Arch Surg.* 1969;98:659-61.
11. Ouriel K, Adams JT. Adenocarcinoma of the small intestine. *Am J Surg.* 1984;147:66-71.
12. Gustafsson BI, Siddique L, Chan A, Dong M, Drozdov I, Kidd M, et al. Uncommon cancers of the small intestine, appendix and colon: an analysis of SEER 1973-2004, and current diagnosis and therapy. *Int J Oncol.* 2008;33:1121-31.
13. Gabos S, Berkel J, Band P, Robson D, Whittaker H. Small bowel cancer in western Canada. *Int J Epidemiol.* 1993;22: 198-206.
14. Gill SS, Heuman DM, Mihas AA. Small intestinal neoplasms. *J Clin Gastroenterol.* 2001;33:267-82.
15. Gerber J, Bergwerk A, Fleischer D. A capsule endoscopy guide for the practicing clinician: technology and troubleshooting. *Gastrointest Endosc.* 2007;66:1188-95.
16. Cave DR, Fleischer DE, Leighton JA, Faigel DO, Heigh RI, Sharma VK, et al. A multicenter randomized comparison of the Endocapsule and the Pillcam SB. *Gastrointest Endosc.* 2008;68:487-94.
17. Hartmann D, Eickhoff A, Damian U, Riemann JF. Diagnosis of small-bowel pathology using paired capsule endoscopy with two different devices: a randomized study. *Endoscopy.* 2007;39:1041-5.
18. Kim HM, Kim YJ, Kim HJ, Park S, Park JY, Shin SK, et al. A Pilot Study of Sequential Capsule Endoscopy Using MiroCam and PillCam SB Devices with Different Transmission Technologies. *Gut Liver.* 2010;4:192-200.
19. Pennazio M, Rondonotti E, de Franchis R. Capsule endoscopy in neoplastic diseases. *World J Gastroenterol.* 2008; 14:5245-53.
20. Lewis BS. How to read wireless capsule endoscopic images: tips of the trade. *Gastrointest Endosc Clin N Am.* 2004;14:11-6.
21. Cobrin GM, Pittman RH, Lewis BS. Increased diagnostic yield of small bowel tumors with capsule endoscopy. *Cancer.* 2006;107:22-7.
22. Rondonotti E, Pennazio M, Toth E, Menchen P, Riccioni ME, De Palma GD, et al. Small-bowel neoplasms in patients undergoing video capsule endoscopy: a multicenter European study. *Endoscopy.* 2008;40:488-95.
23. Flieger D, Keller R, May A, Ell C, Fischbach W. Capsule endoscopy in gastrointestinal lymphomas. *Endoscopy.* 2005;37:1174-80.
24. Spada C, Riccioni ME, Familiari P, Marchese M, Bizzotto A, Costamagna G. Video capsule endoscopy in small-bowel tumours: a single centre experience. *Scand J Gastroenterol.* 2008;43:497-505.
25. Mergener K, Ponchon T, Gralnek I, Pennazio M, Gay G, Selby W, et al. Literature review and recommendations for clinical application of small-bowel capsule endoscopy, based on a panel discussion by international experts. Consensus statements for small-bowel capsule endoscopy, 2006/2007. *Endoscopy.* 2007;39:895-909.

26. Cave D, Legnani P, de Franchis R, Lewis BS. ICCE consensus for capsule retention. *Endoscopy.* 2005;37:1065-7.
27. Van Weyenberg SJ, Van Turenhout ST, Bouma G, Van Waesberghe JH, Van der Peet DL, Mulder CJ, et al. Double-balloon endoscopy as the primary method for small-bowel video capsule endoscope retrieval. *Gastrointest Endosc.* 2010;71:535-41.
28. Li F, Gurudu SR, De Petris G, Sharma VK, Shiff AD, Heigh RI, et al. Retention of the capsule endoscope: a single-center experience of 1000 capsule endoscopy procedures. *Gastrointest Endosc.* 2008;68:174-80.
29. Lin OS, Brandabur JJ, Schembre DB, Soon MS, Kozarek RA. Acute symptomatic small bowel obstruction due to capsule impaction. *Gastrointest Endosc.* 2007;65:725-8.
30. Urbain D, De Looze D, Demedts I, Louis E, Dewit O, Macken E, et al. Video capsule endoscopy in small-bowel malignancy: a multicenter Belgian study. *Endoscopy.* 2006; 38:408-11.
31. Appleyard M, Glukhovsky A, Swain P. Wireless-capsule diagnostic endoscopy for recurrent small-bowel bleeding. *N Engl J Med.* 2001;344:232-3.
32. Clarke JO, Giday SA, Magno P, Shin EJ, Buscaglia JM, Jagannath SB, et al. How good is capsule endoscopy for detection of periampullary lesions? Results of a tertiary-referral center. *Gastrointest Endosc.* 2008;68:267-72.
33. Gay G, Delvaux M, Fassler I. Outcome of capsule endoscopy in determining indication and route for push-and-pull enteroscopy. *Endoscopy.* 2006;38:49-58.
34. Nakamura M, Ohmiya N, Shirai O, Takenaka H, Morishima K, Miyahara R, et al. Route selection for double-balloon endoscopy, based on capsule transit time, in obscure gastrointestinal bleeding. *J Gastroenterol.* 2010;45:592-9.
35. Fischer D, Schreiber R, Levi D, Eliakim R. Capsule endoscopy: the localization system. *Gastrointest Endosc Clin N Am.* 2004;14:25-31.
36. Kim J, Kim YS, Chun HJ, Hyun JH, Cho MY, Suh SO. Laparoscopy-assisted exploration of obscure gastrointestinal bleeding after capsule endoscopy: the Korean experience. *J Laparoendosc Adv Surg Tech A.* 2005;15:365-73.
37. Spada C, Spera G, Riccioni M, Biancone L, Petruzziello L, Tringali A, et al. A novel diagnostic tool for detecting functional patency of the small bowel: the Given patency capsule. *Endoscopy.* 2005;37:793-800.
38. Delvaux M, Ben Soussan E, Laurent V, Lerebours E, Gay G. Clinical evaluation of the use of the M2A patency capsule system before a capsule endoscopy procedure, in patients with known or suspected intestinal stenosis. *Endoscopy.* 2005;37:801-7.
39. Brown G, Fraser C, Schofield G, Taylor S, Bartram C, Phillips R, et al. Video capsule endoscopy in Peutz-Jeghers syndrome: a blinded comparison with barium follow-through for detection of small-bowel polyps. *Endoscopy.* 2006;38:385-90.
40. Mata A, Llach J, Castells A, Rovira JM, Pellise M, Gines A, et al. A prospective trial comparing wireless capsule endoscopy and barium contrast series for small-bowel surveillance in hereditary GI polyposis syndromes. *Gastrointest Endosc.* 2005;61:721-5.
41. Schulmann K, Hollerbach S, Kraus K, Willert J, Vogel T, Moslein G, et al. Feasibility and diagnostic utility of video capsule endoscopy for the detection of small bowel polyps in patients with hereditary polyposis syndromes. *Am J Gastroenterol.* 2005;100:27-37.
42. Caspari R, von Falkenhausen M, Krautmacher C, Schild H, Heller J, Sauerbruch T. Comparison of capsule endoscopy and magnetic resonance imaging for the detection of polyps of the small intestine in patients with familial adenomatous polyposis or with Peutz-Jeghers' syndrome. *Endoscopy.* 2004;36:1054-9.
43. Gupta A, Postgate AJ, Burling D, Ilangovan R, Marshall M, Phillips RK, et al. A prospective study of MR enterography versus capsule endoscopy for the surveillance of adult patients with Peutz-Jeghers syndrome. *AJR Am J Roentgenol.* 2010;195:108-16.
44. Yamamoto H, Sekine Y, Sato Y, Higashizawa T, Miyata T, Iino S, et al. Total enteroscopy with a nonsurgical steerable double-balloon method. *Gastrointest Endosc.* 2001;53: 216-20.
45. Gerson LB, Flodin JT, Miyabayashi K. Balloon-assisted enteroscopy: technology and troubleshooting. *Gastrointest Endosc.* 2008;68:1158-67.
46. Hartmann D, Eickhoff A, Tamm R, Riemann JF. Balloon-assisted enteroscopy using a single-balloon technique. *Endoscopy.* 2007;39:E276.
47. May A, Farber M, Aschmoneit I, Pohl J, Manner H, Lotterer E, et al. Prospective multicenter trial comparing push-and-pull enteroscopy with the single- and double-balloon techniques in patients with small-bowel disorders. *Am J Gastroenterol.* 2010;105:575-81.
48. Akerman PA, Agrawal D, Cantero D, Pangtay J. Spiral enteroscopy with the new DSB overtube: a novel technique for deep peroral small-bowel intubation. *Endoscopy.* 2008; 40:974-8.
49. Khashab MA, Lennon AM, Dunbar KB, Singh VK, Chandrasekhara V, Giday S, et al. A comparative evaluation of single-balloon enteroscopy and spiral enteroscopy for patients with mid-gut disorders. *Gastrointest Endosc.* 2010;72:766-72.
50. Ross A, Mehdizadeh S, Tokar J, Leighton JA, Kamal A, Chen A, et al. Double balloon enteroscopy detects small bowel mass lesions missed by capsule endoscopy. *Dig Dis Sci.* 2008;53:2140-3.
51. Raju GS, Gerson L, Das A, Lewis B. American Gastroenterological Association (AGA) Institute technical review on obscure gastrointestinal bleeding. *Gastroenterology.* 2007;133:1697-717.
52. Pasha SF, Leighton JA, Das A, Harrison ME, Decker GA, Fleischer DE, et al. Double-balloon enteroscopy and capsule endoscopy have comparable diagnostic yield in

small-bowel disease: a meta-analysis. *Clin Gastroenterol Hepatol.* 2008;6:671-6.

53. Chen LH, Chen WG, Cao HJ, Zhang H, Shan GD, Li L, et al. Double-balloon enteroscopy for obscure gastrointestinal bleeding: a single center experience in China. *World J Gastroenterol.* 2010;16:1655-9.
54. Gerson LB, Batenic MA, Ross A, Semrad C. Long-term outcomes after double balloon enteroscopy for obscure gastrointestinal bleeding. *Clin Gastroenterol Hepatol.* 2009.
55. Mitsui K, Tanaka S, Yamamoto H, Kobayashi T, Ehara A, Yano T, et al. Role of double-balloon endoscopy in the diagnosis of small-bowel tumors: the first Japanese multicenter study. *Gastrointest Endosc.* 2009;70:498-504.
56. Almeida N, Figueiredo P, Lopes S, Gouveia H, Leitao MC. Double-balloon enteroscopy and small bowel tumors: a South-European single-center experience. *Dig Dis Sci.* 2009;54:1520-4.
57. Hegde SR, Iffrig K, Li T, Downey S, Heller SJ, Tokar JL, et al. Double-balloon enteroscopy in the elderly: safety, findings, and diagnostic and therapeutic success. *Gastrointest Endosc.* 2010;71:983-9.
58. Bresci G, Parisi G, Bertoni M, Tumino E, Capria A. The role of video capsule endoscopy for evaluating obscure gastrointestinal bleeding: usefulness of early use. *J Gastroenterol.* 2005;40:256-9.
59. Godeschalk MF, Mensink PB, van Buuren HR, Kuipers EJ. Primary balloon-assisted enteroscopy in patients with obscure gastrointestinal bleeding: findings and outcome of therapy. *J Clin Gastroenterol.* 2010;44:e195-200.
60. Viazis N, Papaxoinis K, Vlachogiannakos J, Efthymiou A, Theodoropoulos I, Karamanolis DG. Is there a role for second-look capsule endoscopy in patients with obscure GI bleeding after a nondiagnostic first test? *Gastrointest Endosc.* 2009;69:850-6.
61. Postgate A, Despott E, Burling D, Gupta A, Phillips R, O'Beirne J, et al. Significant small-bowel lesions detected by alternative diagnostic modalities after negative capsule endoscopy. *Gastrointest Endosc.* 2008;68:1209-14.
62. Mensink PB, Haringsma J, Kucharzik T, Cellier C, Perez-Cuadrado E, Monkemuller K, et al. Complications of double balloon enteroscopy: a multicenter survey. *Endoscopy.* 2007;39:613-5.
63. May A, Nachbar L, Pohl J, Ell C. Endoscopic interventions in the small bowel using double balloon enteroscopy: feasibility and limitations. *Am J Gastroenterol.* 2007;102:527-35.
64. Yamamoto H, Kita H, Sunada K, Hayashi Y, Sato H, Yano T, et al. Clinical outcomes of double-balloon endoscopy for the diagnosis and treatment of small-intestinal diseases. *Clin Gastroenterol Hepatol.* 2004;2:1010-6.
65. Tominaga K, Iida T, Nakamura Y, Nagao J, Yokouchi Y, Maetani I. Small intestinal perforation of endoscopically unrecognized lesions during peroral single-balloon enteroscopy. *Endoscopy.* 2008;40:E213-4.
66. Mehdizadeh S, Ross A, Gerson L, Leighton J, Chen A, Schembre D, et al. What is the learning curve associated with double-balloon enteroscopy? Technical details and early experience in 6 US tertiary care centers. *Gastrointest Endosc.* 2006;64:740-50.
67. Gerson LB, Tokar J, Chiorean M, Lo S, Decker GA, Cave D, et al. Complications associated with double balloon enteroscopy at nine US centers. *Clin Gastroenterol Hepatol.* 2009;7:1177-82, 1182.e1-3.
68. Tsujikawa T, Saitoh Y, Andoh A, Imaeda H, Hata K, Minematsu H, et al. Novel single-balloon enteroscopy for diagnosis and treatment of the small intestine: preliminary experiences. *Endoscopy.* 2008;40:11-5.
69. Kawamura T, Yasuda K, Tanaka K, Uno K, Ueda M, Sanada K, et al. Clinical evaluation of a newly developed single-balloon enteroscope. *Gastrointest Endosc.* 2008;68:1112-6.
70. Manabe N, Tanaka S, Fukumoto A, Nakao M, Kamino D, Chayama K. Double-balloon enteroscopy in patients with GI bleeding of obscure origin. *Gastrointest Endosc.* 2006;64:135-40.
71. Matsumoto T, Esaki M, Moriyama T, Nakamura S, Iida M. Comparison of capsule endoscopy and enteroscopy with the double-balloon method in patients with obscure bleeding and polyposis. *Endoscopy.* 2005;37:827-32.
72. Akahoshi K, Kubokawa M, Matsumoto M, Endo S, Motomura Y, Ouchi J, et al. Double-balloon endoscopy in the diagnosis and management of GI tract diseases: Methodology, indications, safety, and clinical impact. *World J Gastroenterol.* 2006;12:7654-9.
73. Zhong J, Ma T, Zhang C, Sun B, Chen S, Cao Y, et al. A retrospective study of the application on double-balloon enteroscopy in 378 patients with suspected small-bowel diseases. *Endoscopy.* 2007;39:208-15.
74. Sun B, Shen R, Cheng S, Zhang C, Zhong J. The role of double-balloon enteroscopy in diagnosis and management of incomplete small-bowel obstruction. *Endoscopy.* 2007;39:511-5.
75. Li F, Osuoha C, Leighton JA, Harrison ME. Double-balloon enteroscopy in the diagnosis and treatment of hemorrhage from small-bowel lymphangioma: a case report. *Gastrointest Endosc.* 2009;70:189-90.
76. May A, Nachbar L, Schneider M, Neumann M, Ell C. Push-and-pull enteroscopy using the double-balloon technique: method of assessing depth of insertion and training of the enteroscopy technique using the Erlangen Endo-Trainer. *Endoscopy.* 2005;37:66-70.
77. Ell C, May A, Nachbar L, Cellier C, Landi B, di Caro S, et al. Push-and-pull enteroscopy in the small bowel using the double-balloon technique: results of a prospective European multicenter study. *Endoscopy.* 2005;37:613-6.
78. Di Caro S, May A, Heine DG, Fini L, Landi B, Petruzziello L, et al. The European experience with double-balloon enteroscopy: indications, methodology, safety, and clinical impact. *Gastrointest Endosc.* 2005;62:545-50.

79. Hadithi M, Heine GD, Jacobs MA, van Bodegraven AA, Mulder CJ. A prospective study comparing video capsule endoscopy with double-balloon enteroscopy in patients with obscure gastrointestinal bleeding. *Am J Gastroenterol.* 2006;101:52-7.
80. Heine GD, Hadithi M, Groenen MJ, Kuipers EJ, Jacobs MA, Mulder CJ. Double-balloon enteroscopy: indications, diagnostic yield, and complications in a series of 275 patients with suspected small-bowel disease. *Endoscopy.* 2006;38:42-8.
81. Monkemuller K, Weigt J, Treiber G, Kolfenbach S, Kahl S, Rocken C, et al. Diagnostic and therapeutic impact of double-balloon enteroscopy. *Endoscopy.* 2006;38:67-72.
82. Gross SA, Stark ME. Initial experience with double-balloon enteroscopy at a US center. *Gastrointest Endosc.* 2008;67: 890-7.
83. Lahat A, Nadler M, Simon C, Lahav M, Novis B, Bar-Meir S. Double balloon enteroscopy: a 2 year experience. *Isr Med Assoc J.* 2009;11:456-9.

9 Solid and Cystic Lesions of Pancreas: Role of Endosonography

Mohammed A Qadeer, Girish Mishra

ABSTRACT

Solid and cystic lesions of the pancreas include a myriad of benign and malignant tumors, of which pancreatic adenocarcinoma is the most important one, as it is the leading cause of mortality amongst all gastrointestinal cancers. It has a poor survival rate due to its late presentation. Solid lesions are usually malignant in nature and include adenocarcinoma, neuroendocrine tumors (NETs), mucinous neoplasms, and metastatic tumors from nearby organs. On the other hand, cystic lesions of the pancreas can range from benign simple cysts to malignant neoplasms. Endoscopic ultrasonography (EUS) has been helpful in delineating the malignant potential of pancreatic lesions to a reasonable extent. EUS also has other therapeutic applications, such as drainage and ablation of the cyst, stereotactic radiotherapy, and intratumoral chemotherapy. The role of EUS as a diagnostic and therapeutic tool for pancreatic lesions will be reviewed in this chapter.

INTRODUCTION

Pancreatic cancer ranks second in incidence and first in mortality amongst the gastrointestinal cancers in the United States.[1] According to the Surveillance, Epidemiology, and End Results (SEER) database, the expected incidence and mortality for pancreatic cancer in the year 2010 was 43,140 and 36,800, respectively.[1] This cancer equally affects both genders. Thus, the prevalence of cancer is relatively stable due to similar incidence and mortality. The overall 5-year survival of patients with pancreatic cancer is less than 5%, which is primarily due to late detection. Only 18% of newly diagnosed cancers were found to be surgically resectable in a study of 799 pancreatic cancer patients.[2] Surgical unresectability at diagnosis was associated with almost 100% mortality by 5 years.[2] On the other hand, surgical resection of cancers smaller than 1 cm resulted in 100% survival at 5 years in a small group of patients.[3] Therefore, early detection and surgical resection of pancreatic cancer is the only long-term curative option. Thus, it is not surprising that every pancreatic lesion is viewed with a suspicion of malignancy.

Endosonography or endoscopic ultrasonography (EUS) was developed about 25 years ago, and continues to play an essential role in the evaluation of pancreatic lesions. EUS has long been used as a diagnostic tool in pancreatic lesions due to excellent imaging obtained because of the close proximity of the scope tip to the pancreas, and the ability to perform fine needle aspiration (FNA) enabling pathological diagnosis. A population-based study revealed that the performance of EUS in patients with pancreatic cancer might improve survival.[4] More recently, EUS-based interventions have been performed for a variety of therapeutic purposes, and this field is still evolving. Thus, EUS is an indispensable tool in the evaluation and management of pancreatic lesions.

Pancreatic lesions can be broadly classified into solid and cystic lesions, although mixed heterogeneous (cystic solid combination) lesions can also be seen. With the widespread use of cross-sectional abdominal imaging, pancreatic lesions are being increasingly recognized at an earlier, asymptomatic stage. Although many of these cystic lesions are benign, it is imperative to identify lesions that are malignant and those who have a malignant potential, as early resection may be curative.

SOLID LESIONS OF PANCREAS

Vast majority of solid lesions of the pancreas are malignant. A malignant lesion was detected in 62% of focal solid lesions seen on cross-sectional imaging in a recent study involving 173 patients presenting without obstructive jaundice.[5] Such lesions included adenocarcinomas (n = 89), neuroendocrine tumors (NETs) (n = 14), mucinous cystadenocarcinomas (n = 1), solid pseudopapillary tumor (n = 2), and metastases (n = 4). The remaining 38% of lesions were all benign; benign cyst (n = 19), pseudocyst (n = 9), abscess (n = 4), chronic pancreatitis (n = 32), and normal pancreas (n = 39). Similarly, another study reported that adenocarcinomas constituted about 80% of lesions, while NETs constituted 11%, lymphomas 3%, and other types 5%.[6]

Most of the solid pancreatic lesions are present in the head of pancreas followed by body and tail. In a database study from the University of Alabama in which 101 patients with suspected pancreatic cancers were evaluated, the location of lesions was as follows: head 65%, body 17%, uncinate process 12%, and tail 6%.[7] Another study evaluating 93 patients found a similar distribution of lesions: head 73%, body 20%, and tail 7%.[6] Thus, solid lesions in the head are more likely to be malignant and need to be evaluated diligently.

Occasionally, malignancy presents only as fullness of pancreas, either focal or diffuse. Although most of these findings are benign, one study noted that up to 9% of such lesions could be malignant.[8] The investigators evaluated 69 cases of pancreatic fullness examined by EUS and found that 19 patients required FNA, of which 6 turned out to be cancers (4 pancreatic cancer, 1 metastatic renal cell cancer, and 1 metastatic colon cancer). Similarly, in another study that evaluated enlarged pancreatic head with and without pancreatic duct dilation, but without common bile duct (CBD) dilation or obstructive jaundice found that 10/110 (9%) had malignancy, while the majority of them had either chronic pancreatitis or normal pancreas.[9] Therefore, all cases of focal and diffuse fullness of the pancreas need further evaluation by EUS ± FNA for further classification.

Unfortunately, adenocarcinoma of pancreas is usually detected late in the disease course unless it grows in close proximity to CBD, when obstructive jaundice manifests early in the disease. EUS is the most accurate diagnostic modality to diagnose cancer of the pancreas. Typical EUS features include an irregular hypoechoic lesion with poor demarcation. Studies have shown that EUS has better sensitivity and specificity in comparison to computed tomography (CT) scan.[10,11] EUS is also comparable or better than CT scan for detection of local spread of the disease (T stage) while CT scan is better in the detection of distant disease.[12,13] EUS has an added advantage over CT scan and magnetic resonance imaging (MRI) due to FNA capability needed for cytological diagnosis.

NETs are typically well-demarcated, hypoechoic, solid, and homogeneous lesions. Up to 10% of these tumors could be cystic, 14% functional, and 16% were 10 mm or smaller.[14] Usually, nonfunctioning NETs are more common and advanced than functioning NETs. The overall 5-year survival has been reported to be 60%. An 11-year study by the Indiana group evaluated 92 patients with NETs and found that non-functioning NETs were usually larger and had cystic features. They also found that patients with malignant NETs were older, had abdominal pain, and larger tumors with irregular margins. The overall sensitivity for EUS diagnosis was 87%, which was higher in malignant lesions compared to benign lesions.[15] Sometimes, NETs can present with diagnostic challenges. A study of 48 NETs from Athens, Greece found that the cytological findings that were most helpful in the diagnosis were the presence of a richly cellular sample with a monotonous, poorly cohesive population of small or medium-sized cells with granular chromatin (salt and pepper) and plasmacytoid morphology.[16] Immunocytochemistry was also found to be very helpful to confirm the diagnosis in majority of these tumors. A rare variant of a pancreatic NETs consist of those in which cystic degeneration has occurred—a cystic islet cell or neuroendocrine neoplasm. Figure 9-1 depicts the MRI, EUS with FNA, and figure 9-2 shows the cytology from such a case.

Other rare tumors of the pancreas include pseudopapillary tumors that are predominantly seen in young women and arise typically in body and tail. These tumors are detected incidentally on cross-sectional imaging of the abdomen. In a pooled multicenter study, the investigators described EUS features of these tumors in 28 patients.[17] Most patients were women (24 out of 28). These tumors had well-defined, echo-poor mass in 86%. About 50% of these tumors were solid, 39% were mixed solid and cystic, and 11% were cystic. EUS-FNA was able to make a correct diagnosis in only 75% of these patients.

The accuracy of EUS with FNA has been well documented mostly from large database registries. In general, the accuracy depends on the presence of an on-site cytotechnologist, technique of FNA, number of passes, and size of the needle. The presence of an on-site cytotechnologist significantly improves the accuracy

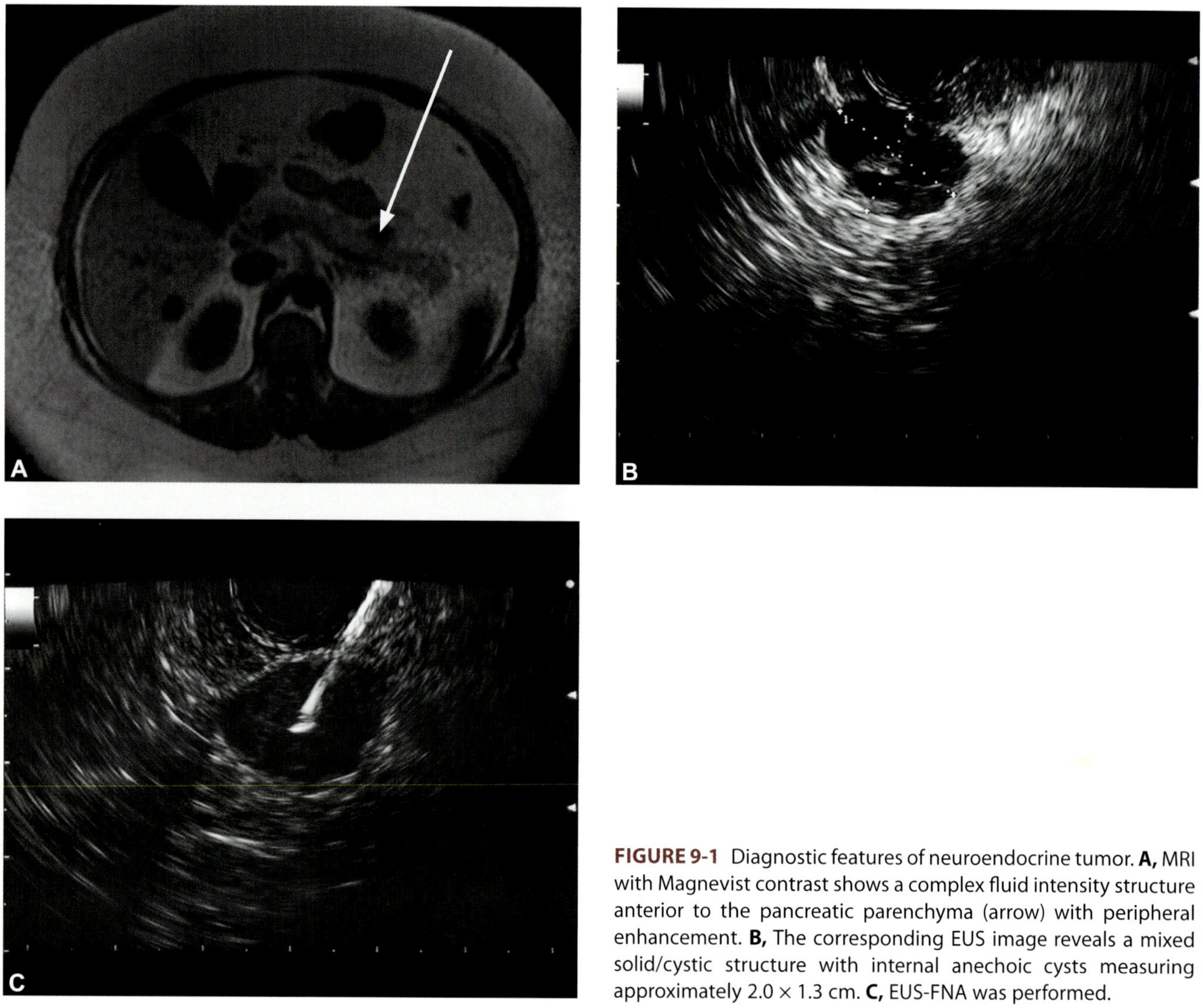

FIGURE 9-1 Diagnostic features of neuroendocrine tumor. **A,** MRI with Magnevist contrast shows a complex fluid intensity structure anterior to the pancreatic parenchyma (arrow) with peripheral enhancement. **B,** The corresponding EUS image reveals a mixed solid/cystic structure with internal anechoic cysts measuring approximately 2.0 × 1.3 cm. **C,** EUS-FNA was performed.

of the FNA. The accuracy of FNA has been reported to be less than 80% in studies that did not have an on-site cytotechnologist, compared to more than 90% in that had an on-site cytotechnologist.[5-7,18,19] Therefore, all the major EUS centers utilize the services of on-site cytotechnologists. In the absence of cytotechnologists, the adequacy of sample is difficult to predict by gross visual assessment of the slide. This was revealed in a study, in which the investigators assessed the correlation of gross visual examination of slide by cytotechnologist and endoscopic technologist to that of final cytopathological result. The kappa coefficient of correlation between gross visualization and the final cytopathological result was only 0.2, suggesting a poor correlation.[20] Therefore, the investigators suggested that at least 6–7 passes should be performed to improve the accuracy and yield in the absence of an on-site cytotechnologist.

Needle size also appears to be important in improving the accuracy of EUS-FNA. In a study of 24 patients,[21] the investigators compared the accuracy of the 25-gauge, 22-gauge, and Trucut™ needles, and found that the overall accuracy for these types of needles were 92, 80, and 54%, respectively. The investigators also found that 25-guage needles performed much better in the head and uncinate lesions compared to the body lesions. Similar results were obtained in another study assessing needle accuracy.[22] Once again, the larger diameter needles performed poorly in head and uncinate lesions; their utility was mainly confined to body, genu, and tail lesions.

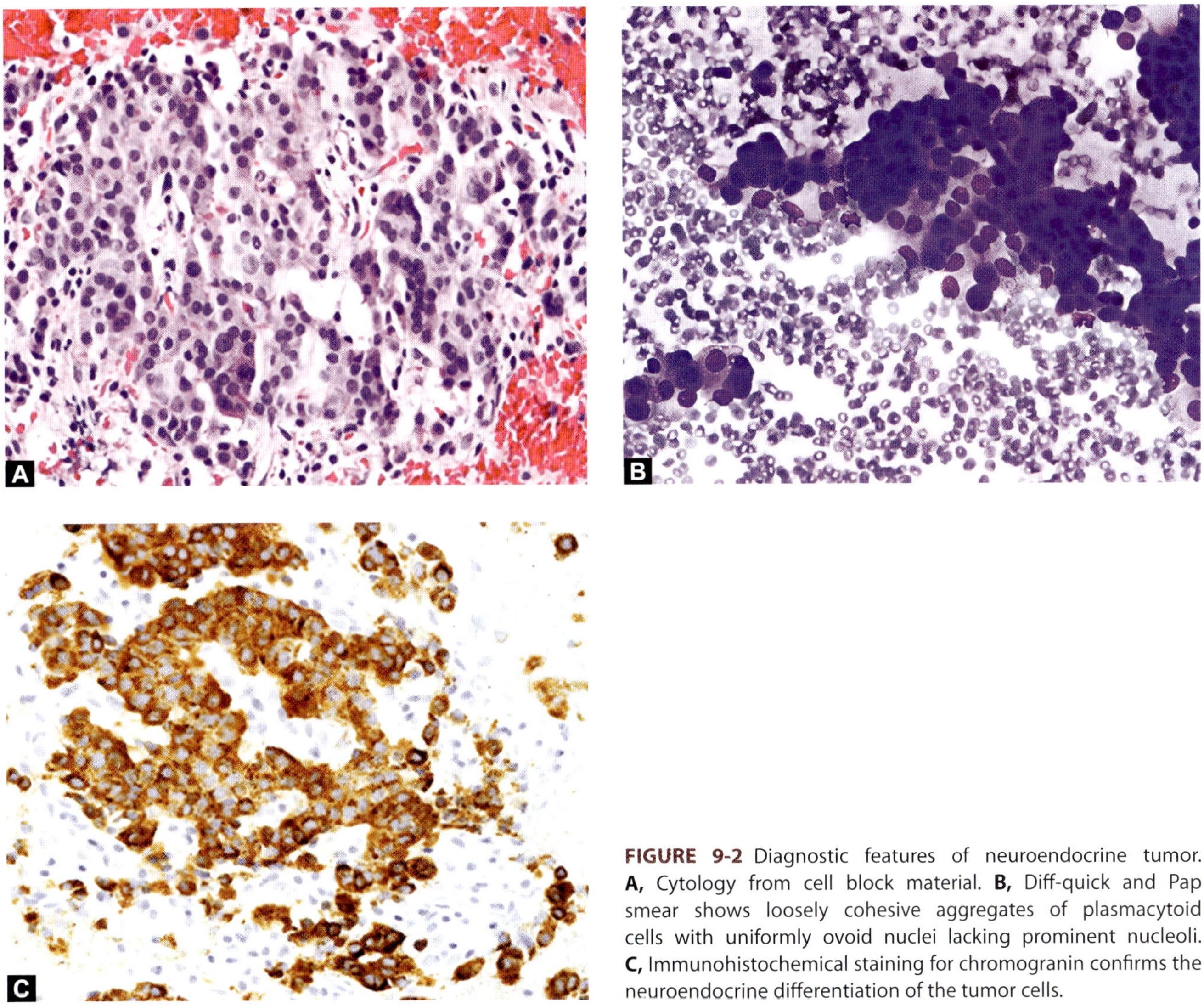

FIGURE 9-2 Diagnostic features of neuroendocrine tumor. **A,** Cytology from cell block material. **B,** Diff-quick and Pap smear shows loosely cohesive aggregates of plasmacytoid cells with uniformly ovoid nuclei lacking prominent nucleoli. **C,** Immunohistochemical staining for chromogranin confirms the neuroendocrine differentiation of the tumor cells.

Although the overall accuracy for diagnosing malignancy by EUS-FNA-based cytological examination may be as high as more than 90% in some studies, the cytological findings can be equivocal in the presence of chronic pancreatitis. Occasionally, mass-like lesions in chronic pancreatitis called pseudotumoral inflammation appear to mimic pancreatic cancer morphology and can be difficult to differentiate from pancreatic cancer, both on EUS and cytology. In such cases, analysis of K-ras mutation in the cytological sample may be helpful in differentiating cancer from chronic pancreatitis. In a prospective study of 178 patients with pancreatic cancer, chronic pancreatitis, or benign lesions, investigators observed that none of the patients with chronic pancreatitis were found to have K-ras mutation, whereas 66% of pancreatic cancer samples revealed this mutation.[23] Therefore, K-ras may be a helpful adjunct in classifying the lesion in patients with a mass lesion against the background of chronic pancreatitis. An additional benign lesion that may further vex the endosonographer and the cytopathologist alike involves discriminating autoimmune pancreatitis. This condition may mimic a pancreatic adenocarcinoma. Figure 9-3 highlights a patient erroneously labeled as suffering from a pancreatic adenocarcinoma who was later successfully treated with steroids for autoimmune pancreatitis with complete resolution of his pancreatic mass.

Another recent advancement has been the use of contrast enhanced harmonic EUS (CEH-EUS). A prototype echoendoscope was used to differentiate benign

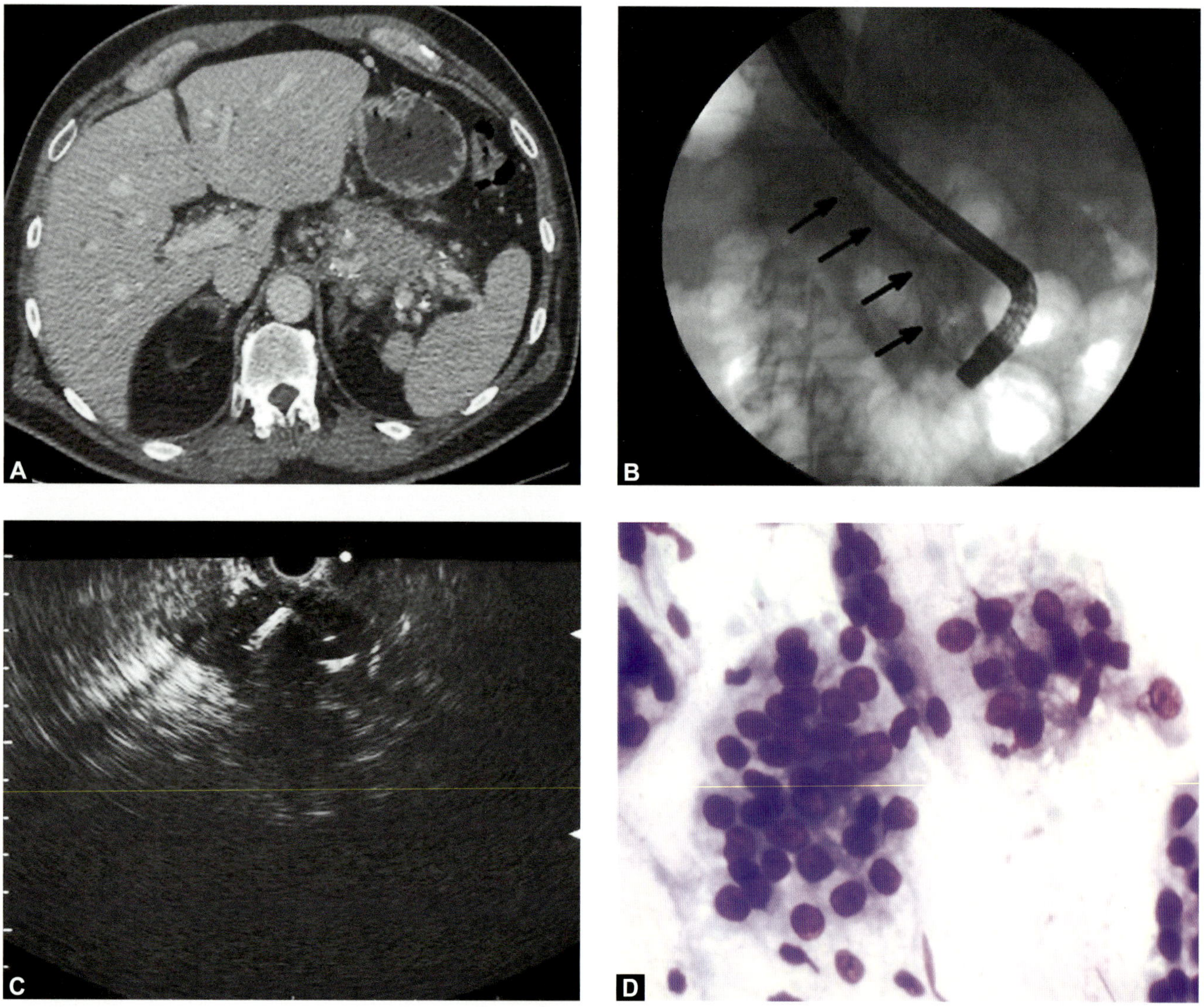

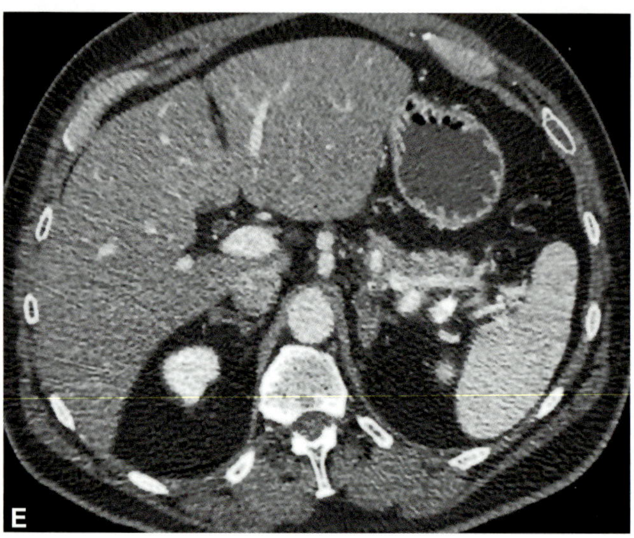

FIGURE 9-3 Pseudotumoral inflammation mimicing pancreatic cancer morphology. **A,** CT scan of the pancreas shows a prominent mass-like lesion throughout the entire pancreatic gland with indistinct borders. **B,** ERCP reveals a distal CBD stricture (arrows). Brushings were negative for malignancy. **C,** EUS-FNA of a hypoechoic lesion in the body of the pancreas. **D,** Cytology revealed reactive cells with small nucleoli but without marked nuclear atypia. The patient was presumed to have autoimmune pancreatitis based on the above clinical profile along with elevations in serum IgG4. He was treated with prednisone for approximately two months. **E,** Repeat CT showed complete resolution of the diffuse pancreatic mass.

from malignant lesions.[24] A second-generation ultrasound contrast dye was injected intravenously during the procedure. The investigators found that EUS had a high sensitivity for identifying cancers. A hypointense signal on CEH-EUS was seen in 18 patients, of whom 16 were adenocarcinomas. The sensitivity, specificity, negative predictive value (NPV), positive predictive value (PPV), and accuracy of hypointensity for diagnosing pancreatic adenocarcinoma were 89, 88, 88, 89, and 88.5%, compared with corresponding values of 72, 100, 77, 100, and 86%, respectively, for EUS-FNA. Interestingly, 4/5 adenocarcinomas that were false-negative at EUS-FNA had a hypointense echo signal suggestive of cancer at CEH-EUS. If confirmed in other studies, this could prove to be a very useful diagnostic tool.

The use of contrast enhanced EUS (CE-EUS) was also evaluated in NETs. The investigators found that it increased the sensitivity of EUS in detecting pancreatic endocrine tumors (PETs). In a study of 62 PETs seen in 41 patients, CE-EUS showed that heterogeneous ultrasonographic texture was most characteristic of malignancy.[25] CE-EUS had a sensitivity of 95% in identifying PETs compared with CT scan (80%) and ultrasound (45%).

CYSTIC LESIONS OF PANCREAS

Unlike solid lesions that are mostly malignant, vast majority of cystic lesions of the pancreas are benign. However, a significant number of cystic lesions can be classified as premalignant or harbor invasive components within the cyst. Thus, it is imperative to correctly identify these premalignant lesions, as they would warrant surgical management. On the other hand, it is equally important to correctly categorize completely benign lesions in order to avoid unnecessary surgery, with its inherent complications and risks. Therefore, diagnosis and management of cystic lesions of the pancreas can be quite challenging.

Cystic lesions of the pancreas are detected incidentally in majority of cases on cross-sectional imaging of the abdomen. Therefore, most of these lesions are asymptomatic. A single institution study over an 8-year period reviewed 24,039 cross-sectional imaging reports (CT and MR) and found that pancreatic cysts were present in 1.2% of patients.[26] Most of these cysts were incidentally noted and about 60% were cystic neoplasms. About 2/3rd of these cystic neoplasms were either malignant or had malignant potential. Another study reviewed 616 consecutive MRI examinations of the abdomen over a 1 year period and found that the prevalence of incidental cysts was 13.5%.[27] More importantly, the investigators also noted that the radiologists reported only 31% of these cysts. In this study, the investigators found that 60% of the cysts were solitary, and 88% were simple. The mean cyst diameter was 7.4 mm (range 2–24 mm).

There is a wide array of pathological disorders presenting as cystic lesions of the pancreas (Table 9-1). The goal is to correctly ascertain the pathology of the cyst with the help of EUS morphology and cyst fluid analysis. EUS features helpful in classifying a cyst include cyst size, cyst wall thickness, internal septations, intramural nodules, echogenicity, and communication with the pancreatic duct. Cyst size is directly proportional to the malignant potential of the pancreatic cysts. This is particularly true of side branch intraductal papillary mucinous neoplasms (IPMNs), where a cyst size greater than 3 cm is usually associated with malignancy, whereas a cyst size less than 3 cm is less likely to be malignant and can be followed up periodically.[28] However, smaller cysts (<2 cm) could also harbor malignancy rarely. A retrospective case series evaluating the pathological findings of asymptomatic cysts revealed that 1 out of 28 asymptomatic cysts (4%) less than 2 cm in diameter had cancer compared with 13 out of 50 cysts (26%) greater than 2 cm in diameter.[29] However, premalignant lesions were almost equally distributed among them, 46% and 38%, respectively. Thus, cyst size has to be evaluated in conjunction with other factors for management decisions.

Cyst wall thickness can differentiate benign from premalignant and malignant cysts. In a retrospective review of 74 macrocystic pancreatic lesions, the investigators noted that the cyst wall thickness was statistically significant on multivariable analysis in differentiating benign from premalignant and malignant cysts.[30] The International Association of Pancreatology formulated consensus guidelines for the management of mucinous cystic neoplasms and IPMNs in which cysts greater than 3 cm were recommended to undergo surgery.[31] For cysts 1-3 cm in size, surgery was recommended, if they were symptomatic or had high-risk stigmata, such as mural nodules, positive cytology, or dilated main pancreatic duct. In the absence of stigmata, MR or CT follow-up was recommended every 6 months. If the cysts were smaller than 1 cm, then MR or CT follow-up was recommended every 12 months. A subsequent study evaluated these guidelines in 77 patients with resected branch duct IPMNs and found that presence of any one stigma had sensitivity, specificity, positive, and negative predictive values of 100, 23, 14, and 100%, respectively, for the presence of underlying malignancy.[32]

TABLE 9-1 Characteristics of Cystic Lesions of the Pancreas

	Pseudocyst	*IPMN*	*Mucinous cystadenoma*	*Serous cystadenoma*	*Cystic endocrine neoplasm*	*Solid pseudopapillary neoplasm*	*Ductal adenocarcinoma with cystic degeneration*
Clinical features	History of moderate to severe pancreatitis	History of pancreatitis, abdominal pain, or found incidentally	Usually found incidentally but can cause abdominal pain and a palpable mass, if large	Usually found incidentally but can cause abdominal pain and a palpable mass, if large	May have clinical features of solid pancreatic endocrine neoplasm	Usually found incidentally; rarely causes abdominal discomfort	Presents with painless jaundice, abdominal/back pain, or rarely pancreatitis
Morphology/ EUS findings	Anechoic, thick walled, rare septations, regional inflammatory nodes may be seen	Dilated main pancreatic duct or side branches; may appear as a septated cyst; may have a solid component	Macrocystic, occasionally septated; peripheral calcifications, solid components, and regional adenopathy when malignant	Microcystic with a honeycomb appearance; rarely has a macrocystic component; central calcification	Unilocular cyst occupies most of the neoplasm	Solid and cystic components	Primarily solid mass with cystic spaces
Fluid characteristics	Thin, muddy brown	Viscous or stringy, clear	Viscous or stringy, clear	Thin, clear to serosanguinous	Thin, clear	Bloody + necrotic debris	Bloody ± debris
Cytology	Neutrophils, macrophages, histiocytes; negative staining for mucin	Mucinous columnar cells with variable atypia; fluid stains positive for mucin	Mucinous columnar cells with variable atypia; fluid stains positive for mucin	Cuboidal epithelial cells that stain positive for glycogen	Monomorphic endocrine cells; stains positive for chromogranin and synaptophysin	Monomorphic cells with round nuclei and eosinophilic or foamy cytoplasms; stains positive for vimentin and α-1 antitrypsin	Malignant adenocarcinoma can be seen, but varying degrees of atypia may be present in the specimen
Malignant potential	None	Yes	Yes	Almost none (rare reports)	Yes	Yes	Already present

IPMN, intraductal papillary mucinous neoplasm; EUS, endoscopic ultrasonography.

Source: Jacobson BC, Baron TH, Adler DG, Davila RE, Egan J, Hirota WK, et al. ASGE guideline: the role of endoscopy in the diagnosis and the management of cystic lesions and inflammatory fluid collections of the pancreas. *Gastrointest Endosc*. 2005;61:363-70.

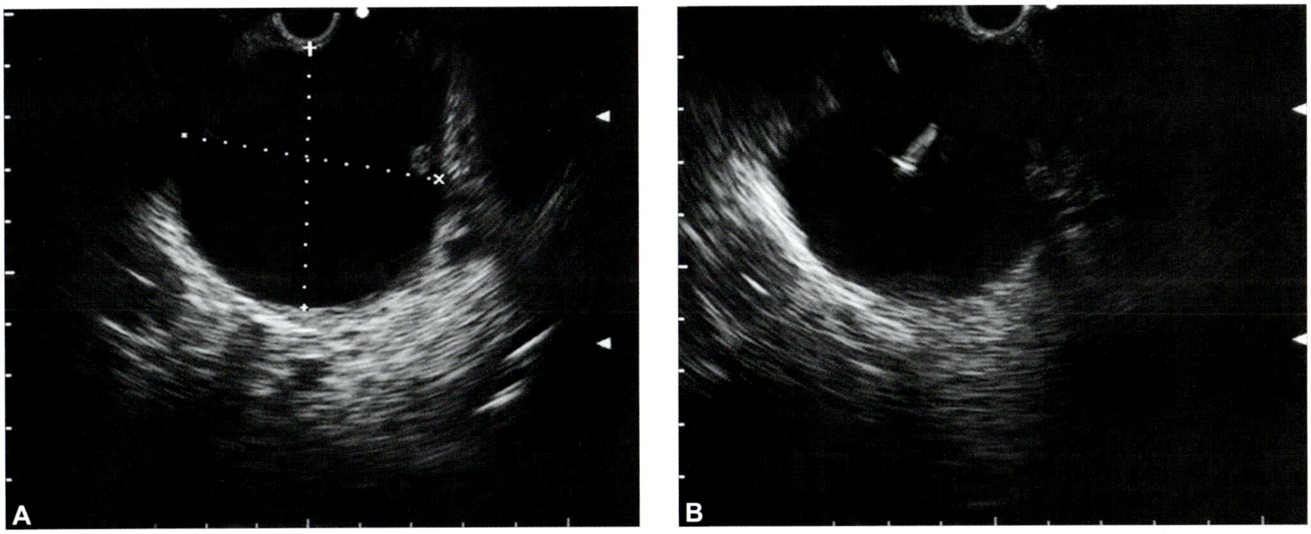

FIGURE 9-4 Pancreatic cyst with mural nodule. **A,** EUS image of a large anechoic 5.0 × 5.0 cm cyst with an intramural nodule, a more worrisome feature. **B,** EUS-FNA of this cyst yielded a very high CEA level (approx. 10,000). Subsequent distal pancreatectomy with splenectomy showed a mucinous cystic neoplasm with focal moderate dysplasia. No invasive carcinoma was seen.

EUS-FNA of the cyst content has become the standard of care for evaluating pancreatic cysts. In general, FNA is performed for cysts greater than 1 cm as the quantity of fluid obtained from cysts less than 1 cm is too scant for any meaningful study. As a general rule, pancreatic cysts should be aspirated completely to reduce the risk of infection and parenteral antibiotics are typically administered at the time of cyst aspiration. Pancreatic duct may be aspirated when IPMNs are suspected.[33,34] If the cyst wall is thick and if mural nodules are present, endoscopists should attempt to aspirate from these specific locations to increase the diagnostic yield (Figure 9 4).

Cyst fluid analysis has two main goals: (a) to differentiate mucinous cysts from serous cysts or inflammatory fluid collections and (b) to diagnose underlying malignancy in mucinous cysts. All the tests on the cyst fluid could be grouped into cytology, tumor markers, biochemical markers, and nuclear DNA-based tests.

Cytological evaluation of the cyst contents may provide useful information for differentiating various types of pancreatic cysts. Frossard et al. used staining features, cellularity, cell pattern, nuclear pattern, mucin stain, periodic acid-Schiff (PAS) stain, and alcian blue stain, and were able to correctly identify the pathology of the cysts.[35] For example, cyst aspirates from mucinous cystic neoplasms may show mucinous epithelial cells, and sometimes adenocarcinoma cells in cases of malignant degeneration of the cyst; glycogen rich cuboidal cells from serous cystic neoplasms; and macrophages, histiocytes, and neutrophils from pseudocysts. The diagnostic accuracy of EUS-FNA varies widely in literature and has been reported to range from 50 to over 90% in reported series.[33-37]

As the EUS-FNA cytology is dependent mostly on exfoliated cells from the cyst wall, utility of cytological brushes through the EUS scope has been assessed to determine incremental benefit over FNA. In one study, the investigators evaluated the efficacy of cytobrush (Echobrush) in 10 cysts greater than 2 cm and found that brushings yielded greater degree of cellularity in 7 out of 10 patients.[38] However, there were two intracystic bleeding episodes associated with the brush that slightly tempered the enthusiasm. In another study, investigators evaluated cytobrush technique in 51 patients and found that FNA yielded greater cellularity compared with brush, but the difference was not statistically significant.[39] However, more cancers were detected by brush than by simple FNA, but the numbers were too small to draw any conclusions.

Simple biochemical tests, such as amylase and lipase may be elevated in pseudocysts and IPMNs; high level usually implies connection of the cyst to the pancreatic ductal system. But these values should be evaluated with caution due to microscopic connection of the ductal system to the cyst wall, resulting in high values in other cysts.[35,37,40]

The role of tumor markers is now firmly established in the diagnosis of pancreatic cysts on the basis of the results of cooperative pancreatic cyst study.[37] The investigators studied carcinoembryonic antigen (CEA), CA 19-9, CA 125, CA 72-4, and CA 15.3 along with EUS features and cytology in 341 patients of whom 112 had final pathological confirmation. Of all the tumor markers, CEA cut-off of 192 ng/mL had the highest area under the curve (0.79) for differentiating mucinous from nonmucinous cystic lesions. Furthermore, the investigators noted that the accuracy of CEA was greater than the accuracy of EUS morphology alone and cytology alone (79, 51, and 59%, respectively). CEA alone was also superior to any combination of tests. Therefore, CEA level is routinely checked on cyst fluid aspirates. It is worth pointing out that although CEA differentiates mucinous from nonmucinous cysts, it is not a sensitive test to differentiate benign from malignant mucinous cysts. About 7% of mucinous cystic neoplasms have a low CEA level (<5 ng/mL), as in almost all the serous cystic neoplasms.[41]

Cyst fluid DNA based tests have entered the realm of EUS only in the last few years. In a multicenter study (Prospective Assessment in Newborns of Diabetes Autoimmunity, PANDA study), Khalid et al. evaluated 113 cysts and found that K-ras mutation, allelic loss amplitude, and high DNA content of the cysts were highly discriminatory in differentiating malignant from benign cysts.[42] More importantly, DNA analysis helped to diagnose all malignant cysts with a negative cytologic evaluation. Thus, DNA evaluation of the cysts was found to be extremely useful in their study. These tests were further evaluated in another study in which the investigators compared the CEA level and the cyst DNA content and found poor correlation between the two markers.[43] Furthermore, combining these two markers increased the sensitivity to 100%. Therefore, it appears that these two markers are complementary rather than supplementary. However, the enthusiasm about the DNA tests was partially tempered by the findings of another study in which the DNA tests were found to have lower test accuracy in comparison to CEA for detecting malignant and mucinous cysts from benign cysts.[44] Moreover, the investigators also noted that there were false-positive and false-negative results with DNA tests. Although this was a much smaller study (n = 20), it is reasonable to await the results of larger studies for validation of earlier studies before introduction into routine practice.

THERAPEUTIC ROLE OF ENDOSCOPIC ULTRASONOGRAPHY

The therapeutic role for EUS has been exploited ever since the 1990s when EUS assisted pseudocyst drainage was first performed.[45] Although pseudocysts can be drained without EUS assistance if a distinct intraluminal bulge is visualized, EUS is invaluable when an intraluminal bulge is not readily apparent. In a study of 60 patients, the investigators compared EUS drainage with conventional transmural drainage and found that 8 patients needed to be cross-overed to EUS for drainage due to non-bulging.[46] However, the overall outcomes were not significantly different between the two methods when comparing only successful conventional transmural drainage with EUS drainage.

Another application for therapeutic endosonography involves pancreatic cyst ablation. Investigators from the Massachusetts General Hospital reported the use of ethanol lavage for pancreatic cysts in 25 patients and found that 8 patients had complete resolution of the cyst on follow-up.[47] The investigators used 5–80% ethanol and lavaged for 3–5 minutes. More importantly, the ethanol lavage was found to be safe and feasible. Another group from Korea went a step further and injected paclitaxel into the cysts following ethanol lavage.[48] In their series of 14 patients, 11 were observed to have complete resolution on follow-up while 2 patients had partial resolution, and one had persistent cyst. In this series, there were 3 complications: 1 acute pancreatitis, 1 hyperamylasemia, and 1 patient with upper abdominal pain.

EUS-guided fiducial placement has proved to be very helpful for guiding high dose focal radiation (stereotactic body radiotherapy) in locally advanced and recurrent pancreatic cancer. In a study of 51 patients, the investigators successfully placed gold fiducials in 90% of patients with a complication rate of 2%.[49] The rate of migration of fiducials was 7%. Thus, EUS assisted fiducial placement was found to be safe and feasible.

A recent study from Italy demonstrated that EUS assisted Nd:yttrium aluminium garnet (YAG) laser can be used for focal ablation of pancreatic tissue.[50] In this study of 8 pigs, the investigators used EUS-Nd:YAG laser to ablate pancreatic tails. The volumes of ablated tissue ranged from 314 to 483 mm^3. There were no procedure related complications. This application may have significant potential for focal ablation of pancreatic malignancies in the future.

EUS assisted injection of intratumoral TNFerade and brachytherapy for locally advanced pancreatic cancers have been described. Chang et al. injected intratumoral TNFerade by EUS guided fine needle injection into the pancreatic tumors as an adjunct to systemic therapy and radiotherapy on weekly intervals for 5 weeks.[51] Three-month follow-up revealed progression-free survival.

The results are still early and the findings of a large multicenter trial are expected in the near future. In patients with locally advanced unresectable pancreatic cancers, Jin et al. implanted radioactive iodine (^{125}I) seeds and noted that there was a significant drop in pain scores at one month.[52] There was seed translocation in only 1 out of 25 patients with rest of the patients tolerating the procedure well. All these are preliminary studies, and it is expected that EUS therapeutics will gain prominence in the future, and add to our therapeutic armamentarium.

COMPLICATIONS OF ENDOSCOPIC ULTRASONOGRAPHY

EUS is generally a very safe procedure. However, a number of complications have been described from various institutions. In a series of 355 consecutive patients who underwent EUS-FNA for solid pancreatic masses, 9 patients (2.5%) had major complications, which included acute pancreatitis, severe abdominal pain, fever, and use of reversal medications.[53] The risk of intracystic hemorrhage during EUS-FNA for pancreatic cysts is reported to be around 6% (3 in 50 patients).[54] Bleeding was noted on EUS as a small hyperechoic area at the puncture site that gradually involved the entire cyst cavity. These patients were given antibiotics and recovered completely. The investigators did not find any clinical history or laboratory predictors for intracystic hemorrhage. The risk of acute pancreatitis following EUS-FNA in a multicenter study was reported to be 0.29%; however, in prospective databases, the risk was 0.64%.[55] The risk of cervical esophageal perforation during EUS is reported to be 3 out of 4,894 patients (0.06%).[56] All these perforations occurred in octogenarians and women, and the curvilinear echoendoscope was used in all 3 patients.

CONCLUSION

Pancreatic lesions, both solid and cystic, comprise a large pool of patients that gastroenterologists encounter. EUS offers unsurpassed value in better characterizing solid and cystic lesions since subtle variations of each are well recognized and documented in the literature. Factorizing the ability to perform FNA with its already established imaging prowess, the role of EUS in managing pancreatic lesions becomes even more critical. The complications of EUS, as for diagnostic EUS and even for performing FNA, are minimal with rare cases of pancreatitis or infections reported when sampling cystic lesions. Tumor marker assays such as CEA and other yet to be identified proteins offer hope for future diagnostic capabilities using EUS-FNA for better pancreatic cyst characterization. Finally, although in its infancy, therapeutic EUS offers great promise and applications in pancreatic and gastro-intestinal malignancies.

REFERENCES

1. Altekruse SF, Kosary CL, Krapcho M, et al., editors. SEER Cancer Statistics Review, 1975-2007, National Cancer Institute. Bethesda, MD, http://seer.cancer.gov/csr/1975_2007/, based on November 2009 SEER data submission, posted to the SEER web site, 2010.
2. Geer RJ, Brennan MF. Prognostic indicators for survival after resection of pancreatic adenocarcinoma. *Am J Surg.* 1993;165:68-72.
3. Ariyama J, Suyama M, Satoh K, Sai J. Imaging of small pancreatic ductal adenocarcinoma. *Pancreas.* 1998;16:396-401.
4. Ngamruengphong S, Li F, Zhou Y, Chak A, Cooper GS, Das A. EUS and survival in patients with pancreatic cancer: a population-based study. *Gastrointest Endosc.* 2010;72:78-83.
5. Krishna NB, LaBundy JL, Saripalli S, Safdar R, Agarwal B. Diagnostic value of EUS-FNA in patients suspected of having pancreatic cancer with a focal lesion on CT scan/MRI but without obstructive jaundice. *Pancreas.* 2009;38:625-30.
6. Fisher L, Segarajasingam DS, Stewart C, Deboer WB, Yusoff IF. Endoscopic ultrasound guided fine needle aspiration of solid pancreatic lesions: performance and outcomes. *J Gastroenterol Hepatol.* 2009;24:90-6.
7. Eloubeidi MA, Jhala D, Chhieng DC, Chen VK, Eltoum I, Vickers S, et al. Yield of endoscopic ultrasound-guided fine-needle aspiration biopsy in patients with suspected pancreatic carcinoma. *Cancer.* 2003;99:285-92.
8. Horwhat JD, Gerke H, Acosta RD, Pavey DA, Jowell PS. Focal or diffuse "fullness" of the pancreas on CT. Usually benign, but EUS plus/minus FNA is warranted to identify malignancy. *JOP.* 2009;10:37-42.
9. Agarwal B, Krishna NB, Labundy JL, Safdar R, Akduman EI. EUS and/or EUS-guided FNA in patients with CT and/or magnetic resonance imaging findings of enlarged pancreatic head or dilated pancreatic duct with or without a dilated common bile duct. *Gastrointest Endosc.* 2008;68:237-42.
10. Gress FG, Hawes RH, Savides TJ, Ikenberry SO, Cummings O, Kopecky K. Role of EUS in the preoperative staging of pancreatic cancer: a large single center experience. *Gastrointest Endosc.* 1999;50:786.
11. Shoup M, Hodul P, Aranha GV, Choe D, Olson M, Leya J, et al. Defining a role for endoscopic ultrasound in staging periampullary tumors. *Am J Surg.* 2000;179:453-6.
12. Brugge WR, Lee MJ, Kelsey PB, Schapiro RH, Warshaw AL. The use of EUS to diagnose portal venous invasion by pancreatic cancer. *Gastrointest Endosc.* 1996;43:561-7.

13. Ahmad NA, Lewis JD, Ginsberg GG, Rosato EF, Morris JB, Kochman ML. EUS in preoperative staging of pancreatic cancer. *Gastrointest Endosc.* 2000;52:463-8.
14. Figueiredo FA, Giovannini M, Monges G, Charfi S, Bories E, Pesenti C, et al. Pancreatic endocrine tumors: a large single-center experience. *Pancreas.* 2009;38:936-40.
15. Pais SA, Al-Haddad M, Mohamadnejad M, Leblanc JK, Sherman S, McHenry L, et al. EUS for pancreatic neuroendocrine tumors: a single-center, 11-year experience. *Gastrointest Endosc.* 2010;71:1185-93.
16. Chatzipantelis P, Salla C, Konstantinou P, Karoumpalis I, Sakellariou S, Doumani I. Endoscopic ultrasound-guided fine-needle aspiration cytology of pancreatic neuroendocrine tumors: a study of 48 cases. *Cancer.* 2008;114:255-62.
17. Jani N, Dewitt J, Eloubeidi M, Varadarajulu S, Appalaneni V, Hoffman B, et al. Endoscopic ultrasound-guided fine-needle aspiration for diagnosis of solid pseudopapillary tumors of the pancreas: a multicenter experience. *Endoscopy.* 2008;40:200-3.
18. Touchefeu Y, Le Rhun M, Coron E, Alamdari A, Heymann MF, Mosnier JF, et al. Endoscopic ultrasound-guided fine-needle aspiration for the diagnosis of solid pancreatic masses: the impact on patient-management strategy. *Aliment Pharmacol Ther.* 2009;30:1070-7.
19. Voss M, Hammel P, Molas G, Palazzo L, Dancour A, O'Toole D, et al. Value of endoscopic ultrasound guided fine needle aspiration biopsy in the diagnosis of solid pancreatic masses. *Gut.* 2000;46:244-9.
20. Nguyen YP, Maple JT, Zhang Q, Ylagan LR, Zhai J, Kohlmeier C, et al. Reliability of gross visual assessment of specimen adequacy during EUS-guided FNA of pancreatic masses. *Gastrointest Endosc.* 2009;69:1264-70.
21. Sakamoto H, Kitano M, Komaki T, Noda K, Chikugo T, Dote K, et al. Prospective comparative study of the EUS guided 25-gauge FNA needle with the 19-gauge Trucut needle and 22-gauge FNA needle in patients with solid pancreatic masses. *J Gastroenterol Hepatol.* 2009;24:384-90.
22. Itoi T, Itokawa F, Sofuni A, Nakamura K, Tsuchida A, Yamao K, et al. Puncture of solid pancreatic tumors guided by endoscopic ultrasonography: a pilot study series comparing Trucut and 19-gauge and 22-gauge aspiration needles. *Endoscopy.* 2005;37:362-6.
23. Bournet B, Souque A, Senesse P, Assenat E, Barthet M, Lesavre N, et al. Endoscopic ultrasound-guided fine-needle aspiration biopsy coupled with KRAS mutation assay to distinguish pancreatic cancer from pseudotumoral chronic pancreatitis. *Endoscopy.* 2009;41:552-7.
24. Napoleon B, Alvarez-Sanchez MV, Gincoul R, Pujol B, Lefort C, Lepilliez V, et al. Contrast-enhanced harmonic endoscopic ultrasound in solid lesions of the pancreas: results of a pilot study. *Endoscopy.* 2010;42:564-70.
25. Ishikawa T, Itoh A, Kawashima H, Ohno E, Matsubara H, Itoh Y, et al. Usefulness of EUS combined with contrast-enhancement in the differential diagnosis of malignant versus benign and preoperative localization of pancreatic endocrine tumors. *Gastrointest Endosc.* 2010;71:951-9.
26. Spinelli KS, Fromwiller TE, Daniel RA, Kiely JM, Nakeeb A, Komorowski RA, et al. Cystic pancreatic neoplasms: observe or operate. *Ann Surg.* 2004;239:651-7.
27. Lee KS, Sekhar A, Rofsky NM, Pedrosa I. Prevalence of incidental pancreatic cysts in the adult population on MR imaging. *Am J Gastroenterol.* 2010;105:2079-84.
28. Sadakari Y, Ienaga J, Kobayashi K, Miyasaka Y, Takahata S, Nakamura M, et al. Cyst size indicates malignant transformation in branch duct intraductal papillary mucinous neoplasm of the pancreas without mural nodules. *Pancreas.* 2010;39:232-6.
29. Fernández-del Castillo C, Targarona J, Thayer SP, Rattner DW, Brugge WR, Warshaw AL. Incidental pancreatic cysts: clinicopathologic characteristics and comparison with symptomatic patients. *Arch Surg.* 2003;138:427-3.
30. Kim SH, Lim JH, Lee WJ, Lim HK. Macrocystic pancreatic lesions: differentiation of benign from premalignant and malignant cysts by CT. *Eur J Radiol.* 2009;71:122-8.
31. Tanaka M, Chari S, Adsay V, Fernandez-del Castillo C, Falconi M, Shimizu M, et al; International Association of Pancreatology. International consensus guidelines for management of intraductal papillary mucinous neoplasms and mucinous cystic neoplasms of the pancreas. *Pancreatology.* 2006;6:17-32.
32. Pelaez-Luna M, Chari ST, Smyrk TC, Takahashi N, Clain JE, Levy MJ, et al. Do consensus indications for resection in branch duct intraductal papillary mucinous neoplasm predict malignancy? A study of 147 patients. *Am J Gastroenterol.* 2007;102:1759-64.
33. Brandwein S, Farrell JJ, Centeno BA, Brugge WR. Detection and tumor staging of malignancy in cystic, intraductal, and solid tumor of the pancreas by EUS. *Gastrointest Endosc.* 2001;53:722-7.
34. Lai R, Stanley MW, Bardales R, Linzie B, Mallery S. Endoscopic ultrasound-guided pancreatic duct aspiration: diagnostic yield and safety. *Endoscopy.* 2002;34:715-20.
35. Frossard JL, Amouyal P, Amouyal G, Palazzo L, Amaris J, Soldan M, et al. Performance of endosonography-guided fine needle aspiration and biopsy in the diagnosis of pancreatic cystic lesions. *Am J Gastroenterol.* 2003;98:1516-24.
36. Williams DB, Sahai AV, Aabakken L, Penman ID, van Velse A, Webb J, et al. Endoscopic ultrasound guided fine needle aspiration biopsy: a large single centre experience. *Gut.* 1999;44:720-6.
37. Brugge WR, Lewandrowski K, Lee-Lewandrowski E, Centeno BA, Szydlo T, Regan S, et al. Diagnosis of pancreatic cystic neoplasms: a report of the cooperative pancreatic cyst study. *Gastroenterology.* 2004;126:1330-6.
38. Al-Haddad M, Raimondo M, Woodward T, Krishna M, Pungpapong S, Noh K, et al. Safety and efficacy of cytology brushings versus standard FNA in evaluating cystic lesions of the pancreas: a pilot study. *Gastrointest Endosc.* 2007;65:894-8.
39. Thomas T, Bebb J, Mannath J, Ragunath K, Kaye PV, Aithal GP. EUS-guided pancreatic cyst brushing: a comparative study in a tertiary referral centre. *JOP.* 2010;11:163-9.

40. Hammel P, Levy P, Voitot H, Levy M, Vilgrain V, Zins M, et al. Preoperative cyst fluid analysis is useful for the differential diagnosis of cystic lesions of the pancreas. *Gastroenterology.* 1995;108:1230-5.
41. O'Toole D, Palazzo L, Hammel P, Ben Yaghlene L, Couvelard A, Felce-Dachez M, et al. Macrocystic pancreatic cystadenoma: the role of EUS and cyst fluid analysis in distinguishing mucinous and serous lesions. *Gastrointest Endosc.* 2004;59:823-9.
42. Khalid A, Zahid M, Finkelstein SD, LeBlanc JK, Kaushik N, Ahmad N, et al. Pancreatic cyst fluid DNA analysis in evaluating pancreatic cysts: a report of the PANDA study. *Gastrointest Endosc.* 2009;69:1095-102.
43. Sawhney MS, Devarajan S, O'Farrel P, Cury MS, Kundu R, Vollmer CM, et al. Comparison of carcinoembryonic antigen and molecular analysis in pancreatic cyst fluid. *Gastrointest Endosc.* 2009;69:1106-10.
44. Sreenarasimhaiah J, Lara LF, Jazrawi SF, Barnett CC, Tang SJ. A comparative analysis of pancreas cyst fluid CEA and histology with DNA mutational analysis in the detection of mucin producing or malignant cysts. *JOP.* 2009;10:163-8.
45. Siefert H, Dietrich C, Schmitt T, Caspary W, Wehrmann T. Endoscopic ultrasound-guided one-step transmural drainage of cystic abdominal lesions with a large channel echoendoscope. *Endoscopy.* 2000;32:255-9.
46. Park DH, Lee SS, Moon SH, Choi SY, Jung SW, Seo DW, et al. Endoscopic ultrasound-guided versus conventional transmural drainage for pancreatic pseudocysts: a prospective randomized trial. *Endoscopy.* 2009;41:842-8.
47. Gan SI, Thompson CC, Lauwers GY, Bounds BC, Brugge WR. Source. Ethanol lavage of pancreatic cystic lesions: initial pilot study. *Gastrointest Endosc.* 2005;61:746-52.
48. Oh HC, Seo DW, Lee TY, Kim JY, Lee SS, Lee SK, et al. New treatment for cystic tumors of the pancreas: EUS-guided ethanol lavage with paclitaxel injection. *Gastrointest Endosc.* 2008;67:636-42.
49. Sanders MK, Moser AJ, Khalid A, Fasanella KE, Zeh HJ, Burton S, et al. EUS-guided fiducial placement for stereotactic body radiotherapy in locally advanced and recurrent pancreatic cancer. *Gastrointest Endosc.* 2010;71:1178-84.
50. Di Matteo F, Martino M, Rea R, Pandolfi M, Rabitti C, Masselli GM, et al. EUS-guided Nd:YAG laser ablation of normal pancreatic tissue: a pilot study in a pig model. *Gastrointest Endosc.* 2010;72:358-63.
51. Chang KJ, Senzer N, Chung T, Hecht JR, Vogel S, Rosemurgy A, et al. A novel gene transfer therapy against pancreatic cancer (TNFerade) delivered by endoscopic ultrasound (EUS) and percutaneous guided fine needle injection (FNI). *Gastrointest Endosc.* 2004;59:P92.
52. Jin Z, Du Y, Li Z, Jiang Y, Chen J, Liu Y. Endoscopic ultrasonography-guided interstitial implantation of iodine 125 seeds combined with chemotherapy in the treatment of unresectable abdominal carcinoma: a prospective study. *Endoscopy.* 2008;40:314-20.
53. Eloubeidi MA, Tamhane A, Varadarajulu S, Wilcox CM. Frequency of major complications after EUS-guided FNA of solid pancreatic masses: a prospective evaluation. *Gastrointest Endosc.* 2006;63:622-9.
54. Varadarajulu S, Eloubeidi MA. Frequency and significance of acute intracystic hemorrhage during EUS-FNA of cystic lesions of the pancreas. *Gastrointest Endosc.* 2004; 60:631-5.
55. Eloubeidi MA, Gress FG, Savides TJ, Wiersema MJ, Kochman ML, Ahmad NA, et al. Acute pancreatitis after EUS-guided FNA of solid pancreatic masses: a pooled analysis from EUS centers in the United States. *Gastrointest Endosc.* 2004;60:385-9.
56. Eloubeidi MA, Tamhane A, Lopes TL, Morgan DE, Cerfolio RJ. Cervical esophageal perforations at the time of endoscopic ultrasound: a prospective evaluation of frequency, outcomes, and patient management. *Am J Gastroenterol.* 2009;104:53-6.

10 Endoscopic Therapy for Ampullary and Pancreatic Neoplasms

Alessandro Repici, Cesare Hassan, Daniel de Paula Pessoa Ferreira

ABSTRACT

Ampullary neoplasms are largely uncommon and benign neoplasms are managed either by endosocopic resection or surgery. Endoscopy has been helpful in detecting ampullary neoplasms, their extent, and surveillance. Endoscopic papillectomy offers a curative option for ampullary neoplasms. On the other hand, only 15% of pancreatic neoplasms can be managed with curative intent, while majority of them are managed palliatively because of their late presentation and presence of fewer therapeutic options. Endoscopy is helpful in the successful drainage of the biliary system as well as pain management. Celiac plexus block (CPB) and neurolysis have emerged as a tool for pain relief by disrupting the pancreatic afferent signaling to the spinal cord in an attempt to reduce abdominal pain and improvement in the patient's quality of life. Obstructive jaundice is the most common symptom caused by pancreatic cancer, occurring in approximately 70–80% of patients at the time of diagnosis; endoscopic approaches have proved to be safe and effective for biliary drainage (BD) in such situations. The traditional approach for the palliation of malignant gastric outlet obstruction (GOO) has been gastrojejunostomy; however, endoscopic self-expandable metal stent (SEMS) placement has become more routine in recent times.

ENDOSCOPIC THERAPY FOR AMPULLARY NEOPLASMS

INTRODUCTION

Ampullary neoplasms are rare with a reported prevalence of 0.04–0.12% in autopsy studies (Figure 10-1).[1,2] Although most of them are benign adenomas, these lesions have the potential to undergo malignant transformation to ampullary cancer.[3] Despite most of these malignancies being sporadic, some hereditary diseases have been associated with a higher risk for ampullary cancers. The strongest genetic predisposition is for familial adenomatous polyposis (FAP) syndrome with a prevalence of ampullary cancer of 3–12%, which represents a 100–200% increased risk.[4]

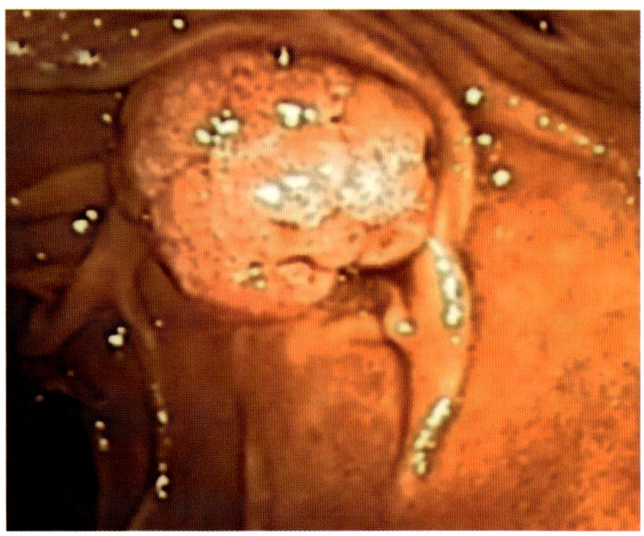

FIGURE 10-1 Ampullary neoplasms: Gross appearance.

SURGICAL APPROACH

For a long time, the only feasible treatment modality for curative therapy has been radical surgery. The negative aspects of the surgical approach are the associated high morbidity and mortality, whereas its greatest advantage is the low recurrence rate.[5,6] Transduodenal ampullectomy is the surgical option carrying lower morbidity (14–27%)[5] and mortality (0–4%)[7] as well as preserving more functional pancreatic tissue. However, it is associated with higher recurrence rates (17-32%).[8] On the other hand, pancreaticoduodenectomy (Whipple's procedure) has the benefit of a very low recurrence rate, but it carries a high perioperative mortality rate ranging from 2 to 9% and a very significant postoperative complication rate (up to 41%).[5,9] Considering that most ampullary tumors are benign, both the surgical approaches frequently result in overtreatment.[10] Consequently, because of the lower morbidity and mortality, endoscopic treatment has achieved increasing consensus as the first-choice therapy for ampullary adenomas, subsequent surgery being not precluded by previous endoscopic resection.[11]

BIOPSIES

Although conventional endoscopy may identify warning features of malignancy and chromoendoscopy, magnifying and narrow band imaging (NBI) may reasonably predict histology. Based only on the endoscopic appearance, it is very difficult to distinguish an ampullary adenoma from an ampullary carcinoma, carcinoid tumors, gangliocytic paragangliomas, or hamartomas.[10] Therefore, tissue sampling for definitive diagnosis is a prerequisite for appropriate management of these lesions. A minimum of 6 biopsies have been recommended to increase histologic confirmation.[12] Unfortunately, endoscopic biopsy of ampullary tumors carries an alarming false-negative rate of 14–42% for detecting carcinoma *in situ* and invasive carcinoma.[4,11] This means that preoperative biopsy showing only a benign histology does not exclude the presence of malignancy; a careful examination of the ampullectomy specimen being vital.[10,13] In selected cases, brush cytology may offer additional information to biopsy for the detection of malignancy.[14]

INDICATIONS FOR ENDOSCOPIC PAPILLECTOMY

At present, there is no consensus on when an ampullary adenoma should remain in surveillance or should be resected endoscopically or surgically. However, some decisive factors, such as the patient's general condition, available expertise, tumor histology, and endoscopic appearance should be simultaneously assessed to guide the treatment.[13] Despite unfavorable tumor characteristics, the clinical context (i.e., a debilitated patient with significant comorbidities) can recommend an endoscopic approach, as well as patients refusing surgery.[9,13] Conventional endoscopic features, such as ulceration, friability, firmness, and non-lifting sign suggest a possible malignancy, and such lesions should be considered for surgical resection even in the absence of malignancy on biopsy specimens.[15] When planning the treatment of ampullary tumors, endoscopic ultrasonography (EUS) was found to be more accurate than computed tomography (CT) and magnetic resonance imaging (MRI) in the overall assessment of the T stage of ampullary neoplasms (EUS 78%, CT 24%, and MRI 46%).[16]

There is no definitive consensus regarding the maximum tumor size or diameter indicating a safe endoscopic treatment. Several authors recommend that lesions greater than 4–5 cm should be sent for surgical resection, because of the high risk of either complications or incomplete resection; however, selected cases of successful endoscopic removal of ampullary lesions of greater size have also been reported.[15-17]

High-grade dysplasia unequivocally indicates the need for resection, because of the high risk of malignant progression or already prevalent cancer.[7,18] However, it does not represent a contraindication for endoscopic papillectomy. Several authors also recommend that endoscopic resection should be limited to patients without evidence of invasive cancer.[16,17] However, endoscopic papillectomy has been reported as a successful alternative to radical surgery in selected cases of early, localized intramucosal ampullary adenocarcinoma, as well as in lesions with intraductal growth.[12]

Endoscopic resection is generally indicated as first-line therapy in patients with benign ampullary tumors, however, the final treatment decision should be based on histologic findings of the endoscopically resected specimen.[13] When an invasive carcinoma is diagnosed, a definitive surgical approach is recommended in order to achieve complete resection, including removal of the frequently affected lymph nodes.

TECHNIQUES

The term "ampullectomy" refers to resection of the entire ampulla of Vater, requiring surgical reimplantation of the distal common bile ducts and pancreatic ducts. Technically, when endoscopic resections are performed, only tissue from the papilla is removed, and thus, the term "papillectomy" is more appropriate, although both terms are often used in the literature to describe the endoscopic approach.[19]

Endoscopic ampullectomy is performed with a standard duodenoscope to ensure better visualization of the papillary lesion and to provide access to the biliary ducts. Pancreatic or biliary sphincterotomies are frequently performed in order to assist the drainage of pancreaticobiliary ducts, to simplify duct accesses, and for post-papillectomy surveillance. However, it is still controversial whether these maneuvers should be performed at all, much less before or after the papillectomy.[12] Some authors have proposed a submucosal injection with isotonic saline, epinephrine, and hydroxypropyl methylcellulose to elevate the tumor immediately before papillectomy.[20-22] However, the edema induced by the injection may hinder access to the biliary and pancreatic ducts, increasing the risk of post-ampullectomy pancreatitis.[13]

Endoscopic resection is traditionally performed with a standard "braided" polypectomy snare, although fine-wire snares specifically designed for papillary resection are available.[16] There are no data comparing the utility or documenting the superiority of one type of snare over the other. Both pure cutting- and blended-currents have been applied during endoscopic papillectomy. The former has been associated with a lower risk of bleeding, while the latter with a higher risk of pancreatitis;[13] at the moment neither having been proven to be superior. Power settings have also not been standardized.[1]

En bloc resection is the preferred technique to guide the pathologist in assessing tumor margins, and it should be performed when the lesion can be completely ensnared. It also has the advantages of potentially shortening the procedure time and requiring less electrocautery. To facilitate the ensnarement of a larger lesion, the use of an intraductal balloon catheter has been proposed.[23] Lesions larger than 2 cm in diameter may frequently require piecemeal papillectomy, although successful en bloc resection of a 6 cm ampullary adenoma by endoscopic submucosal dissection technique has been reported.[24]

Although ablative therapies [argon plasma coagulation, Nd:YAG (yttrium aluminium garnet) laser, monopolar or bipolar electrocoagulation] should not be routinely used alone in attempt to remove the entire tumor, they are useful to destroy remaining adenomatous tissue after papillectomy. Disadvantages of this method are the risk of pancreatitis or stenosis and the impossibility to get samples for pathologic analysis.[1,12]

At present, the routine placement of a prophylactic pancreatic stent (5 F stents) after papillectomy is adopted by most endoscopists (Figure 10-2). This practice is supported by the fact that several studies have shown a lower incidence of post-papillectomy pancreatitis in patients who underwent pancreatic stent placement (0–9.6 vs. 17–25%).[25,26] However, some authors advocate pancreatic stents only when the pancreatic duct does not drain properly after papillectomy.[1] Most pancreatic stents will spontaneously migrate out of the pancreatic duct within 2 weeks of insertion. This is usually confirmed with an abdominal X-ray at 2 weeks.[12] A stent that remains *in situ* should be removed endoscopically.[25,27,28] Although, theoretically, cholangitis can occur after endoscopic papillectomy, its rare occurrence does not justify routine prophylactic biliary stenting.[17] Nasobiliary drainage could be a valid alternative.[1]

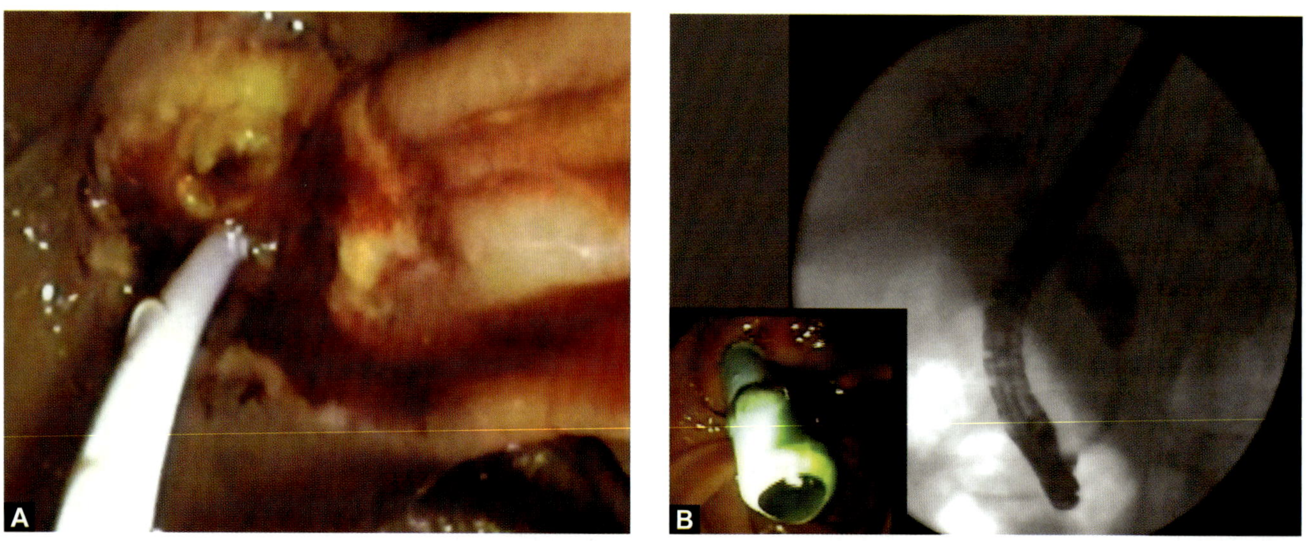

FIGURE 10-2 Prophylactic pancreatic stent after papillectomy.

COMPLICATIONS

Complications related to endoscopic papillectomy are divided into early (acute pancreatitis, bleeding, and perforation) and late (post-papillectomy stenosis).[10] Delayed bleeding after papillectomy is common, occurring in 2–16% of patients, and is usually managed conservatively or by endoscopic re-intervention.[21,28] Pancreatitis arises in 0–8% of the cases and can be treated with sphincterotomy and stents, as previously discussed. Perforation after papillectomy has been reported in 0–4%[16,17,25] and may be successfully managed with combined hemoclips and antibiotics.[25] Death due to endoscopic ampullary resection has been rarely reported.

Because of the 23% (range 10–58%) morbidity and the 0.4% (range 0–7%) mortality rates, endoscopic papillectomy represents a "high-risk" procedure. For this reason, a period of postprocedure inpatient observation should be considered for detection and treatment of any immediate or slightly delayed complications.[1]

OUTCOMES

Endoscopic resection of benign ampullary tumors is curative in over 85% of patients, whilst the overall success is only 46% in patients with intraductal growth.[13,20] Recurrence rates range from 0 to 33%, with large size, genetic predisposition, final histology, presence of intraductal tumor, and the expertise of the endoscopist representing as predisposing factors. The application of adjuvant thermal ablation can reduce the recurrence rate, although associated with an increased morbidity.[1]

SURVEILLANCE AFTER ENDOSCOPIC TREATMENT

Although there is no consensus on the appropriate interval, endoscopic surveillance for early detection of residual or recurrent neoplastic tissue is recommended after endoscopic papillectomy. Using a duodenoscope, multiple biopsies should be performed from the site of resected ampulla, even in the presence of apparent normal tissue. Residual or recurrent adenoma is treated by repeat resection or thermal ablative therapy. Surgery is indicated in case of invasive carcinoma or intraductal tumor extension that cannot be resected endoscopically.[12,13]

The duration of surveillance intervals depends on a number of factors: tumor size, histologic findings, and a history of FAP. For benign lesions less than 3 cm, with clear resection margins (R0), the initial surveillance examination should be performed at 3–6 months after the resection, and after that, at 6–12 month intervals up to 2 years and then, if 2 consecutive biopsies have shown no residual adenomatous tissue, it can be extended to every 2 years.[17,25,27] For lesions greater than 3 cm, piecemeal resected, with positive margins, or containing high-grade dysplasia, a shorter surveillance interval (2–3 months) is to be recommended.[17,27] Endoscopic retrograde cholangio-pancreatography (ERCP) is also indicated in the suspicion of intraductal tumor involvement. Patients with FAP should undergo annual surveillance indefinitely.[29]

ENDOSCOPIC THERAPY FOR PANCREATIC NEOPLASMS

INTRODUCTION

Pancreatic ductal adenocarcinoma (PC) is the second most common gastrointestinal cancer, with an incidence ranging 8–12 per 100,000 per year, and it is now the fourth leading cause of cancer-related death in the United States, with an estimate of some 35,000 deaths per year, and the fifth in Europe. Up to 80–85% of patients have incurable disease at the time of diagnosis.[30,31] The average age of diagnosis is 60–65 years, with 10% of cases indicated as "early onset," occurring in people aged less than 50 years. The incidence of PC is slightly higher in males than females.

The disease presents in a subtle way, with symptoms including weight loss, anorexia, fatigue, abdominal pain, newly diagnosed diabetes mellitus, jaundice, pruritus, and nausea, which are nonspecific and typically occur late in the course of the disease. In most series, the possibility of curative surgical resection is approximately 15–20% and even after the curative surgery attempt, the 5-year survival rate remains between 3 and 5%. Since most of the pancreatic cancer patients will have disease progression or recurrence, palliation therapy is necessary. The goal of palliative therapies is to alleviate symptoms, decrease hospitalizations, improve quality of life, and potentially improve morbidity and mortality.[32,33]

ENDOSCOPIC PALLIATION FOR BILIARY OBSTRUCTION

Obstructive jaundice is the most common symptom caused by pancreatic cancer, occurring in approximately 70–80% of patients at the time of diagnosis.[34] Untreated biliary obstruction leads to jaundice, pruritus, coagulopathy, eventually to cholangitis, and to death due to liver failure.[35] It has already been demonstrated that biliary surgical bypass increased survival when compared to exploratory laparotomy alone, some studies, however, suggest that biliary release also improves other factors, such as anorexia, fatigue, insomnia, cognition, and overall quality of life.[36-40]

Before the implementation of endoscopic and radiological therapy, surgery was the only means to decompress the biliary tree. Two randomized trials published in the 1980s compared the efficacy, safety, survival, overall complications, and hospitalization time of endoscopic drainage with those of conventional surgical bypass.[40,41] Apart from the overall hospitalization time that was shorter among the stented group, no significant differences were found among these therapies. A larger randomized trial showed lower procedure-related mortality (3 vs. 14%) and a lower complication rate (11 vs. 29%) with endoscopic therapy, despite equivalent technical success and overall survival.[42] A recent meta-analysis showing no differences in mortality rates between the two procedures, recommended endoscopic bypass as the best treatment for patients surviving less than 6 months, whereas surgical bypass should be considered for those surviving longer.[43]

The endoscopic approach also proved to be safer and more effective than the transhepatic approach when using plastic stents,[44] however, there is no data with metal stents. For this reason, despite both techniques being available in most institutions, endoscopic therapy is generally preferred, reserving the percutaneous transhepatic route for cases of endoscopic failure.

STENT CHOICE

Once an endoscopic drainage for advanced PC has been chosen, a further controversy relies on the type of stent to be applied. The patency of plastic stents is well-known to be limited to 3 months, so that in the case of prolonged survival, repeated endoscopic procedures may be needed to avoid post-stenting occlusion of the biliary tree. For this reason, adoption of metallic stents has been advocated. Metallic stents are expected to result into a longer patency, but they are expensive and can be occluded by tumor ingrowth or overgrowth. Several trials compared the efficacy and safety of different types of stents for endoscopic drainage of inoperable PC. A recent meta-analysis showed that self-expanding metal stents (SEMS) were associated with a significantly reduced risk of recurrent biliary obstruction at 4 months (RR 0.44, 95% CI 0.3, 0.63) or prior to death, or end of study (RR 0.52, 95% CI 0.39–0.69) as compared to plastic stents, although they did not appear to be superior in terms of technical success, therapeutic success, mortality, or complications.[45] Despite the unequivocal evidence of a higher efficacy, the use of metal stents in patients with advanced PC is still limited. This appears to be related to a substantially higher initial cost of this type of stent as compared to the plastic ones. However, a recent cost-effectiveness analysis showed a favorable incremental cost-effectiveness ratio of metal stents, being $1,820 per ERCP prevented. On the other hand, when considering the relatively high cost of metal stents, plastic stents should be preferred in any patient whose life expectancy is shorter than 6 months.[45]

Plastic stents are widely used, mainly because of low cost. Among the plastic stents, the 10 F have significantly longer patency compared with 7 and 8 F,[46,47] and equivalent patency compared with the 11.5 F diameter,[48] usually representing the preferred choice. Determining the optimal interval for stent exchange remains debatable. Since the mean time of occlusion is 3–5 months, some experts recommend exchanging every 3 months, whereas others prefer to wait for the earliest clinical symptoms or signs of stent occlusion.[49]

Several different types of biliary metal stents are available, varying in shape, design, and metal alloy. Some randomized clinical trials compared the various types of metal stents for the treatment of malignant biliary obstruction and found no differences in ease of placement, occlusion rates, and overall patency.[50,51] One of the few differences found was the lower patency rates with early stent occlusion and increased rates of cholangitis, when the 6 mm stent was used for treatment of distal malignant biliary strictures, which contraindicates its use in such cases.[52]

The covered metal stent was developed to prevent tumor ingrowth which was the main cause of stent occlusion when using an uncovered metal stent, occurring in 35–55% of the cases.[53,54] Isayama et al. compared the efficacy of the covered with the uncovered metal stent in a randomized study, showing that the placement of the covered type resulted in a significantly longer patency and a lower incidence of obstruction than the uncovered metal stent.[55] Although, the use of a covered metal stent decreases stent occlusion, prolonged stent placement is associated with other complications such as, cholecystitis, pancreatitis, and stent migration.[56]

For patients with plastic stents, treatment options include replacement with other plastic stent or SEMS. Patients with prior history of multiple or premature plastic stent occlusion seem to be at risk for future plastic stent dysfunction and may benefit from earlier SEMS placement.[57,58] Recanalization of occluded metal stents can be achieved endoscopically with insertion of a plastic stent within the occluded SEMS, insertion of a second SEMS, and mechanical cleaning (catheter irrigation or use of stone-extraction balloons) of the occluded stent lumen. Overall, success rates for re-establishing biliary drainage (BD) are over 80%, although, the mechanical cleaner has a lower efficacy.[59] Diathermic ablation of the ingrown tissue is generally not recommended, as it carries a high risk of bleeding, ductal injury with perforation, stent fragmentation and, moreover, the effect is only temporary.[60,61]

STENTING TECHNIQUES

To identify the precise site and extension of the lesion, it is imperative to obtain a successful BD. A detailed cholangiogram obtained during the stent placement procedure at endoscopic ERCP is important to study the biliary tract and obstruction, and also provides useful information for planning correct stent deployment. Before endoscopy, a magnetic resonance cholangiopancreatography (MRCP) or a thin-section CT scan can be helpful to characterize the lesion, especially when evaluating strictures involving the hepatic confluence or intrahepatic ducts.[62] Deep selective cannulation of the common bile duct is necessary before placement of biliary stents. A guidewire must then pass across the stricture into the obstructed bile ducts to maintain access and facilitate device exchange. Multiple guidewires should be placed if multiple stents are expected. Hydrophilic guidewires can advance easily through tight and tortuous strictures. In addition, curved guidewires may assist in negotiating difficult strictures.[51]

Tissue sampling, when indicated, may be obtained from the stricture before stenting.[62-64] Although, the specificity and positive predictive value for standard ERCP-sampling techniques [transpapillary wire-guided brush cytology, endoluminal forceps biopsy, or transductal fine needle aspiration (FNA)] are almost 100%, the sensitivity is low-to-moderate ranging from 15 to 70%.[65] Combining two or more techniques has been shown to increase sensitivity, cancer detection rate varying from 55 to 73% with the combination of biopsy and brushings and from 62 to 82% with the combination of biopsy, brushings, and FNA.[66,67] Intraductal endoscopic visualization of the biopsy target during peroral cholangioscopy or peroral pancreatoscopy might enhance the diagnostic value of ERCP by improving target selection and tissue acquisition.[68]

It remains controversial whether endoscopic biliary sphincterotomy (EBS) should be performed prior to metal or plastic stent deployment. EBS may facilitate stent insertion and also helps in preventing the development of pancreatitis from stent-related occlusion of the pancreatic duct. On the other hand, EBS is also independently associated with pancreatitis, bleeding, and perforation. A recent prospective study showed that there was more stent migration among patients undergoing EBS prior to stent placement and a higher risk of complications.[69] In contrast, a smaller case series reported that biliary sphincterotomy seemed to reduce the risk of post-ERCP pancreatitis in patients with proximal malignant biliary strictures.[70] Nevertheless, the decision to perform a biliary sphincterotomy before stent placement is often left to the discretion of the therapeutic endoscopist.

Dilation of the stricture with mechanical or pneumatic catheters may be rarely required to allow stent delivery. When a very high-grade stenosis is present, the standard endoscopic dilation devices occasionally fail. In this situation, a plastic stent retrieval device (Soehendra Stent Retriever; Wilson-Cook) has been used to pass through strictures, allowing subsequent stenting with over 90% success rates.[71,72]

The most widely used technique for plastic biliary stent deployment involves advancing a stiff polyethylene guide catheter over the guidewire. The plastic stent is then advanced over the complex guidewire; guide catheter using an outer pusher catheter as a three-layer system. The guide catheter and guidewire are then withdrawn, leaving the stent in position (Figure 10-2). SEMS are delivered within an outer, narrower, constraining delivery system that is advanced over a stricture, traversing the guidewire. When the delivery catheter is in position (confirmed fluoroscopically), the constraining outer catheter is removed to allow SEMS deployment and full expansion. The successful placement rate of a plastic or metal stent at ERCP is over 90% in experienced centers.[73-75]

ENDOSCOPIC ULTRASONOGRAPHY-GUIDED BILE DUCT DRAINAGE

Although ERCP is successful in accessing the bile and pancreatic ducts in 90% of patients with unresectable malignant biliary obstruction, failure to achieve BD still occurs.[76] Traditionally, such patients underwent percutaneous drainage using ultrasound and radiological guidance, and endoscopic (non-ultrasonography) transmural drainage; however, these methods carry a high complication rate and could be associated with fistula formation and recurrent cholangitis.[77]

In 1996, Wiersema et al. first described EUS-guided cholangiography, and five years later, Giovannini et al. demonstrated the feasibility of EUS-BD.[78,79] Since then, dedicated accessories allowed to create bilio- or pancreato-digestive anastomosis and EUS-guided pancreatic drainage (EUS-PD).

Usually, EUS-BD has been indicated for patients with advanced malignant obstruction. Few studies have described the application of EUS-BD for preoperative decompression of the biliary tree,[80,81] despite the preoperative enforcement of this maneuver is still controversial.[37]

There are currently two main EUS approaches to access the bile duct: either cholangioduodenostomy (draining the extrahepatic common bile duct from the duodenum) or hepaticogastrostomy (draining the left biliary ductal system from the stomach), however, the basic techniques are similar. A needle-knife catheter, a 19-gauge or a 22-gauge FNA needle under EUS guidance can be used to achieve the initial puncture. After the bile is aspirated, contrast is injected to obtain a cholangiogram under fluoroscopy. Once confirmed to be in the bile duct (or its main left branches, if accessed from the stomach), a 0.035 or 0.021-inch guidewire is inserted into the bile duct via the FNA needle or catheter. At this moment, every effort should be made to advance the guidewire across the stricture into the duodenum to allow transpapillary stenting using the standard ERCP based approach. This EUS-guided "rendezvous" technique appears to be safer than placing a transmural biliary stent. If this is not possible, the new tract is dilated using a biliary catheter or a papillary balloon dilator. Finally, a biliary plastic stent (up to 10 F, size is dependent on location) or SEMS is inserted through the choledochoduodeno/gastrostomy site into the bile duct.[37,76]

The overall technical success rate was about 90% in patients submitted to and approximately 80% in hepaticogastrostomy.[82] Obstructive jaundice release was successfully achieved in all patients, once the stents were placed. The rate of procedure-related complications was approximately 20% in EUS-BD, including focal bile peritonitis, bleeding, pneumoperitoneum, infection caused by occlusion/migration of the stent, and death. An exceptionally long patency (mean 211.8 days using 7–8.5 F plastic stent) of choledochoduodenostomy has been reported.[82] It is worth mentioning that this procedure involves no risk of pancreatitis because of lack of influence on the pancreatic duct during procedures.

ENDOSCOPIC PALLIATION FOR GASTRIC OUTLET OBSTRUCTION

Gastric outlet obstruction (GOO) may occur in patients with advanced pancreatic, gastric or ampullary carcinomas, lymphomas, or metastases. The traditional approach for the palliation of malignant GOO has been gastrojejunostomy, however recently, endoscopic SEMS placement has become a routine practice.[83,84]

The area of stenosis is generally reached using a therapeutic upper endoscope, or in some cases with a colonoscope.[85] The length of the stricture is normally determined using contrast fluoroscopy of the duodenum during the procedure. Once the stenosis is reached, a guidewire is passed through the stricture and advanced at least 20 cm distal to the obstructing area. The stent length should be 3–4 cm longer than the stenosis to provide an adequate stent margin after placement, although, some authors choose the stent length just 1–2 cm longer than the stricture.[85,86] After that, assisted by fluoroscopy, the SEMS delivery system is passed over the guidewire through the working channel of the endoscope, aiming to align the stent straddling the stricture. Once the alignment is correct, the stent is then deployed in the distal end first, followed by the proximal end. Next, luminal patency is carefully confirmed advancing the endoscope through it, which also facilitates stent expansion.[86] In addition, a hydrostatic stent dilation during the initial procedure can occasionally be performed to manage insufficient expansion.[85]

There is no consensus on which stent, covered or uncovered, is the best option for malignant GOO, since uncovered stents have recurrent obstruction, as tumor ingrowth is common[87,88] and the covered stents' migration was found to be unacceptably high (over 20%).[89,90] However, it was reported that reintervention is more commonly required after covered stent placement.[91]

Biliary obstruction occurs in 2–8% of patients after stent placement in the proximal duodenum.[92-94] It is often difficult or even impossible to cannulate the papilla through the stent mesh. For that reason, several authors advocate to stent the common bile duct, prior to stent placement in the proximal duodenum.[95]

Complication rates range from 11 to 43%,[95,96] although, severe complications are rare.[32] Immediate and early complications include problems with sedation, aspiration, stent dysfunction, perforation, and

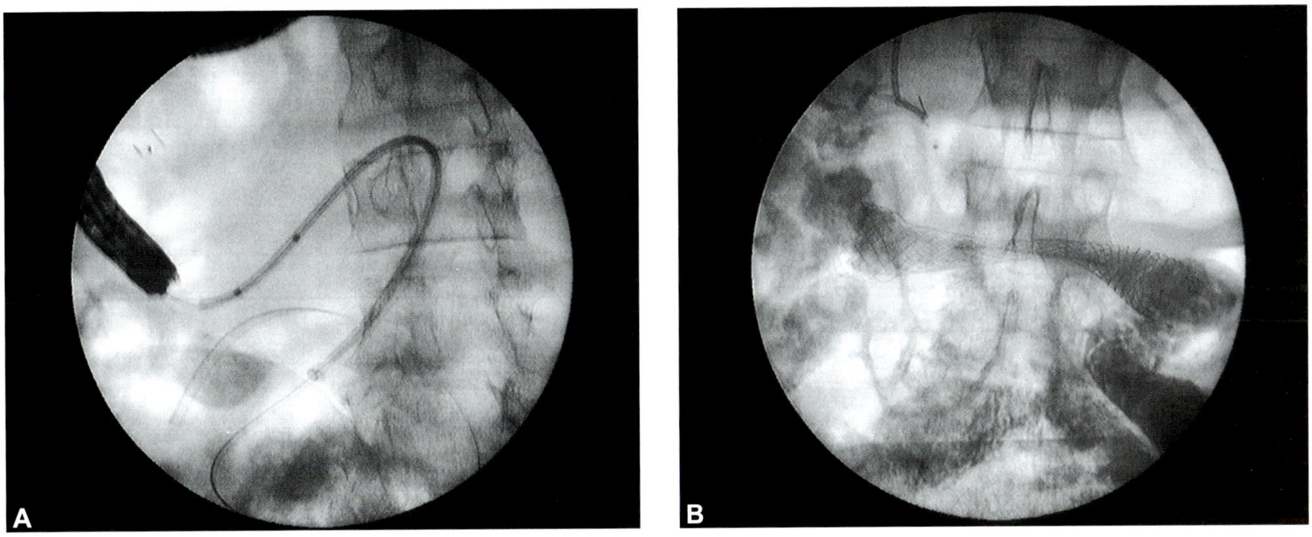

FIGURE 10-3 Self-expanding metal stent for gastric outlet obstruction.

bleeding. Late complications include stent obstruction, stent migration, perforation, and fistula formation.[97] Recurrence of obstructive symptoms, due to tumor ingrowth, more commonly, and tumor overgrowth, is reported in 33.3% of cases.[98] It is successfully treated with placement of a covered stent in the new stenotic area.[99,100] Stent migration is cited in 3.8–6.3% of patients.[101]

Technical success for endoscopic stenting of the duodenum with SEMS is reported in 92–100% of cases,[102] although, clinical success rates are usually lower with reports ranging from 79 to 91% (Figure 10-3).

ENDOSCOPIC PALLIATION FOR ABDOMINAL PAIN: CELIAC PLEXUS NEUROLYSIS

Abdominal pain is a common and debilitating problem for patients with pancreatic cancer. It is often a difficult symptom to manage and a key point in the palliative treatment of this malignancy.[103] The final common pathway of any pathologic process producing pain in the pancreas is believed to pass through the celiac plexus.[104] Celiac plexus block (CPB) and celiac plexus neurolysis (CPN) then emerged to disrupt the pancreatic afferent signaling to the spinal cord in an attempt to reduce abdominal pain and so improve patient quality of life.[105]

CPB and neurolysis were traditionally performed by percutaneous, posterior approach under CT or ultrasound-guidance, or during surgery. However, since 1996, when Wiersema et al.[106] reported EUS-guided transgastric CPN, EUS has been increasingly used to control abdominal pain in patients with unresectable pancreatic cancer.

The celiac ganglia are located at the origin of the celiac artery, which is easily identified at endosonography. The relative proximity of the celiac ganglia to the posterior gastric wall ensures an accurate passage of the injecting needle into the ganglia, thereby, potentially increasing the effectiveness of the block. Technically, to proceed CNP, the EUS operator must identify the take-off of the celiac artery and inject bupivacaine (0.25%) followed by ethyl alcohol (98%), utilizing a 19- or 22-gauge FNA needle on either side of the vessel or on the area just at the angle above the celiac artery take-off from the aorta.[107] Alternatively, a recently developed fenestrated 20-gauge needle proposes a much smoother injection making it easier to administer the solution. While CPN uses an anesthetic with a sclerosing agent such as alcohol or phenol, CPB involves injecting an anesthetic with a steroid into the celiac plexus region.[108]

The majority of EUS-guided CPN studies demonstrate effectiveness in abdominal pain relief due to pancreatic cancer varying from about 70–94%.[109] In a very recent meta-analyses comprising a total of 119 patients with inoperable pancreatic cancer, EUS-guided CPN was successful in alleviating abdominal pain in about 73% of patients.[110] However, the extent of pain relief has been inconsistent. In a pilot study, pain relief lasting for a median of 10 weeks was achieved in 88% of patients undergoing EUS-CPN.[109] Contradictorily, another study reported initial pain exacerbation lasting a mean duration of 2.2 days in 34% of the patients who had EUS-CPN, but at follow-up, those patients experienced greater pain relief.[111] On multivariate analysis, the benefit of EUS-CPN was independent of morphine use, chemotherapy, and radiation.[112] The EUS guided neurolysis can be performed on either one or both sides of the aorta, although Sahai et al. recently compared bilateral injection with central single injection approach, and demonstrated the superiority of the bilateral method in reducing the pain score (70 vs. 46%; $p = 0.0016$).[113] The location of tumor may also be important, making a difference in the effectiveness of CPN. In a study performed by Catalano et al.,[114] CPN was more effective in patients with pancreatic cancer located in the body or tail of the pancreas as compared to patients with the tumors located in the head of pancreas.

Although EUS-guided CPN did not improve survival, it was associated with improved pain control, decreased narcotic usage, reduced constipation, besides lower complications rate and higher cost-effectiveness; when compared to other modalities of CPN. All these facts have consolidated this procedure as a safe and effective option for controlling pain in patients with pancreatic cancer and tolerance to narcotic analgesics.

REFERENCES

1. Pandolfi M, Martino M, Gabbrielli A. Endoscopic treatment of ampullary adenomas. *JOP.* 2008;9:1-8.
2. Stolte M, Pscherer C. Adenoma-carcinoma sequence in the papilla of Vater. *Scand J Gastroenterol.* 1996;31:376-82.
3. Agoff SN, Crispin DA, Bronner MP, Dail DH, Hawes SE, Haggitt RC. Neoplasms of the ampulla of Vater with concurrent pancreatic intraductal neoplasia: a histological and molecular study. *Mod Pathol.* 2001;14:139-46.
4. Heinrich S, Clavien PA. Ampullary cancer. *Curr Opin Gastroenterol.* 2010;26:280-5.
5. Beger HG, Treitschke F, Gansauge F, Harada N, Hiki N, Mattfeldt T. Tumor of the ampulla of Vater: experience with local or radical resection in 171 consecutively treated patients. *Arch Surg.* 1999;134:526-32.
6. Branum GD, Pappas TN, Meyers WC. The management of tumors of the ampulla of Vater by local resection. *Ann Surg.* 1996;224:621-7.
7. de Castro SM, van Heek NT, Kuhlmann KF, Busch OR, Offerhaus GJ, van Gulik TM, et al. Surgical management of neoplasms of the ampulla of Vater: local resection or pancreatoduodenectomy and prognostic factors for survival. *Surgery.* 2004;136:994-1002.
8. Farnell MB, Sakorafas GH, Sarr MG, Rowland CM, Tsiotos GG, Farley DR, et al. Villous tumors of the duodenum: reappraisal of local vs. extended resection. *J Gastrointest Surg.* 2000;4:13-21.
9. Neoptolemos JP, Talbot IC, Carr-Locke DL, Shaw DE, Cockleburgh R, Hall AW, et al. Treatment and outcome in 52 consecutive cases of ampullary carcinoma. *Br J Surg.* 1987;74:957-61.
10. Hernandez LV, Catalano MF. Endoscopic papillectomy. *Curr Opin Gastroenterol.* 2008;24:617-22.
11. Bohnacker S, Soehendra N, Maguchi H, Chung JB, Howell DA. Endoscopic resection of benign tumors of the papilla of Vater. *Endoscopy.* 2006;38:521-5.
12. Standards of Practice Committee, Adler DG, Qureshi W, Davila R, Gan SI, Lichtenstein D. The role of endoscopy in ampullary and duodenal adenomas. *Gastrointest Endosc.* 2006;64:849-54.
13. Nguyen NQ, Binmoeller KF. Endoscopic ampullectomy. *Tech Gastrointest Endosc.* 2010;12:53-60.
14. Bardales RH, Stanley MW, Simpson DD, Baker SJ, Steele CT, Schaefer RF, et al. Diagnostic value of brush cytology in the diagnosis of duodenal, biliary, and ampullary neoplasms. *Am J Clin Pathol.* 1998;109:540-8.
15. Cheng CL, Sherman S, Fogel EL, McHenry L, Watkins JL, Fukushima T, et al. Endoscopic snare papillectomy for tumors of the duodenal papillae. *Gastrointest Endosc.* 2004;60:757-64.
16. Cannon ME, Carpenter SL, Elta GH, Nostrant TT, Kochman ML, Ginsberg GG, et al. EUS compared with CT, magnetic resonance imaging, and angiography and the influence of biliary stenting on staging accuracy of ampullary neoplasms. *Gastrointest Endosc.* 1999;50:27-33.
17. Binmoeller KF, Boaventura S, Ramsperger K, Soehendra N. Endoscopic snare excision of benign adenomas of the papilla of Vater. *Gastrointest Endosc.* 1993;39:127-31.
18. Seifert E, Schulte F, Stolte M. Adenoma and carcinoma of the duodenum and papilla of Vater: a clinicopathologic study. *Am J Gastroenterol.* 1992;87:37-42.
19. Han J, Kim MH. Endoscopic papillectomy for adenomas of the major duodenal papilla (with video). *Gastrointest Endosc.* 2006;63:292-301.
20. Bohnacker S, Seitz U, Nguyen D, Thonke F, Seewald S, deWeerth A. Endoscopic resection of benign tumors of the duodenal papilla without and with intraductal growth. *Gastrointest Endosc.* 2005;62:551-60.
21. Desilets DJ, Dy RM, Ku PM, Hanson BL, Elton E, Mattia A, et al. Endoscopic management of tumors of the major duodenal papilla: refined techniques to improve outcome and avoid complications. *Gastrointest Endosc.* 2001;54:202-8.
22. Eswaran SL, Sanders M, Bernadino KP, Ansari A, Lawrence C, Stefan A, et al. Success and complications of endoscopic removal of giant duodenal and ampullary polyps: a comparative series. *Gastrointest Endosc.* 2006;64:925-32.
23. Aiura K, Imaeda H, Kitajima M, Kumai K. Balloon-catheter-assisted endoscopic snare papillectomy for benign tumors of the major duodenal papilla. *Gastrointest Endosc.* 2003;57:743-7.
24. Fukushima H, Yamamoto H, Nakano H, Nakazawa K, Sunada K, Wada S, et al. Complete en bloc resection of a large ampullary adenoma with a focal adenocarcinoma by using endoscopic submucosal dissection (with video). *Gastrointest Endosc.* 2009;70:592-5.
25. Norton ID, Gostout CJ, Baron TH, Geller A, Petersen BT, Wiersema MJ. Safety and outcome of endoscopic snare

excision of the major duodenal papilla. *Gastrointest Endosc.* 2002;56:239-43.

26. Fazel A, Quadri A, Catalano MF, Meyerson SM, Geenen JE. Does a pancreatic duct stent prevent post-ERCP pancreatitis? A prospective randomized study. *Gastrointest Endosc.* 2003;57:291-4.
27. Baillie J. Endoscopic ampullectomy. *Am J Gastroenterol.* 2005;100:2379-81.
28. Catalano MF, Linder JD, Chak A, Sivak MV Jr, Raijman I, Geenen JE, et al. Endoscopic management of adenoma of the major duodenal papilla. *Gastrointest Endosc.* 2004;59:225-32.
29. Cordero-Fernandez C, Garzon-Benavides M, Pizarro-Moreno A, García-Lozano R, Márquez-Galán JL, López Ruiz T, et al. Gastroduodenal involvement in patients with familial adenomatous polyposis. Prospective study of the nature and evolution of polyps: evaluation of the treatment and surveillance methods applied. *Eur J Gastroenterol Hepatol.* 2009;21:1161-7.
30. Jemal A, Siegel R, Ward E, Murray T, Xu J, Thun MJ. Cancer Statistics, 2007. *CA Cancer J Clin.* 2007;57:43-66.
31. Ferlay J, Autier P, Boniol M, Heanue M, Colombet M, Boyle P. Estimates of the cancer incidence and mortality in Europe in 2006. *Ann Oncol.* 2007;18:581-92.
32. Kruse EJ. Palliation in pancreatic cancer. *Surg Clin N Am.* 2010;90:355-64.
33. Sanders M, Papachristou GI, McGrath KM, Slivka A. Endoscopic palliation of pancreatic cancer. *Gastroenterol Clin N Am.* 2007;36:455-76.
34. Lillemoe KD, Pitt HA. Palliation. Surgical and otherwise. *Cancer.* 1996;78:605-14.
35. Flamm CR, Mark DH, Aronson N. Evidence-based assessment of ERCP approaches to managing pancreaticobiliary malignancies. *Gastrointest Endosc.* 2002;56:S218-25.
36. Puli SR, Reddy JB, Bechtold ML, Antillon MR, Brugge WR. EUS-guided celiac plexus neurolysis for pain due to chronic pancreatitis or pancreatic cancer pain: a meta-analysis and systematic review. *Dig Dis Sci.* 2009;54:2330-7.
37. Irisawa A, Hikichi T, Shibukawa G, Takagi T, Wakatsuki T, Takahashi Y, et al. Pancreatobiliary drainage using the EUS-FNA technique: EUS-BD and EUS-PD. *J Hepatobiliary Pancreat Surg.* 2009;16:598-604.
38. Abraham NS, Barkun JS, Barkun AN. Palliation of malignant biliary obstruction: a prospective trial examining impact on quality of life. *Gastrointest Endosc.* 2002;56:835-41.
39. Sarr MG, Cameron JL. Surgical management of unresectable carcinoma of the pancreas. *Surgery.* 1982;91:123-33.
40. Shepherd HA, Royle G, Ross AP, Diba A, Arthur M, Colin-Jones D. Endoscopic biliary endoprosthesis in the palliation of malignant obstruction of the distal common bile duct: a randomized trial. *Br J Surg.* 1988;75:1166-8.
41. Andersen JR, Sorensen SM, Kruse A, Rokkjaer M, Matzen P. Randomised trial of endoscopic endoprosthesis versus operative bypass in malignant obstructive jaundice. *Gut.* 1989;30:1132-5.
42. Smith AC, Dowsett JF, Russell RC, Hatfield AR, Cotton PB. Randomised trial of endoscopic stenting versus surgical bypass in malignant low bile duct obstruction. *Lancet.* 1994;344:1655-60.
43. Taylor MC, McLeod RS, Langer B. Biliary stenting versus bypass surgery for the palliation of malignant distal bile duct obstruction: a meta-analysis. *Liver Transpl.* 2000;6:302-8.
44. Speer AG, Cotton PB, Russel RC, Mason RR, Hatfield AR, Leung JW, et al. Randomized trial of endoscopic versus percutaneous stent insertion in malignant obstructive jaundice. *Lancet.* 1987;2:57-62.
45. Moss AC, Morris E, Leyden J, MacMathuna P. Do the benefits of metal stents justify the costs? A systematic review and meta-analysis of trials comparing endoscopic stents for malignant biliary obstruction. *Eur J Gastroenterol Hepatol.* 2007;19:1119-24.
46. Speer AG, Cotton PB, MacRae KD. Endoscopic management of malignant biliary obstruction. Stents of 10 French gauge are preferable to stents of 8 French gauge. *Gastrointest Endosc.* 1988;34:412-7.
47. Pedersen FM. Endoscopic management of malignant biliary obstruction. Is stent size of 10 French gauge better than 7 French gauge? *Scand J Gastroenterol.* 1993;28:185-9.
48. Pereira-Lima JC, Jakobs R, Maier M, Benz C, Kohler B, Riemann JF. Endoscopic biliary stenting for the palliation of pancreatic cancer: results, survival predictive factors, and comparison of 10-French with 11.5-French gauge stents. *Am J Gastroenterol.* 1996;91:2179-84.
49. Hawes RH. Diagnostic and therapeutic uses of ERCP in pancreatic and biliary tract malignancies. *Gastrointest Endosc.* 2002;56:S201-5.
50. Dumonceau JM, Cremer M, Auroux J, Delhaye M, Devière J. A comparison of Ultraflex Diamond stents and Wallstents for palliation of distal malignant biliary strictures. *Am J Gastroenterol.* 2000;95:670-6.
51. Shah RJ, Howell DA, Desilets DJ, Sheth SG, Parsons WG, Okolo P 3rd, et al. Multicenter randomized trial of the spiral Z-stent compared with the Wallstent for malignant biliary obstruction. *Gastrointest Endosc.* 2003;57:830-6.
52. Howell DA, Sanders MK, Bernadino KP, Lawrence C, Kortan PP, May G, et al. Randomized controlled trial (RCT) of a new nitinol non-foreshortening self-expanding metal stent (SEMS) for malignant biliary obstruction: an international multi-center comparison in two diameters to Wallstent. *Gastrointest Endosc.* 2006;63:AB298.
53. Davids PHP, Groen AK, Rauws EA, Tytgat GN, Huibregtse K. Randomized trial of self-expanding metal stents versus polyethylene stents for distal malignant biliary obstruction. *Lancet.* 1992;340:1488-92.
54. Kubota Y, Mukai H, Nakaizumi A, Tanaka K, Okabe Y, Sakagami T, et al. Covered Wallstent for palliation of malignant common bile duct stricture: prospective multicenter evaluation. *Dig Endosc.* 2005;17:218-23.
55. Isayama H, Komatsu Y, Tsujino T, Sasahira N, Hirano K, Toda N, et al. A prospective randomised study of "covered"

versus "uncovered" diamond stents for the management of distal malignant biliary obstruction. *Gut.* 2004;53:729-34.
56. Nakai Y, Isayama H, Komatsu Y, Toda N, Sasahira N, Yamamoto N, et al. Efficacy and safety of covered Wallstent in patients with distal malignant biliary obstruction. *Gastrointest Endosc.* 2005;62:742-8.
57. Matsuda Y, Shimakura K, Akamatsu T. Factors affecting the patency of stents in malignant biliary obstructive disease: univariate and multivariate analysis. *Am J Gastroenterol.* 1991;86:843-9.
58. Menon K, Romagnuolo J, Barkun AN. Expandable metal biliary stenting in patients with recurrent premature polyethylene stent occlusion. *Am J Gastroenterol.* 2001;96: 1435-40.
59. Bueno JT, Gerdes H, Kurtz RC. Endoscopic management of occluded biliary Wallstents: a cancer center experience. *Gastrointest Endosc.* 2003;58:879-84.
60. Cremer M, Deviere J, Sugai B, Baize M. Expandable biliary metal stents for malignancies: endoscopic insertion and diathermic cleaning for tumor ingrowth. *Gastrointest Endosc.* 1990;36:451-7.
61. Ell C, Fleig WE, Hochberger J. Broken biliary metal stent after repeated electrocoagulation for tumor ingrowth. *Gastrointest Endosc.* 1992;38:197-9.
62. Costamagna G, Pandolfi M. Endoscopic stenting for biliary and pancreatic malignancies. *J Clin Gastroenterol.* 2004;38: 59-67.
63. Kubota Y, Takaoka M, Tani K, Ogura M, Kin H, Fujimura K, et al. Endoscopic transpapillary biopsy for diagnosis of patients with pancreatobiliary ductal strictures. *Am J Gastroenterol.* 1993;88:1700-4.
64. Howell DA, Parsons WG, Jones MA, Bosco JJ, Hanson BL. Complete tissue sampling of biliary strictures at ERCP using a new device. *Gastrointest Endosc.* 1996;43:498-502.
65. Ferrari Júnior AP, Lichtenstein DR, Slivka A, Chang C, Carr-Locke DL. Brush cytology during ERCP for the diagnosis of biliary and pancreatic malignancies. *Gastrointest Endosc.* 1994;40:140-5.
66. Jailwala J, Fogel EL, Sherman S, Gottlieb K, Flueckiger J, Bucksot LG, et al. Triple tissue sampling at ERCP in malignant biliary obstruction. *Gastrointest Endosc.* 2000; 51:383-90.
67. de Bellis M, Sherman S, Fogel EL, Cramer H, Chappo J, McHenry L Jr, et al. Tissue sampling at ERCP in suspected malignant biliary strictures (Part 2). *Gastrointest Endosc.* 2002;56:720-30.
68. Iqbal S, Stevens PD. Cholangiopancreatoscopy for targeted biopsies of the bile and pancreatic ducts. *Gastrointest Endosc Clin N Am.* 2009;19:567-77.
69. Artifon EL, Sakai P, Ishioka S, Marques SB, Lino AS, Cunha JE, et al. Endoscopic sphincterotomy before deployment of covered metal stent is associated with greater complication rate: a prospective randomized control trial. *J Clin Gastroenterol.* 2008;42:815-9.
70. Tarnasky PR, Cunningham JT, Hawes RH, Hoffman BJ, Uflacker R, Vujic I, et al. Transpapillary stenting of proximal biliary strictures: does biliary sphincterotomy reduce the risk of postprocedure pancreatitis? *Gastrointest Endosc.* 1997;45:46-51.
71. van Someren RN, Benson MJ, Glynn MJ, Ashraf W, Swain CP. A novel technique for dilating difficult malignant biliary strictures during therapeutic ERCP. *Gastrointest Endosc.* 1996;43:495-8.
72. Brand B, Thonke F, Obytz S, Binmoeller KF, Rathod V, Seitz U, et al. Stent retriever for dilation of pancreatic and bile duct strictures. *Endoscopy.* 1999;31:142-5.
73. Prat F, Chapat O, Ducot B, Ponchon T, Pelletier G, Fritsch J, et al. A randomized trial of endoscopic drainage methods for inoperable malignant strictures of the common bile duct. *Gastrointest Endosc.* 1998;47:1-7.
74. Schmassmann A, von Gunten E, Knuchel J, Scheurer U, Fehr HF, Halter F. Wallstents versus plastic stents in malignant biliary obstruction: effects of stent patency of the first and second stent on patient compliance and survival. *Am J Gastroenterol.* 1996;91:654-9.
75. Kaassis M, Boyer J, Dumas R, Ponchon T, Coumaros D, Delcenserie R, et al. Plastic or metal stents for malignant stricture of the common bile duct? Results of a randomized prospective study. *Gastrointest Endosc.* 2003;57:178-82.
76. Al-Haddad M, Eloubeidi MA. Interventional EUS for the diagnosis and treatment of locally advanced pancreatic cancer. *JOP.* 2010;11:1-7.
77. Lameris JS, Stoker J, Nijs HG, Zonderland HM, Terpstra OT, van Blankenstein M, et al. Malignant biliary obstruction: percutaneous use of self-expandable stents. *Radiology.* 1991;179:703-7.
78. Wiersema MJ, Sandusky D, Carr R, Wiersema LM, Erdel WC, Frederick PK. Endosonography-guided cholangiopancreatography. *Gastrointest Endosc.* 1996;43:102-6.
79. Giovannini M, Moutardier V, Pesenti C, Bories E, Lelong B, Delpero JR. Endoscopic ultrasound-guided bilioduodenal anas-tomosis: a new technique for biliary drainage. *Endoscopy.* 2001;33:898-900.
80. Puspok A, Lomoschitz F, Dejaco C, Hejna M, Sautner T, Gangl A. Endoscopic ultrasound guided therapy of benign and malignant biliary obstruction: a case series. *Am J Gastroenterol.* 2005;100:1743-7.
81. Fujita N, Noda Y, Kobayashi G, Ito K, Obana T, Horaguchi J, et al. Histological changes at an endosonography-guided biliary drainage site: a case report. *World J Gastroenterol.* 2007;13:5512-5.
82. Yamao K, Bhatia V, Mizuno N, Sawaki A, Ishikawa H, Tajika M, et al. EUS-guided choledochoduodenostomy for palliative biliary drainage in patients with malignant biliary obstruction: results of long-term follow-up. *Endoscopy.* 2008;40:340-2.
83. Adler DG, Baron TH. Endoscopic palliation of malignant gastric outlet obstruction using self-expanding metal stents: experience in 36 patients. *Am J Gastroenterol.* 2002;97:72-8.
84. Lopera JE, Brazzini A, Gonzales A, Castaneda-Zuniga WR. Gastroduodenal stent placement: current status. *Radiographics.* 2004;24:1561-73.

85. Jeurnink SM, Repici A, Luigiano C, Pagano N, Kuipers EJ, Siersema PD. Use of a colonoscope for distal duodenal stent placement in patients with malignant obstruction. *Surg Endosc.* 2009;23:562-7.
86. Gaidos JK, Draganov PV. Treatment of malignant gastric outlet obstruction with endoscopically placed self-expandable metal stents. *World J Gastroenterol.* 2009;15:4365-71.
87. Nevitt AW, Vida F, Kozarek RA, Traverso LW, Raltz SL. Expandable metallic prostheses for malignant obstructions of gastric outlet and proximal small bowel. *Gastrointest Endosc.* 1998;47:271-6.
88. Yates MR, Morgan DE, Baron TH. Palliation of malignant gastric and small intestinal strictures with self-expandable metal stents. *Endoscopy.* 1998;30:266-72.
89. Jung GS, Song HY, Kang SG, Huh JD, Park SJ, Koo JY, et al. Malignant gastroduodenal obstructions: treatment by means of a covered expandable metallic stent-initial experience. *Radiology.* 2000;216:758-63.
90. Park KB, Do YS, Kang WK, Choo SW, Han YH, Suh SW, et al. Malignant obstruction of gastric outlet and duodenum: palliation with flexible covered metallic stents. *Radiology.* 2001;219:679-83.
91. Maetani I, Ukita T, Tada T, Shigoka H, Omuta S, Endo T. Metallic stents for gastric outlet obstruction: reintervention rate is lower with uncovered versus covered stents, despite similar outcomes. *Gastrointest Endosc.* 2009;69:806-12.
92. Maetani I, Akatsuka S, Ikeda M, Tada T, Ukita T, Nakamura Y, et al. Self-expandable metallic stent placement for palliation in gastric outlet obstructions caused by gastric cancer: a comparison with surgical gastrojejunostomy. *J Gastroenterol.* 2005;40:932-7.
93. Telford JJ, Carr-Locke DL, Baron TH, Tringali A, Parsons WG, Gabbrielli A, et al. Palliation of patients with malignant gastric outlet obstruction with the enteral Wallstent: outcomes from a multicenter study. *Gastrointest Endosc.* 2004;60:916-20.
94. Laasch HU, Martin DF, Maetani I. Enteral stents in the gastric outlet and duodenum. *Endoscopy.* 2005;37:74-81.
95. Lopes CV, Pesenti C, Bories E, Caillol F, Giovannini M. Self-expandable metallic stents for palliative treatment of digestive cancer. *J Clin Gastroenterol.* 2008;42:991-6.
96. Masci E, Viale E, Mangiavillano B, Contin G, Lomazzi A, Buffoli F, et al. Enteral self-expandable metal stent for malignant luminal obstruction of the upper and lower gastrointestinal tract: a prospective multicentric study. *J Clin Gastroenterol.* 2008;42:389-94.
97. Baron TH, Harewood GC. Enteral self-expandable stents. *Gastrointest Endosc.* 2003;58:421 33.
98. Cho YK, Kim SW, Hur WH, Nam KW, Chang JH, Park JM, et al. Clinical outcomes of self-expandable metal stent and prognostic factors for stent patency in gastric outlet obstruction caused by gastric cancer. *Dig Dis Sci.* 2010;55:668-74.
99. Kim TO, Kang DH, Kim GH, Heo J, Song GA, Cho M, et al. Self-expandable metallic stents for palliation of patients with malignant gastric outlet obstruction caused by stomach cancer. *World J Gastroenterol.* 2007;13:916-20.
100. Nassif T, Prat F, Meduri B, Fritsch J, Choury AD, Dumont JL, et al. Endoscopic palliation of malignant gastric outlet obstruction using self-expandable metallic stents: results of a multicenter study. *Endoscopy.* 2003;35:483-9.
101. Feretis C, Benakis P, Dimopoulos C, Manouras A, Tsimbloulis B, Apostolidis N. Duodenal obstruction caused by pancreatic head carcinoma: palliation with self-expandable endoprostheses. *Gastrointest Endosc.* 1997;46:161-5.
102. Ly J, O'Grady G, Mittal A, Plank L, Windsor JA. A systematic review of methods to palliate malignant gastric outlet obstruction. *Surg Endosc.* 2010;24:290-7.
103. Ammann RW, Muellhaupt B. The natural history of pain in alcoholic chronic pancreatitis. *Gastroenterology.* 1999;116:1132-40.
104. Vera-Portocarrero L, Westlund KN. Role of neurogenic inflammation in pancreatitis and pancreatic pain. *Neurosignals.* 2005;14:158-65.
105. Bradley EL 3rd, Bem J. Nerve blocks and neuroablative surgery for chronic pancreatitis. *World J Surg.* 2003;27:1241-8.
106. Wiersema MJ, Wiersema LM. Endosonography guided celiac plexus neurolysis (EUS CPN) in patients with pain due to intraabdominal malignancy (IAM). *Gastrointest Endosc.* 1996;4:A565.
107. Ashida R, Chang KJ. Interventional EUS for the treatment of pancreatic cancer. *J Hepatobiliary Pancreat Surg.* 2009;16:592-7.
108. Collins D, Penman I, Mishra G, Draganov P. EUS-guided celiac block and neurolysis. *Endoscopy.* 2006;38:935-9.
109. Wiersema MJ, Wiersema LM. Endosonography-guided celiac plexus neurolysis. *Gastrointest Endosc.* 1996;44:656-62.
110. Kaufman M, Singh G, Das S, Concha-Parra R, Erber J, Micames C, et al. Efficacy of endoscopic ultrasound-guided celiac plexus block and celiac plexus neurolysis for managing abdominal pain associated with chronic pancreatitis and pancreatic cancer. *J Clin Gastroenterol.* 2010;44:127-34.
111. Gleeson FC, Levy MJ, Papachristou GI, Pelaez-Luna M, Rajan E, Clain JE, et al. Frequency of visualization of presumed celiac ganglia by endoscopic ultrasound. *Endoscopy.* 2007;39:620-4.
112. Gunaratnam NT, Sarma AV, Norton ID, Wiersema MJ. A prospective study of EUS-guided celiac plexus neurolysis for pancreatic cancer pain. *Gastrointest Endosc.* 2001;54:316-24.
113. Sahai AV, Lemelin V, Lam E, Paquin SC. Central vs. bilateral endoscopic ultrasound-guided celiac plexus block or neurolysis: a comparative study of short-term effectiveness. *Am J Gastroenterol.* 2009;104:326-9.
114. Catalano M, Ahmed U, Chauhan S. Celiac Plexus Neurolysis (CPN) in the treatment of refractory pain of pancreatic cancer (PCA): site specific response to therapy. *Gastrointest Endosc.* 2005;1:AB273.

11 Biliary Tumors: Early Detection and Endotherapy

Guido Costamagna, Ivo Boškoski, Paola Cesaro, Pietro Familiari

ABSTRACT

Biliary tumors are associated with a high morbidity and mortality rate. Majority of these tumors include gallbladder adenocarcinoma and cholangiocarcinoma (CCA). Even with recent advances in medical imaging, most of these tumors are often diagnosed at advanced stages. The radiological imaging consists of computed tomography (CT) scan, magnetic resonance imaging (MRI), magnetic resonance cholangiopancreatography (MRCP), and CT/positron emission tomography (PET) for characterizing these tumors. Endoscopy based imaging technology includes endoscopic retrograde cholangiopancreatogram (ERCP), peroral cholangioscopy (POCS), endoscopic ultrasonography (EUS), intraductal ultrasonography (IDUS), confocal laser endomicroscopy (CLE), and optical coherence tomography (OCT). Endoscopy also provides therapeutic options, including endoscopic stenting, intraluminal high dose brachytherapy, and photodynamic therapy. This chapter discusses in depth regarding diagnostic modalities and therapeutic options in patients with biliary tumors.

INTRODUCTION

Malignant biliary tumors, including neoplasms of the bile ducts and the gallbladder, are difficult clinical problems, encountered not infrequently by gastroenterologist and endoscopists. The estimated incidence of malignant biliary tumors in the United States is 9,760 new cases per year, and in the majority of cases, they are represented by gallbladder adenocarcinomas (with an annual incidence of 2.5 cases per 100,000 people);[1] the incidence of cholangiocarcinoma (CCA) is around 1 case per 100,000 people/year.[2] Early detection of biliary tumors is crucial for a curative treatment. Surgical resection is the only radical and effective therapy for these cancers. The median survival of patients with inoperable CCA is of 6.7–11.6 months, compared to 37.4–42.9 months for resected patients.[3,4] However, despite the progresses in the field of noninvasive imaging, the vast majority of biliary tumors are diagnosed in advanced stages, when any radical surgical resection is inevitably precluded. These patients are often destined only to palliation of biliary obstruction. Endoscopy plays a central role in the management of patients with malignant biliary stricture, both for diagnosis and staging of lesions and for palliation of bile duct obstruction. The most recent endoscopic techniques for early detection, staging, and endoscopic treatment of biliary tumors are discussed in this chapter.

CLINICAL FEATURES

Besides mild and vague symptoms in early stage disease, the usual manifestation of biliary tumors is sudden onset of jaundice due to biliary obstruction, sometimes with nausea, asthenia, and unexplained weight loss. Patients with biliary tumors are more frequently in the seventh or eighth decade of life. Colicky pain is usually absent in case of malignant lesions, in contrast with gallstone diseases of the gallbladder and bile ducts, as the biliary obstruction is progressive and slow. Unfortunately, majority of patients presenting with jaundice already have an advanced stage disease. Gallbladder carcinoma usually invades the biliary tree at a later stage, when palliation is the only possible approach. In case of CCA, biliary obstruction might occur earlier, and as a consequence, CCAs are sometimes suitable for surgical resection. Laboratory findings in early stage biliary tumors can be unremarkable or with unexplained high hepatobiliary enzyme levels, along with other abnormalities on blood tests during standard health checks. As for tumor markers, although there is no specific one, carbohydrate antigen CA 19-9 and carcinoembryonic antigen (CEA) may support the diagnosis of biliary tumors.[5] However, neither of them is sensitive nor specific enough to be used for screening purposes, as they can be elevated in the presence of other malignancies (e.g., pancreas and stomach) or benign conditions, such as cholangitis or hepatolithiasis.[6]

RADIOLOGICAL IMAGING

The current cross-sectional noninvasive modalities, such as computed tomography (CT scan) and magnetic resonance (MR) with cholangiopancreatography (MRCP) are fundamental tools for the diagnosis and staging of biliary tumors. Common findings in the CT scan are intrahepatic bile duct dilation usually associated with biliary masses. In the last decade, MRCP has emerged as an alternative diagnostic technology to endoscopic retrograde cholangiopancreatogram (ERCP). MRCP can yield images almost comparable to those from ERCP. MRCP can differentiate the origin of a filling defect or a stenosis of the biliary tree, study the hepatic parenchyma, the biliary tree (cholangiographic mapping), vessels, and lymph nodes. Positron emission tomography (PET) with 18F-fluoro-2-deoxy-D-glucose (FDG) combined with multidetector row helical CT scanner (FDG-PET/CT) has been recently introduced, and is a useful tool for evaluation of biliary cancers.[7-9] The flaw in all these noninvasive diagnostic tools is the inability of tissue sampling. However, when endoscopic or radiological palliation of jaundice is the only therapeutic chance for the patients, histology is usually not strictly necessary. In contrast, it becomes fundamental when radiotherapy or chemotherapy has been planned, or in case of surgery. Nevertheless, there are a variety of clinical situations in which the benign or malignant nature of the biliary stricture cannot reasonably be discriminated. Besides benign postoperative lesions of the biliary tree and gallstone disease, attention should be paid to sclerosing cholangitis and immunoglobulin G4 (IgG4)-related cholangitis, with or without pancreatic involvement.[10] The IgG4-associated cholangitis is a highly steroid-responsive process. Other steroid-responsive dominant bile duct lesions, sometimes mimicking infiltrating hilar CCA without pancreatic abnormalities, have also been reported. Therefore, in the differential diagnosis of biliary tumors, tissue sampling is of milestone value.

Primary sclerosing cholangitis is a well-known chronic inflammatory disease associated with an increased risk of biliary cancer. A neoplasm should be always searched and reasonably excluded in patients with primary sclerosing cholangitis and dominant biliary strictures.

ENDOSCOPIC IMAGING AND EARLY DETECTION

Despite the recent refinement of noninvasive imaging modalities, there are some clinical scenarios in which an endoscopic approach is requested for the diagnosis. Endoscopy can offer diagnostic imaging, tissue sampling, and at the same time can be therapeutic. Direct cholangioscopy can either be used for direct visualization of the biliary mucosa and for tissue sampling as well. The list of emerging, purely diagnostic endoscopic tools include intraductal ultrasound (IDUS), digital imaging analysis, fluorescence *in situ* hybridization (FISH), confocal laser endomicroscopy (CLE), and optical coherence tomography (OCT). Since all these procedures are operator dependent, there is a need for skilled endoscopists and significant expertise for these techniques in order to avoid postprocedure complications and misdiagnosis. Complications related to diagnostic or therapeutic endoscopic procedures of the biliary tree are gut and biliary perforations, bleeding, pancreatitis, cholangitis, and complications related to sedation and/or anesthesia.

Endoscopic Retrograde Cholangiopancreatography

Until the advent of MRCP, direct cholangiography was the gold standard diagnostic procedure for biliary tumors. ERCP is an invasive procedure but has the advantage of being diagnostic (direct cholangiography and tissue sampling) and therapeutic at the same time. Direct cholangiography visualizes the presence, the level, and in some cases, the extension of biliary obstruction and can suggest the cause of obstruction. However, ERCP is associated with specific complications and should no longer be used for purely diagnostic purposes. On cholangiography, characteristics suggestive of biliary malignancy include filing defects, irregular margins, and an abrupt transition from normal duct to stricture, also known as shouldering (Figure 11-1).[11] The presence of a hilar stricture should in any case raise the suspicion of malignancy. The site, the appearance, and the location of a stricture can also suggest malignancy. Tissue sampling

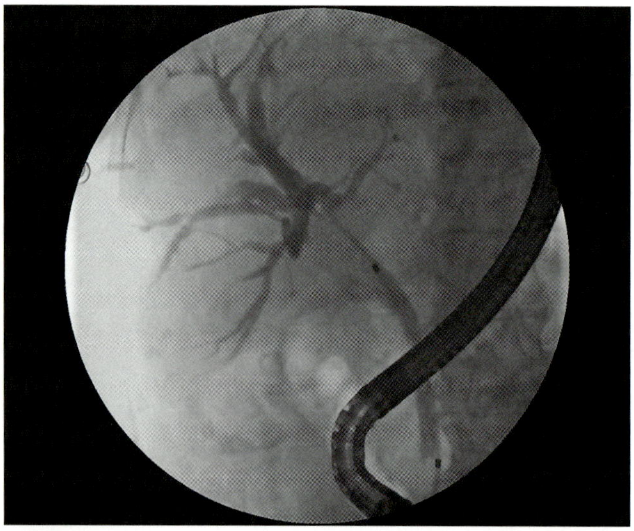

FIGURE 11-1 Cholangiogram in hilar cholangiocarcinoma.

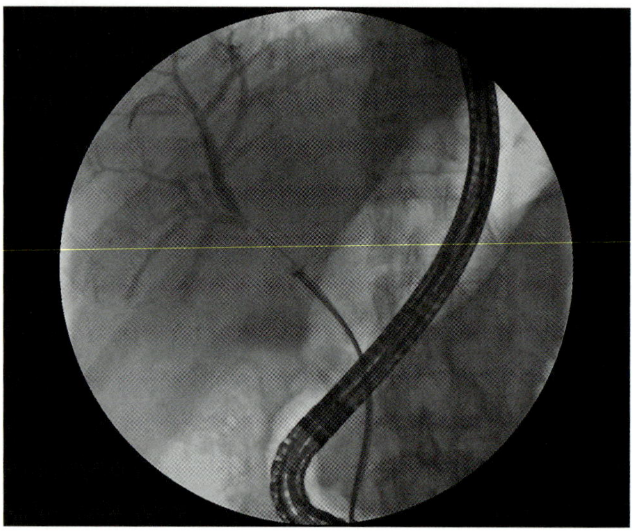

FIGURE 11-2 Endobiliary biopsies.

can be useful in doubtful cases and before radiotherapy or chemotherapy, or surgery. ERCP techniques for tissue sampling are brushing, endobiliary biopsies (Figure 11-2), fine needle aspiration, and bile juice aspiration for cytology. It is expected that the ideal sampling technique is highly sensitive and 100% specific, which means few false-negative results without any false-positive tissue samples. Specificity for ERCP tissue sampling (both biliary mucosal biopsy and brushing) is 100% (malignant specimens are never obtained from a benign biliary stricture). The sensitivity of biliary brushing alone for the diagnosis of CCA ranges between 50 and 60%.[12-14] Combination of biliary brushing with endoscopic biopsies can increase sensitivity to 70%.[15,16] Sensitivity increases when pathologists consider cytologic atypia equal to cancer, but in this way, there is a decrease in specificity. In turn, decreased specificity can lead to erroneous interpretation, and the patient can undergo unnecessary surgery or chemotherapy. When a biliary malignancy is suspected and a tissue diagnosis is required, it is reasonable to perform an ERCP first.[17] Finally, combination of ERCP and endoscopic ultrasonography (EUS) guided tissue acquisition may be required in cases where the differential diagnosis is between biliary stricture due to biliary mass vs. pancreatic tumor.[17]

Peroral Cholangioscopy and Spyglass

The desire of direct visualization of the biliary tree gave birth to the idea for cholangioscopy.[18,19] This examination can be done percutaneously or perorally. In the past years, there have been significant technologic improvements in the design, optical resolution, and maneuverability of peroral cholangioscopes, so that this examination has assumed a role in the diagnosis of biliary lesions. Primary indications for peroral cholangioscopy (POCS) include evaluation of filling defects by direct visualization of the biliary mucosa, tissue sampling of biliary strictures under direct vision, and treatment of difficult choledocholithiasis. Filling defects on ERCP can be due to various benign and malignant causes that may have characteristic cholangiographic features but are not specific enough for management decisions.[11] Besides tissue sampling, recently a narrow band imaging system has been developed for high-contrast observation of mucosal structures and vascular patterns of biliary tumors.[20,21] In a single center Japanese study, it was found that the addition of POCS to ERCP raises the accuracy, sensitivity, and specificity to 93.4, 100, and 86.8%, respectively.[22] At present, the availability of POCS is limited to high costs of instrumentation and the necessity of two well-trained endoscopists. Spyglass Spyscope® is a single operator miniature endoscope that was introduced in 2007[4] (Figure 11-3). This instrument allows either diagnostic or therapeutic procedures, evaluation of strictures with indeterminate nature, and filling defects, but also tissue sampling and bile stone therapy (electrohydraulic or laser lithotripsy). The Spyglass has increased maneuverability that allows four-way tip direction and allows 4-quadrant directed biopsies. The initially reported sensitivity and specificity of Spyglass biopsy to diagnose malignancy were 71 and 100%, respectively.[4]

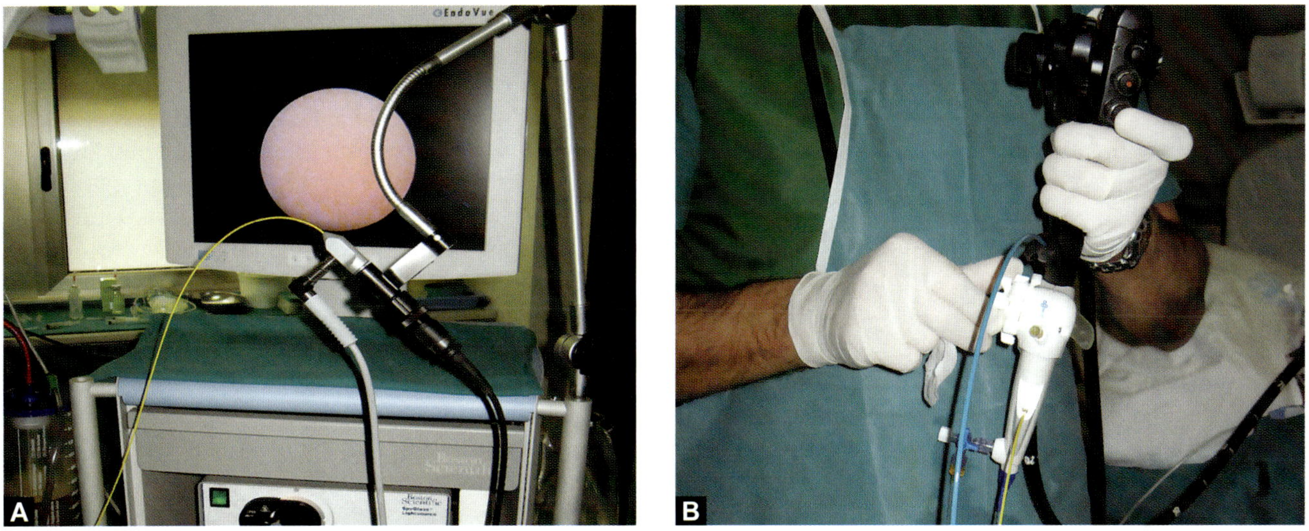

FIGURE 11-3 The Spyglass Spyscope®. **A,** Single operator equipment. **B,** The operator is maneuvering the tip of the Spyglass.

Endoscopic Ultrasonography

EUS is a well-established procedure for diagnosis and staging of malignancies of the pancreaticobiliary (PB) system. EUS offers a fine analysis of tumors and fine needle aspiration (FNA) of masses and lymph nodes. EUS is also suitable for tumor staging. It enables evaluation of liver involvement, the relation with the portal vein and hepatic arteries and vascular invasion, the presence of lymph nodes, and defines extension. Once the biliary mass or stricture has been identified, a tissue sampling from the lesion can be obtained for cytology using FNA. The reported accuracy of EUS-FNA for diagnosis of CCA varies from 79 to 91%, with a sensitivity ranging from 77 to 89% and specificity of 100%.[23-25] Sensitivity of 47 and 25% of EUS-FNA has been found in two other studies without any clear reason for the disparities in the results, even if the majority of the lesions were of the distal biliary tree.[17,26] Hilar CCA is usually more difficult to be visualized and sampled at EUS than distal biliary tract tumors. For malignant hilar biliary strictures, EUS-FNA has been always used after a negative ERCP sampling.[17,23-27] Recently, a newly developed forward-viewing linear EUS has been used for direct imaging of the hilar region and performing FNA as a first diagnostic choice tool.[28,29] These instruments allow to achieve a scanning direction rectangular to the direction of insertion of the echoendoscope. This produces an ultrasound image with an angle quite different from the conventional linear EUS, which may be advantageous in the evaluation of the hilum.[29] Generally, the sensitivity of EUS-FNA is lower for proximal compared to distal biliary strictures. However, further studies investigating EUS-FNA of biliary masses are needed to clarify these differences. The use of EUS and EUS-FNA is, however, optimal for lesions in the mid- or distal bile duct. Furthermore, in case, it is impossible to visualize hilar lesions by EUS, IDUS can be helpful. It is expected that in the near future, EUS will become a tool for direct administration of drugs and placement of devices, and biological agents would be able to diagnose and treat. The future applications of EUS include delivery of cytotoxic agents, such as chemotherapy, gene therapy, and radioactive seeds.

Intraductal Ultrasonography

IDUS probes are high frequency ultrasound probes used for staging of biliary strictures. The IDUS probe is placed into the common bile duct over a 0.035-inch guide wire, and under ERCP guidance. The currently used IDUS probes have a very small diameter, and consequently a biliary sphincterotomy is not strictly necessary for the insertion. Unfortunately, tissue sampling is impossible with IDUS. On normal IDUS image, the bile duct wall has 2 or 3 sonographic layers, while malignant biliary strictures often appear as a hypoechoic mass of the bile duct wall with irregular margins, papillary surface, and disrupted architecture of the duct.[30,31] The accuracy of IDUS for determining the nature of bile duct strictures has been estimated as of 89% compared to 76% of the EUS in the same patients.[30] In patients with biliary strictures and no mass detected on a CT, it has been found that IDUS increases the diagnostic accuracy of ERCP from 58 to 90%.[32] The diagnostic sensitivity and specificity of IDUS in determination of the nature of biliary strictures have been found to be 90 and 93%, respectively.[33] IDUS is suggestive for malignancy in case of a polypoid mass greater than 8 mm, even in case the wall layers are preserved; in any case, directed biopsy specimens of the mass should be obtained.

Cytological Evaluation: Digital Image Analysis and Fluorescence *In Situ* Hybridization

The application of advanced cytologic techniques for the detection of chromosomal instability may be promising in the early detection of biliary tumors. Techniques, such as digital image analysis (DIA) and FISH may improve the accuracy of nonsurgical diagnosis of biliary strictures. DIA is a specialized technique of cytologic analysis that quantifies abnormalities of nuclear DNA (aneuploidy or tetraploidy) by using spectrophotometric principles.[34] The results are categorized as diploid (DNA index between 0.95 and 1.10), aneuploid (DNA index between 1.11 and 1.89), or tetraploid (DNA index between 1.90 and 2.10).[35] Aneuploid and tetraploid results are considered positive for malignancy. FISH uses fluorescently-labeled DNA probes to chromosomal centromeres or unique loci to detect cells which have numeric or structural abnormalities indicative of malignancy.[36] The UroVysion probe set targets the centromere regions of chromosome 3 (CEP 3), chromosome 7 (CEP 7), chromosome 17 (CEP 17), and band 9p21 (P16/CDKN2A gene). A patient's specimen is considered positive for malignancy, if five or more cells show gain of two or more of all four probes (polysomy), or if ≥10 cells show three copies of chromosome 7 or 3 and two or fewer copies of the other probes. Using these techniques, small numbers of tumor cells can be analyzed in contrast to flow cytometry, where a larger number of cells are required for analysis.[37] Although aneuploid/aneusomic cells are generally considered markers of malignancy, premalignant lesions, such as colonic adenomas, have also been shown to demonstrate these findings.[38-40] In contrast, inflammatory processes that involve the bile ducts can increase cellular proliferation but usually do not produce aneuploid/aneusomic cell populations.[41] Furthermore, not all cancers display aneuploid/aneusomic cell populations, and it is estimated that only 80% of biliary malignant strictures demonstrate these genetic aberrations, thereby setting an expected upper limit for diagnostic sensitivity of 80% for DIA and FISH.[42]

Confocal Laser Endomicroscopy

CLE offers realtime *in vivo* microscopic tissue examination that may increase the sensitivity for detection of biliary malignancies and helps in performing targeted biopsies. CLE is a new endoscopic modality developed to obtain very high-resolution images of the mucosal layer of the GI tract. It is based on tissue illumination with a low power laser, with subsequent detection of the fluorescence light reflected from the tissue through a pinhole. The term "confocal" refers to the alignment of both illumination and collection systems in the same focal plane.[43,44] The laser light is focused at a selected depth in the tissue of interest and the reflected light is then refocused onto the detection system by the same lens. Only returning light refocused through the pinhole is detected. The light reflected and scattered at other geometric angles from the illuminated object or refocused out of plane with the pinhole is excluded from detection. This dramatically increases the spatial resolution of confocal endomicroscopy, thus, providing an "optical biopsy," in other terms, a histological examination of the superficial layer of the GI tract.[45,46] Confocal imaging can be based on tissue reflectance or tissue fluorescence. The confocal devices based on tissue reflectance do not require any contrast agents, but available prototypes have numerous technical problems and relatively low resolution, which significantly compromise *in vivo* imaging and clinical utility. In contrast, confocal endomicroscopy based on tissue fluorescence uses local and/or intravenous contrast agents and generates high-quality images comparable to traditional histological examination.[46,47] The latest model of Cellvizio confocal miniprobes created for GI tract applications include CholangioFlex probes, designed for use during ERCP (Figure 11-4). These probes require an endoscope accessory channel of at least 1.2 mm and generate dynamic (12 frames per second) images. The depth of imaging for CholangioFlex probes is 40–70 μm. The maximal field of view for CholangioFlex probes is 325 μm with lateral resolution of 3.5 mm. The fluorescent contrasts for confocal endomicroscopy in the biliary tract is fluorescein that is administered intravenously. Intravenously delivered fluorescein distributes throughout the extracellular matrix of the surface epithelium and lamina propria but does not stain the cell nuclei.[43] Fluorescein is usually administered within 5 minutes of imaging; however, the dose and timing of contrast administration have not yet been standardized. After the contrast administration, the tip of the confocal miniprobe is positioned in

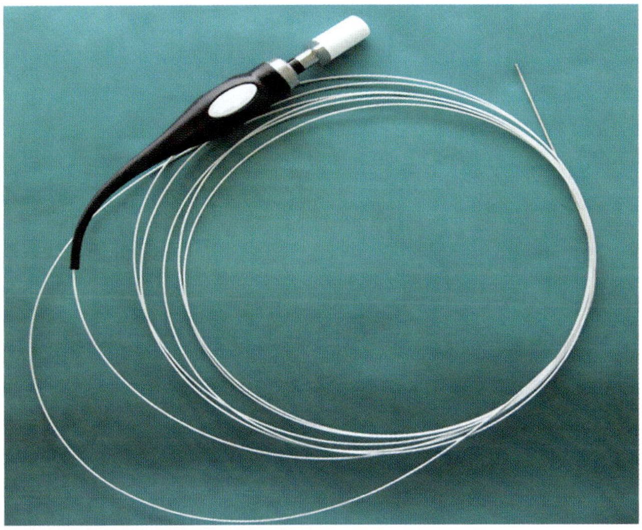

FIGURE 11-4 Confocal miniprobes.

gentle contact with the area of interest to obtain high-resolution confocal images. Accumulated images can be saved for postprocedural analysis. There is no uniform terminology of CLE findings. To standardize the image interpretation criteria of CLE findings in the PB system and develop a descriptive classification of CLE findings in the PB system, investigators from 6 centers (2 European and 4 USA) met at a consensus conference in Miami, Florida.[48] A longitudinal registry of 130 patients undergoing ERCP with CLE was launched to assess indeterminate PB strictures using the CholangioFlex probe after fluorescein injection. Clinical ERCP (when used), tissue sampling and CLE (video recordings) data were collected prospectively. Follow-up was 30 days, until confirmation of malignancy, or 1 year. The investigators subsequently met to validate the Miami Classification (MC) through blinded review of CLE videos of proven malignant and benign cases. Between December 2008 and July 2009, 77 subjects were enrolled in the ongoing longitudinal registry. Twenty-four out of these 77 had confirmed PB malignancy through July 2009 and qualified for inclusion in this preliminary analysis, 3 additional subjects with benign pathology after 1-year follow-up served as negative controls. Sixty-one CLE videos from the 27 subjects were randomized, blindly assessed, and scored using the MC as follows: thick (≥20 μm) or thin (≤20 μm) dark or white bands, ± branching, ± flow, reversal of flow; epithelial structures, dark glands, interstitial fluorescein leakage (Figure 11-5). Single image interpretation criteria had relatively low sensitivity (from 42 to 67%), but with 100% positive predictive value (PPV) for malignancy. The combination of two or more criteria (especially epithelial structures, thick white bands, and dark clumps) significantly increased the sensitivity (from 88 to 96%) with 100% specificity, 100% PPV, and 50–75% negative predictive value (NPV). In conclusion, CLE can offer a significant potential in improving the diagnostic accuracy of PB malignant strictures.

Optical Coherence Tomography

OCT is an optical imaging technique that produces high-resolution cross-sectional images of tissue *in vivo*.[49,50] OCT is analogous to ultrasound imaging but uses infrared light rather than acoustic energy. OCT could be useful in clinical situations in which conventional biopsy specimens are technically difficult to obtain. Cross-sectional images of tissue obtained with current OCT technology have an axial resolution (≈10 μm) that is 10-fold better than that of available high-frequency ultrasound imaging devices. OCT images can be obtained with a catheter device that is inserted through the accessory channel of a conventional endoscope.[51-53] Although a 20 MHz intraductal US probe has a maximum penetration depth of approximately 10 mm, OCT has a penetration depth of approximately 1 mm. By comparison, a conventional biopsy typically provides histological information to a depth of less than 1 mm. The OCT system for imaging uses low-coherence illumination from a superluminescent diode that operates at 1.27 mm center wavelength with an optical bandwidth of 37 nm full-width half-maximum. OCT in the biliary tract increases the sensitivity of ERCP combined with intraductal cytology to detect malignancy from 67 to 84%.[54] However, there are only few *in vivo* pilot studies with a limited number of patients evaluating the feasibility of intraductal biliary OCT during ERCP.

ENDOTHERAPY OF BILIARY TUMORS

The only curative therapy for early stage biliary tumors is radical surgical resection. Unfortunately, only a small number of patients with biliary tumors are candidates for surgery at the time of diagnosis. In patients with unresectable disease, the prognosis is very poor; the progression of the disease and the debilitation of the patient are very rapid, mostly due to biliary obstruction. Biliary decompression is important in these patients, as it prolongs survival and leaves space for chemotherapy and radiotherapy. Palliative biliary decompression can be done surgically, radiologically, or endoscopically. The

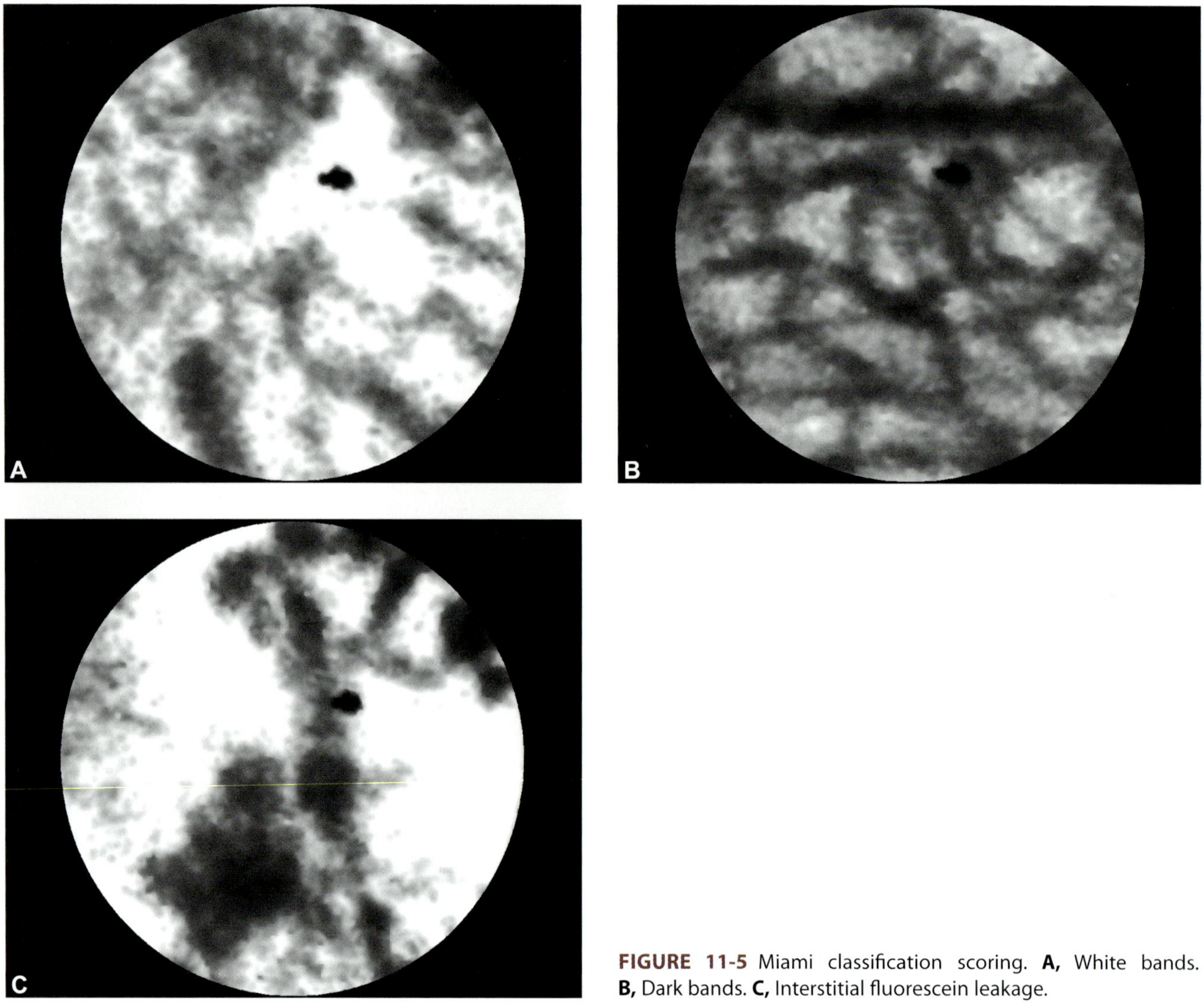

FIGURE 11-5 Miami classification scoring. **A,** White bands. **B,** Dark bands. **C,** Interstitial fluorescein leakage.

primary aim of endoscopic palliation in biliary cancers is to relieve obstructive jaundice, pruritus, cholangitis, and pain. An ideal endoscopic palliation includes improved quality of life via minimal invasiveness, low procedure-related complications, short hospitalization, and low costs. Endotherapy of biliary tumors consists of placement of biliary endoprothesis, nasobiliary probes for successive brachytherapy, and for intraluminal photodynamic therapy (PDT).

Endoscopic Biliary Stenting

Endoscopic biliary stenting consists of placement of one or more endoprostheses bypassing the biliary stricture. Before any endoscopic intervention, an MRCP is useful to assess the biliary anatomy, to determine the site of stricture, and to plan the treatment, especially in biliary strictures (Figure 11-6).[55] A single stent can guarantee complete biliary drainage in the majority of patients with a stricture of the common bile duct (Figure 11-7). A single stent might also guarantee an adequate palliation in case of strictures, which interrupts the main biliary confluence; it is enough to drain 25–30% of the hepatic parenchyma to relieve jaundice.[56,57] Multiple stents might be necessary for a complete biliary drainage, especially in patients with complex hilar strictures and acute cholangitis to drain as much hepatic parenchyma as possible and to prevent abscess formation. Important changes have occurred in the last three decades in design, development, and composition of stents. Stents evolved from plastic

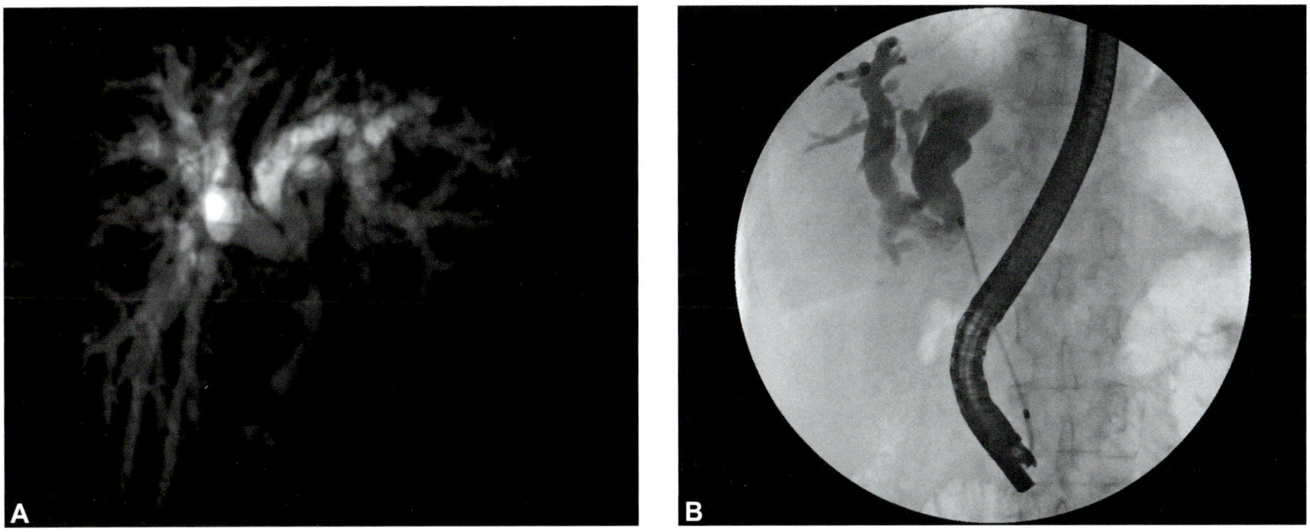

FIGURE 11-6 Malignant biliary stricture. **A,** MRCP image. **B,** Cholangiographic image.

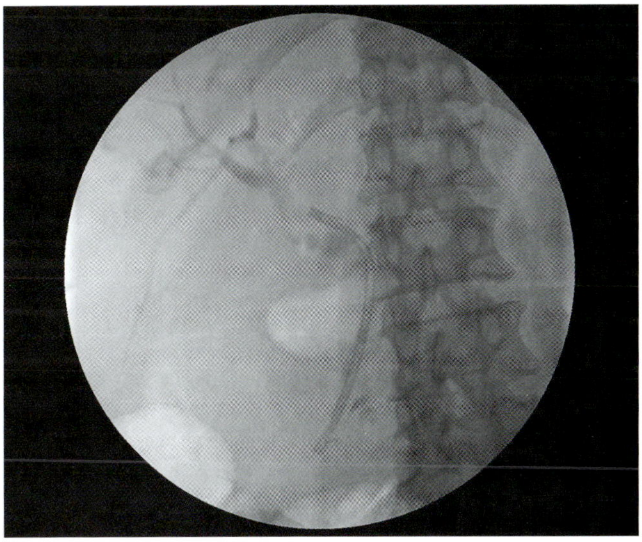

FIGURE 11-7 Plastic endoprothesis in a malignant stricture of the main biliary duct.

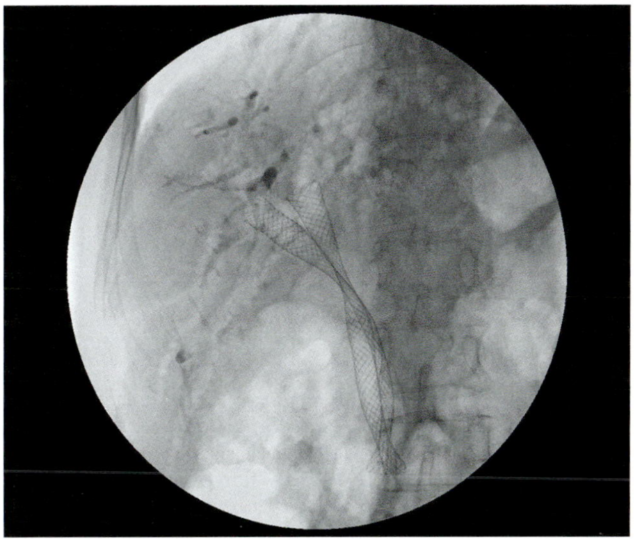

FIGURE 11-8 Two nitinol self-expandable metal stents in malignant hilar stricture.

(polyethylene), through stainless steel, and nitinol self-expandable metal stents (SEMS) (Figure 11-8). There is also a variety of stents in developmental phase, as those covered with various antitumor agents or nano silver particles that can avoid bacterial adherence and biliary occlusion by sludge.[58] Till date, in the clinical practice, only plastic and metal stents are used. Metal stents are more expensive than plastic ones but have larger diameter (8 and 10 mm vs. 3.8 mm of plastic stents) that provides a better bile flow.[59] The mean patency rate of plastic stents is 2–3 months while, of SEMS is 9 months. The larger diameter of metallic stents should guarantee better biliary drainage, specially, if sludge or lithiasis is present over the stricture, and should prevent hemobilia. Metal stents can be either covered or uncovered. Covered SEMS are designed to prevent tumor ingrowth through the meshes of the stent. Materials used for covered SEMS are silicone, polyurethane, and expanded polytetrafluoroethylene. In patients with malignant biliary obstruction, the decision to place a plastic or metal stent depends on a variety of criteria, including the patient's general health conditions, estimated survival, the quality of life, the type and site of the stricture, and the local expertise. SEMS placement is considered cost-effective in patients with an estimated survival of more than 6 months. Furthermore, SEMS placement is recommended in patients who might benefit from chemo- or radiotherapy, because the longer patency of SEMS can guarantee an adequate prosecution of the treatment. In a retrospective analysis on 101 patients, who underwent multiple SEMS placement for malignant hilar strictures, the investigators found a satisfactory (1 year) mean survival, independent of the type of malignancy, presence of metastases, age, and gender.[60] Preoperative biliary drainage is no longer recommended in good surgical candidates. However, it can be useful when neoadjuvant treatments have been planned, in case of cholangitis, or in case surgery has to be delayed.

Drug-eluting Stents

Drug-eluting stents are devices with incorporated anti-tumor agents designed to improve the stent patency, reducing risk of tumor ingrowth and prolonging patient's survival. Stents covered with a paclitaxel-incorporated membrane are currently under investigation.[61] Antitumor agents should be loaded, retained, and released in a controlled manner in a way to achieve correct delivery that usually occurs by simple diffusion into the mucosal and submucosal layers. It is expected that the stents of the future are incorporated with drugs and antibiotics to prevent acid, pepsin and pancreatic enzymes related damage, prevention of biofilms formation, and to avoid stent clogging. It seems that drug-eluting stents are a promising treatment method for bile duct cancers that can exploit the tumor's nature to grow along the lumen and to spread submucosally.

Intraluminal High-dose Brachytherapy

The first report of intraluminal brachytherapy with iridium-192 for extrahepatic bile duct carcinoma was published in 1979.[62] Iridium-192 is a gamma emitter used for radiation therapy. Contrary to low-dose brachytherapy, high-dose rate intraluminal brachytherapy (HDR-ILBT) offers the possibility to administrate high-dose radiation (30–50 Gy) in a short time, within the range of 1–1.5 cm, reducing all the effects of external beam radiotherapy. Currently, low-dose brachytherapy for biliary tumors is considered an obsolete treatment. HDR-ILBT can be administered percutaneously or endoscopically. The endoscopic approach consists of placement of nasobiliary tubes during ERCP. Iridium-192 wires of homogeneous linear activity are subsequently placed through these tubes (Figure 11-9). HDR-ILBT has been evaluated alone

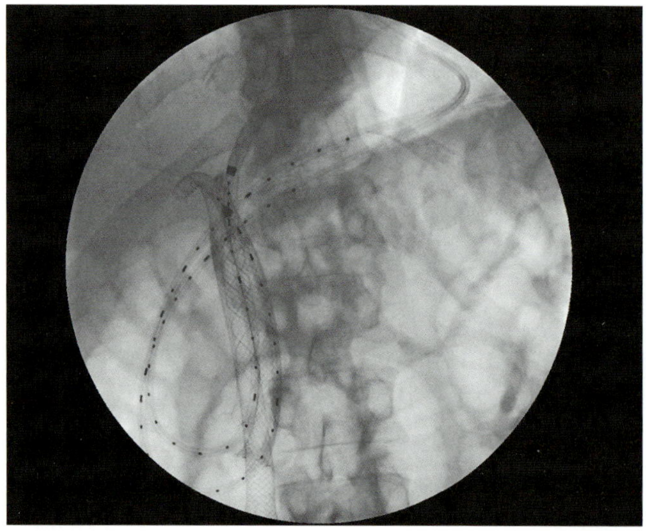

FIGURE 11-9 Iridium-192 wires of homogeneous linear activity placed through nasobiliary tubes and self-expandable metal stents in patient with malignant hilar stricture.

or in association with external beam irradiation and/or chemotherapy in a relatively small number of studies showing prolonged survival and improvement in the quality of life.[63-66] The most frequent complication of intraluminal brachytherapy is cholangitis occurring in 0–44% of patients treated in combination with metallic stenting.[66] Complications observed in patients treated with combined external and internal radiation therapy are gastric and duodenal obstruction, ulcerations, and bleeding.[65,67,68] In patients who previously received SEMS for biliary malignancies, a prolonged stent patency has been found after brachytherapy.[64,69] The local control of tumor prolongs the palliation of jaundice by preventing ingrowth and overgrowth, delaying the fatal complications from progressive obstructive jaundice. Furthermore, combination of brachytherapy and chemotherapy gives promising results in terms of survival in patients with unresectable CCA.[70,71] In order to assess all the benefits of HDR-ILBT, there is a need of further prospective randomized trials.

Photodynamic Therapy

PDT is another palliative treatment that consists of intravenous administration of a photosensitizing drug (sodium porfimer 2 mg/kg body weight, known as photofrin) that preferentially accumulates in malignant cells. Subsequently, a laser light is administered on the neoplastic tissue. This leads to the formation of free oxygen radicals in the tumor tissue leading to ischemic necrosis of the tumor cells that reaches a depth ranging from 4 to 6 mm.[72] Improvements in the quality of life, survival, and biliary drainage in patients with inoperable CCA have been reported in several studies after PDT.[72-74] The role of PDT as neoadjuvant therapy has been evaluated in another study, giving 1-year recurrence-free survival rate of 83% and down staging tumors from inoperable to operable.[75] Generally, side effects of the procedure are the same of biliary endoscopy, with the addition of induced phototoxicity from direct sunlight exposure during the first few weeks after therapy.[72,76] PDT is usually a well-tolerated procedure with a reported 30-day mortality of about 2%.[77] Complications as biloma, hemobilia, and mild-to-moderate epigastric discomfort have also been reported. Contraindications to PDT include porphyria, recent use of photosensitizing or dermatoxic drugs, previously placed coated metal stents, and the presence of severe hepatic or renal failure.

CONCLUSION

The estimated incidence of malignant biliary tumors in the United States is 9,760 new cases per year. Usual signs and symptoms of biliary tumors at gradual onset are of jaundice, sometimes nausea, asthenia, and unexplained weight loss. The key point of clinical approach in biliary tumors is distinguishing benign from malignant lesion; therefore, tissue sampling is of milestone value. In most cases, these tumors are diagnosed at a later stage, when palliation is the only possible approach. All patients with biliary tumors should, however, be well evaluated for the possibility of surgical resection.

REFERENCES

1. Jemal A, Siegel R, Ward E, Hao Y, Xu J, Thun MJ. Cancer statistics, 2009. *CA Cancer J Clin.* 2009;59:225-49.
2. Gallery MR MW. Bile duct cancer. In: Cameron JL, editor. Current surgical therapy. 6th ed. Baltimore: Mosby; 1998;455.
3. Roayaie S, Guarrera JV, Ye MQ, Thung SN, Emre S, Fishbein TM, et al. Aggressive surgical treatment of intrahepatic cholangiocarcinoma: predictors of outcomes. *J Am Coll Surg.* 1998;187:365-72.
4. Chen YK, Pleskow DK. SpyGlass single operator peroral cholangiopancreatoscopy system for the diagnosis and therapy of bile-duct disorders: a clinical feasibility study (with video). *Gastrointest Endosc.* 2007;65:832-41.
5. Chen CY, Shiesh SC, Tsao HC, Lin XZ. The assessment of biliary CA 125, CA 19-9 and CEA in diagnosing cholangiocarcinoma—the influence of sampling time and hepatolithiasis. *Hepatogastroenterology.* 2002;49:616-20.
6. Maestranzi S, Przemioslo R, Mitchell H, Sherwood RA. The effect of benign and malignant liver disease on the tumour markers CA19-9 and CEA. *Ann Clin Biochem.* 1998;35:99-103.
7. Petrowsky H, Wildbrett P, Husarik DB, Hany TF, Tam S, Jochum W, et al. Impact of integrated positron emission tomography and computed tomography on staging and management of gallbladder cancer and cholangiocarcinoma. *J Hepatol.* 2006;45:43-50.
8. Anderson CD, Rice MH, Pinson CW, Chapman WC, Chari RS, Delbeke D. Fluorodeoxyglucose PET imaging in the evaluation of gallbladder carcinoma and cholangiocarcinoma. *J Gastrointest Surg.* 2004;8:90-7.
9. Chikamoto A, Tsuji T, Takamori H, Kanemitsu K, Uozumi H, Yamashita Y, et al. The diagnostic efficacy of FDG-PET in the local recurrence of hilar bile duct cancer. *J Hepatobiliary Pancreat Surg.* 2006;13:403-8.
10. Bjornsson E, Chari ST, Smyrk TC, Lindor K. Immunoglobulin G4 associated cholangitis: description of an emerging clinical entity based on review of the literature. *Hepatology.* 2007;45:1547-54.
11. Park MS, Kim TK, Kim KW, Park SW, Lee JK, Kim JS, et al. Differentiation of extrahepatic bile duct cholangiocarcinoma from benign stricture: findings at MRCP versus ERCP. *Radiology.* 2004;233:234-40.
12. de Bellis M, Sherman S, Fogel EL, Cramer H, Chappo J, McHenry L Jr, et al. Tissue sampling at ERCP in suspected malignant biliary strictures (Part 2). *Gastrointest Endosc.* 2002;56:720-30.
13. Mansfield JC, Griffin SM, Wadehra V, Matthewson K. A prospective evaluation of cytology from biliary strictures. *Gut.* 1997;40:671-7.
14. Venu RP, Geenen JE, Kini M, Hogan WJ, Payne M, Johnson GK, et al. Endoscopic retrograde brush cytology. A new technique. *Gastroenterology.* 1990;99:1475-9.
15. Howell DA, Beveridge RP, Bosco J, Jones M. Endoscopic needle aspiration biopsy at ERCP in the diagnosis of biliary strictures. *Gastrointest Endosc.* 1992;38:531-5.
16. Jailwala J, Fogel EL, Sherman S, Gottlieb K, Flueckiger J, Bucksot LG. Triple-tissue sampling at ERCP in malignant biliary obstruction. *Gastrointest Endosc.* 2000;51:383-90.
17. Rösch T, Hofrichter K, Frimberger E, Meining A, Born P, Weigert N, et al. ERCP or EUS for tissue diagnosis of biliary strictures? A prospective comparative study. *Gastrointest Endosc.* 2004;60:390-6.
18. Kozarek RA. Direct cholangioscopy and pancreatoscopy at time of endoscopic retrograde cholangiopancreatography. *Am J Gastroenterol.* 1988;83:55-7.
19. Rösch W, Koch H. Peroral cholangioscopy in choledochoduodenostomy—patients using the pediatric fiberscope. *Endoscopy.* 1978;10:195-8.
20. Igarashi Y, Okano N, Satou D, Miura T, Miki M. Peroral cholangioscopy using a new thinner videoscope (CHF-B260). *Digestive Endoscopy.* 2005;17:S63-6.
21. Gupta R, Lakhtakia S, Santosh D, Anuradha S, Tandan M, Ramchandani M, et al. Narrow band imaging cholangio-

scopy in hilar cholangiocarcinoma. *Indian J Gastroenterol.* 2010;29:78-80.

22. Fukuda Y, Tsuyuguchi T, Sakai Y, Tsuchiya S, Saisyo H. Diagnostic utility of peroral cholangioscopy for various bile-duct lesions. *Gastrointest Endosc.* 2005;62:374-82.
23. Fritscher-Ravens A, Broering DC, Knoefel WT, Rogiers X, Swain P, Thonke F, et al. EUS-guided fine-needle aspiration of suspected hilar cholangiocarcinoma in potentially operable patients with negative brush cytology. *Am J Gastroenterol.* 2004;99:45-51.
24. Eloubeidi MA, Chen VK, Jhala NC, Eltoum IE, Jhala D, Chhieng DC, et al. Endoscopic ultrasound-guided fine needle aspiration biopsy of suspected cholangiocarcinoma. *Clin Gastroenterol Hepatol.* 2004;2:209-13.
25. DeWitt J, Misra VL, Leblanc JK, McHenry L, Sherman S. EUS-guided FNA of proximal biliary strictures after negative ERCP brush cytology results. *Gastrointest Endosc.* 2006;64:325-33.
26. Lee JH, Salem R, Aslanian H, Chacho M, Topazian M. Endoscopic ultrasound and fine-needle aspiration of unexplained bile duct strictures. *Am J Gastroenterol.* 2004; 99:1069-73.
27. Byrne MF, Gerke H, Mitchell RM, Stiffler HL, McGrath K, Branch MS, et al. Yield of endoscopic ultrasound-guided fine-needle aspiration of bile duct lesions. *Endoscopy.* 2004;36:715-9.
28. Voermans RP, Eisendrath P, Bruno MJ, Le MO, Deviere J, Fockens P. Initial evaluation of a novel prototype forward-viewing US endoscope in transmural drainage of pancreatic pseudocysts (with videos). *Gastrointest Endosc.* 2007;66:1013-7.
29. Larghi A, Lecca PG, Ardito F, Rossi ED, Fadda G, Nuzzo G, et al. Evaluation of hilar biliary strictures by using a newly developed forward-viewing therapeutic echoendoscope: preliminary results of an ongoing experience. *Gastrointest Endosc.* 2009;69:356-60.
30. Menzel J, Poremba C, Dietl KH, Domschke W. Preoperative diagnosis of bile duct strictures—comparison of intraductal ultrasonography with conventional endosonography. *Scand J Gastroenterol.* 2000;35:77-82.
31. Tamada K, Nagai H, Yasuda Y, Tomiyama T, Ohashi A, Wada S, et al. Transpapillary intraductal US prior to biliary drainage in the assessment of longitudinal spread of extrahepatic bile duct carcinoma. *Gastrointest Endosc.* 2001;53:300-7.
32. Stavropoulos S, Larghi A, Verna E, Battezzati P, Stevens P. Intraductal ultrasound for the evaluation of patients with biliary strictures and no abdominal mass on computed tomography. *Endoscopy.* 2005;37:715-21.
33. Farrell RJ, Agarwal B, Brandwein SL, Underhill J, Chuttani R, Pleskow DK. Intraductal US is a useful adjunct to ERCP for distinguishing malignant from benign biliary strictures. *Gastrointest Endosc.* 2002;56:681-7.
34. Sebo TJ. Digital image analysis. *Mayo Clin Proc.* 1995;70: 81-2.
35. Baron TH, Harewood GC, Rumalla A, Pochron NL, Stadheim LM, Gores GJ, et al. A prospective comparison of digital image analysis and routine cytology for the identification of malignancy in biliary tract strictures. *Clin Gastroenterol Hepatol.* 2004;2:214-9.
36. Kipp BR, Stadheim LM, Halling SA, Pochron NL, Harmsen S, Nagorney DM, et al. A comparison of routine cytology and fluorescence in situ hybridization for the detection of malignant bile duct strictures. *Am J Gastroenterol.* 2004; 99:1675-81.
37. Persons DL, Takai K, Gibney DJ, Katzmann JA, Lieber MM, Jenkins RB. Comparison of fluorescence in situ hybridization with flow cytometry and static image analysis in ploidy analysis of paraffin-embedded prostate adenocarcinoma. *Hum Pathol.* 1994;25:678-83.
38. Kristal AR, Baker MS, Flaherty MJ, Feng Z, Ylvisaker TJ, Feld AD, et al. A pilot study of DNA aneuploidy in colorectal adenomas and risk of adenoma recurrence. *Cancer Epidemiol Biomarkers Prev.* 1995;4:347-52.
39. van den Ingh HF, Griffioen G, Cornelisse CJ. DNA aneuploidy in colorectal adenomas. *Br J Cancer.* 1987;55:351.
40. Banner BF, Chacho MS, Roseman DL, Coon JS. Multiparameter flow cytometric analysis of colon polyps. *Am J Clin Pathol.* 1987;87:313-8.
41. Yeaton P, Kiss R, Deviere J, Salmon I, Bourgeois N, Pasteels JL, et al. Use of cell image analysis in the detection of cancer from specimens obtained during endoscopic retrograde cholangiopancreatography. *Am J Clin Pathol.* 1993;100:497-501.
42. Moreno Luna LE, Kipp B, Halling KC, Sebo TJ, Kremers WK, Roberts LR, et al. Advanced cytologic techniques for the detection of malignant pancreatobiliary strictures. *Gastroenterology.* 2006;131:1064-72.
43. Polglase AL, McLaren WJ, Skinner SA, Kiesslich R, Neurath MF, Delaney PM. A fluorescence confocal endomicroscope for in vivo microscopy of the upper- and the lower-GI tract. *Gastrointest Endosc.* 2005;62:686-95.
44. Goetz M, Kiesslich R, Dienes HP, Drebber U, Murr E, Hoffman A, et al. In vivo confocal laser endomicroscopy of the human liver: a novel method for assessing liver microarchitecture in real time. *Endoscopy.* 2008;40:554-62.
45. Wang TD, Van Dam J. Optical biopsy: a new frontier in endoscopic detection and diagnosis. *Clin Gastroenterol Hepatol.* 2004;2:744-53.
46. Aisenberg J. Gastrointestinal endoscopy nears "the molecular era." *Gastrointest Endosc.* 2008;68:528-30.
47. Kiesslich R, Neurath MF. Chromoendoscopy and other novel imaging techniques. *Gastroenterol Clin North Am.* 2006;35:605-19.
48. Chen C, Shah R, Pleskow D, Chuttani R, Slivka A, Stevens P, et al. Miami classification (MC) of probe-based confocal laser endomicroscopy (pCLE) findings in the pancreaticobiliary (PB) system for evaluation of indeterminate strictures: interim results from an international multicenter registry. 71 ed. New Orleans LA; 2010.
49. Huang D, Swanson EA, Lin CP, Schuman JS, Stinson WG, Chang W, et al. Optical coherence tomography. *Science.* 1991;254:1178-81.
50. Tearney GJ, Brezinski ME, Bouma BE, Boppart SA, Pitris C, Southern JF, et al. In vivo endoscopic optical biopsy with optical coherence tomography. *Science.* 1997;276:2037-39.

51. Gladkova ND, Petrova GA, Nikulin NK, Radenska-Lopovok SG, Snopova LB, Chumakov YP, et al. In vivo optical coherence tomography imaging of human skin: norm and pathology. *Skin Res Technol.* 2000;6:6-16.
52. Bouma BE, Tearney GJ, Compton CC, Nishioka NS. High-resolution imaging of the human esophagus and stomach in vivo using optical coherence tomography. *Gastrointest Endosc.* 2000;51:467-74.
53. Sivak MV Jr, Kobayashi K, Izatt JA, Rollins AM, Ung-Runyawee R, Chak A, et al. High-resolution endoscopic imaging of the GI tract using optical coherence tomography. *Gastrointest Endosc.* 2000;51:474-9.
54. Arvanitakis M, Hookey L, Tessier G, Demetter P, Nagy N, Stellke A, et al. Intraductal optical coherence tomography during endoscopic retrograde cholangiopancreatography for investigation of biliary strictures. *Endoscopy.* 2009;41:696-701.
55. Hintze RE, bou-Rebyeh H, Adler A, Veltzke-Schlieker W, Felix R, Wiedenmann B. Magnetic resonance cholangiopancreatography-guided unilateral endoscopic stent placement for Klatskin tumors. *Gastrointest Endosc.* 2001;53:40-6.
56. Dowsett JF, Vaira D, Hatfield AR, Cairns SR, Polydorou A, Frost R, et al. Endoscopic biliary therapy using the combined percutaneous and endoscopic technique. *Gastroenterology.* 1989;96:1180-6.
57. Baer HU, Rhyner M, Stain SC, Glauser PW, Dennison AR, Maddern GJ, et al. The effect of communication between the right and left liver on the outcome of surgical drainage for jaundice due to malignant obstruction at the hilus of the liver. *HPB Surg.* 1994;8:27-31.
58. Leung JW, Lau GT, Sung JJ, Costerton JW. Decreased bacterial adherence to silver-coated stent material: an in vitro study. *Gastrointest Endosc.* 1992;38:338-40.
59. Levy MJ, Baron TH, Gostout CJ, Petersen BT, Farnell MB. Palliation of malignant extrahepatic biliary obstruction with plastic versus expandable metal stents: an evidence-based approach. *Clin Gastroenterol Hepatol.* 2004;2:273-85.
60. Tringali A, Boskoski I, Mutignani M, Amiliari P, Perri V, Costamagna G. Endoscopic palliation of malignant hilar biliary strictures by self-expandable metal stents: clinical results and patency evaluation. 71 ed. 2010. p. AB309.
61. Suk KT, Kim JW, Kim HS, Baik SK, Oh SJ, Lee SJ, et al. Human application of a metallic stent covered with a paclitaxel-incorporated membrane for malignant biliary obstruction: multicenter pilot study. *Gastrointest Endosc.* 2007;66:798-803.
62. Ikeda H, Kuroda C, Uchida H, Miyata Y, Masaki N, Shigematsu Y, et al. Intraluminal irradiation with iridium-192 wires for extrahepatic bile duct carcinoma—a preliminary report (author's transl). *Nippon Igaku Hoshasen Gakkai Zasshi.* 1979;39:1356-8.
63. Shin HS, Seong J, Kim WC, Lee HS, Moon SR, Lee IJ, et al. Combination of external beam irradiation and high-dose-rate intraluminal brachytherapy for inoperable carcinoma of the extrahepatic bile ducts. *Int J Radiat Oncol Biol Phys.* 2003;57:105-12.
64. Bruha R, Petrtyl J, Kubecova M, Marecek Z, Dufek V, Urbanek P, et al. Intraluminal brachytherapy and selfexpandable stents in nonresectable biliary malignancies—the question of long-term palliation. *Hepatogastroenterology.* 2001;48:631-7.
65. Fritz P, Brambs HJ, Schraube P, Freund U, Berns C, Wannenmacher M. Combined external beam radiotherapy and intraluminal high dose rate brachytherapy on bile duct carcinomas. *Int J Radiat Oncol Biol Phys.* 1994;29:855-61.
66. Kocak Z, Ozkan H, Adli M, Garipagaoglu M, Kurtman C, Cakmak A. Intraluminal brachytherapy with metallic stenting in the palliative treatment of malignant obstruction of the bile duct. *Radiat Med.* 2005;23:200-7.
67. Kamada T, Saitou H, Takamura A, Nojima T, Okushiba SI. The role of radiotherapy in the management of extrahepatic bile duct cancer: an analysis of 145 consecutive patients treated with intraluminal and/or external beam radiotherapy. *Int J Radiat Oncol Biol Phys.* 1996;34:767-74.
68. Takamura A, Saito H, Kamada T, Hiramatsu K, Takeuchi S, Hasegawa M, et al. Intraluminal low-dose-rate 192Ir brachytherapy combined with external beam radiotherapy and biliary stenting for unresectable extrahepatic bile duct carcinoma. *Int J Radiat Oncol Biol Phys.* 2003;57:1357-65.
69. Kubota Y, Takaoka M, Kin H, Ogura M, Yamamoto S, Tsuji K, et al. Endoscopic irradiation and parallel arrangement of Wallstents for hilar cholangiocarcinoma. *Hepatogastroenterology.* 1998;45:415-9.
70. Morganti AG, Trodella L, Valentini V, Montemaggi P, Costamagna G, Smaniotto D, et al. Combined modality treatment in unresectable extrahepatic biliary carcinoma. *Int J Radiat Oncol Biol Phys.* 2000;46:913-9.
71. McMasters KM, Tuttle TM, Leach SD, Rich T, Cleary KR, Evans DB, et al. Neoadjuvant chemoradiation for extrahepatic cholangiocarcinoma. *Am J Surg.* 1997;174:605-8.
72. Berr F, Wiedmann M, Tannapfel A, Halm U, Kohlhaw KR, Schmidt F, et al. Photodynamic therapy for advanced bile duct cancer: evidence for improved palliation and extended survival. *Hepatology.* 2000;31:291-8.
73. Ortner MA. Photodynamic therapy in cholangiocarcinomas. *Best Pract Res Clin Gastroenterol.* 2004;18:147-54.
74. Wiedmann M, Caca K, Berr F, Schiefke I, Tannapfel A, Wittekind C, et al. Neoadjuvant photodynamic therapy as a new approach to treating hilar cholangiocarcinoma: a phase II pilot study. *Cancer.* 2003;97:2783-90.
75. Kiesslich T, Wolkersdorfer G, Neureiter D, Salmhofer H, Berr F. Photodynamic therapy for non-resectable perihilar cholangiocarcinoma. *Photochem Photobiol Sci.* 2009;8:23-30.
76. Zoepf T, Jakobs R, Arnold JC, Apel D, Riemann JF. Palliation of nonresectable bile duct cancer: improved survival after photodynamic therapy. *Am J Gastroenterol.* 2005;100:2426-30.
77. Rumalla A, Baron TH, Wang KK, Gores GJ, Stadheim LM, de Groen PC. Endoscopic application of photodynamic therapy for cholangiocarcinoma. *Gastrointest Endosc.* 2001;53:500-4.

12 Endoscopic Imaging of Colorectal Polyps and Cancer

Anna M Buchner, Douglas K Rex

ABSTRACT

Conventional white light colonoscopy is widely accepted as a primary method of screening and the standard method of surveillance for premalignant colorectal lesions and cancer. However, conventional colonoscopy has a substantial miss rate and is operator dependent with regard to detection of premalignant lesions and even cancer. Conventional colonoscopy also results in resection of lesions that are not premalignant, thereby, producing unnecessary costs and risks to patients. Recent developments in endoscopic imaging have focused on these two issues of improving lesion detection and characterizing histology of detected lesions in real time. Attempts to improve detection have generally been unsuccessful, though high-definition optics appears promising in this regard. On the other hand, diagnosis of the histology of detected lesions has proven feasible using a variety of methods. This chapter will review the new developments in endoscopic imaging of colorectal polyps and cancer.

INTRODUCTION

Colorectal cancer is the second most common cause of cancer-related deaths in the US and develops in most cases via a progression from low-grade dysplasia to high-grade one and then to invasive carcinoma. Colorectal lesions harboring dysplasia can be either polypoid (Paris classification type I lesions), flat, or depressed (Paris classification type II lesions).[1] Lesions with these shapes may be either conventional adenomas or may be serrated. Conventional adenomas and serrated lesions have distinct endoscopic appearances and different molecular profiles.[1] Any given endoscopic technique would be expected to have less sensitivity for either conventional adenomas or serrated lesions, when they have flat or depressed morphology (as opposed to polypoid shape) or when they are located on the proximal sides of fold and flexures, etc.

Preneoplastic lesions may not be detected during colonoscopy and even experienced gastroenterologists can miss advanced adenomas and a mean of up to 30% of all adenomas.[2-4] Furthermore, some studies confirmed the development of colorectal cancer, especially in the right site of the colon, despite colonoscopy that apparently cleared the colon of precancerous lesions.[5-7]

A variety of factors diminish the effectiveness of colonoscopy, and some of these are relatively specific to the proximal colon. Bowel preparation tends to be worse in the proximal colon, though this can be overcome by so-called "split dosing" (giving half the preparation the evening before and half on the day of colonoscopy) or giving the entire preparation on the day of examination. In addition, certain lesions, which are endoscopically subtle in appearance, are distributed more towards the proximal colon. These include flat and depressed lesions as well as serrated lesions.

In this regard, a recent study of 1,819 veterans who underwent colonoscopy reported an overall prevalence of 9.35% nonpolypoid adenomas of flat or depressed endoscopic appearance, and 0.82% of all patients were found to have nonpolypoid adenomas with high-grade dysplasia or cancer.[8] Similarly, two recent studies from a single center found dramatic variation among groups of gastroenterologists in their detection of proximal colon serrated lesions, suggesting large miss rates for these lesions among many endoscopists.[9-10] The subtle endoscopic appearances of many flat adenomas and many serrated lesions suggest an opportunity for endoscopic image enhancement technologies that highlight these lesions for endoscopic detection.

TABLE 12-1 Methods of Endoscopic Imaging of Colorectal Polyps and Neoplasia

Method	*Technology*	*Aims*
Expanded colonoscopic systems	Wide angle and hooded colonoscopies, third eye retroscopy	To increase detection
Broad field enhancement technologies	Dye-based chromoendoscopy and virtual chromoendoscopy: NBI, OBI, i-Scan, and autofluorescence	To increase mucosal contrast and detection of flat and depressed lesions
Point field enhancement technologies	Confocal laser endomicroscopy (eCLE, pCLE), endocytoscopy	*In vivo* histology

New modalities are generally directed towards either enhancing detection of precancerous colorectal lesions and cancer or towards characterization (and thereby, realtime histologic diagnosis) of already detected lesions. Detection enhancement modalities include field enhancement technologies, such as traditional dye-based chromoendoscopy and virtual chromoendoscopy with narrow band imaging (NBI), optimal band imaging (OBI)–Fujinon intelligent color enhancement (FICE) system and i-Scan, as well as expanded field of view colonoscopic systems with wide angle views or use of cap-fitted colonoscopies or third eye retroscope (TER) device (Table 12-1). Diagnosis enhancement modalities include chromoendoscopy and virtual chromoendoscopy modalities mentioned above, and also novel point enhancement technologies, such as confocal laser endomicroscopy (CLE) or endocystoscopy (ECS) that actually provide virtual histology.

EXPANDED FIELD OF VIEW METHODS

Over the last decade, awareness of potentially missed flat and subtle lesion led to increased efforts to improve the quality of colonoscopy achieved with longer and careful inspection between and behind folds, appropriate lavaging and suctioning to achieve better visualization, appropriate distention, and spending adequate time for effective inspection. Several expanded field of view methods have been investigated, including wide angle colonoscopy, cap-assisted colonoscopy, and retrograde third eye endoscopy device.

Wide Angle Colonoscopy

The role of wide angle (>170°) colonoscopies has been evaluated in recent randomized trials.[11-13] There was no obvious advantage of improved detection of colorectal lesions, though it shortened withdrawal time without affecting adenoma detection rates.[11] Tribonias et al.[14] demonstrated an increase in the overall polyp detection when newer high-definition (HD) wide angle colonoscopies were used with no significant differences in the detection rate of adenomas.

Cap-assisted Colonoscopy

The use of hooded colonoscopy or cap-assisted colonoscopy is considered a method that could potentially facilitate the inspection between folds and thus, improve detection of adenomas.[15-22]

The reported results are mixed, some studies demonstrating an overall advantage in adenoma detection with the use of hooded colonoscope,[15] and others not confirming the improvement of adenoma detection rates.[18,19] The most recent randomized, tandem colonoscopy trial[19] demonstrated reduced miss rates for all adenomas, especially small adenomas when cap-fitted colonoscopy was utilized. However, the use of hooded colonoscopes has not been widely adopted yet.

Third Eye Retroscope Device Method

TER device is a catheter-based imaging system, which is passed through the accessory channel of the colonoscope. It provides a second image directed towards the proximal side of the folds and viewed simultaneously alongside the forward viewing image provided by the colonoscope. The proximal side of the folds is a common location of adenomas, missed frequently by optical colonoscopy.[23-25] Recent prospective open-label multicenter study confirmed that polyp detection rates improved significantly with TER, especially after 15 procedures, when the mean additional detection rate for adenomas was 25%.[25] Additional detection rates with TER for medium-size and large adenomas were greater than for smaller lesions, suggesting this device can increase detection rates of clinically significant adenomas without detriment to procedure time or procedure complications.[25]

In another nonrandomized trial,[26] TER allowed detection of 13.2% additional polyps, including 11% additional adenomas. Additional detection rates with TER for adenomas 6 mm or larger and 10 mm or larger were 25 and 33.3%, respectively. Finally, a recent prospective randomized controlled multicenter study[27] compared adenoma detection rates among patients undergoing either standard colonoscopy (SC) followed by TER or TER followed by SC. Net additional detection rates with TER were 29.8% for polyps and 23.2% for adenomas. The relative risk of missing with SC compared with TER was 2.56 for polyps ($p < 0.001$) and 1.92 for adenomas ($p = 0.029$). These results are promising and may lead to adoption of this technology in general practice with time.

IMPROVED RESOLUTION AND CONTRAST IMAGE-ENHANCED FIELD OF VIEW METHODS

Some technologies could improve detection by either improved image resolution or highlighting lesions that are endoscopically subtle. Contrast-enhanced image endoscopy includes image-enhanced endoscopy (IEE) technologies, such as dye-based IEE with chromoendoscopy and electronic equipment-based IEE with NBI, FICE, and i-Scan with spectral estimation technologies, and autofluorescence imaging (AFI).[26]

High-resolution and High-definition Endoscopy System

High-resolution endoscopes (HRE) have incorporated high-density charged couple device (CCD) (600,000–1,000,000 pixels per CCD). These colonoscopes sometimes are equipped with a movable lens for magnification endoscopy, in which the focal distance is controlled to allow detailed examination of the mucosal surface at a close range (<3 mm). High magnification can provide enlargement of the image up to 150× as compared with 30× with standard endoscopes. HD system can display up to 1,080 scanning lines on a screen compared to standard definition (SD) analogue system, which can generate up to 576 scanning lines. These HD endoscopes with high CCDs combined with HD 1,080-line television monitors, produce images with increased spatial resolution.[28]

HD imaging system was utilized in recent trials, all achieving very high adenoma detection rates above 50% in average risk screening patients[29-31] and among high-risk patients.[32]

In a large cohort of 2,430 patients, the use of HD colonoscopy was associated with a higher adenoma detection rate in comparison to SD colonoscopy.[33] This higher rate was most apparent for smaller adenomas (<10 mm) and adenomas in the left colon. Other colonoscopic studies comparing SD white light endoscopy with HD white light endoscopy have demonstrated mixed results.[14,32,34,35] Pellise et al.[34] demonstrated no statistically significant difference in detection of adenomas (HD: 26%, SD: 25%) and all polyps (HD: 43%, SD: 38%) using an HD colonoscope vs. a SD colonoscope in 639 patients undergoing routine colonoscopy. However, the study was underpowered to detect small differences between groups in a population with a prevalence of adenomas of less than 30%, typical of average risk individuals. Similarly, in a study by East et al.[32] involving patients undergoing routine colonoscopies by a dedicated and highly experienced endoscopist, adenoma detection rate was higher with HD colonoscopy (71 vs. 60%), but this trend did not reach statistical significance in the small group of 58 HD patients and 72 SD patients.

Further studies are needed to determine whether the use of HD system independently increases adenoma detection. Additional potential advantages of HD systems are that their combined use with image enhancement technologies, such as chromoendoscopy/NBI/AFI techniques may lead to better detection of flat and subtle lesions as well as differentiation between neoplastic and nonneoplastic lesions.

Dye-based Chromoendoscopy in Detection and Characterization

Chromoendoscopy is the application of topical or vital dyes during colonoscopy to detect subtle gastrointestinal lesions and to define surface patterns (Figure 12-1) that have been associated with specific histologies. The colorectal lesions are enhanced either by active mucosal uptake of absorptive stains (e.g., methylene blue) or accumulation of contrast stains in the colonic pits and ridges (e.g., indigo carmine). Kudo pit pattern classification for colonic lesions has become broadly utilized to define colonic lesions.[36] Type 1 (round pits) and type 2 (stellate pits) represent nonneoplastic lesions, whereas type 3 (tubular pits), type 4 (gyrus like pits), and type 5 (irregular pits) correspond to neoplastic lesions. The main value of chromocolonoscopy technique appears to be the detection of small and flat lesions not seen by conventional colonoscopy and distinction between neoplastic and nonneoplastic lesions during ongoing colonoscopy.[8,37-41] Three randomized controlled trials compared pancolonic chromoendoscopy with

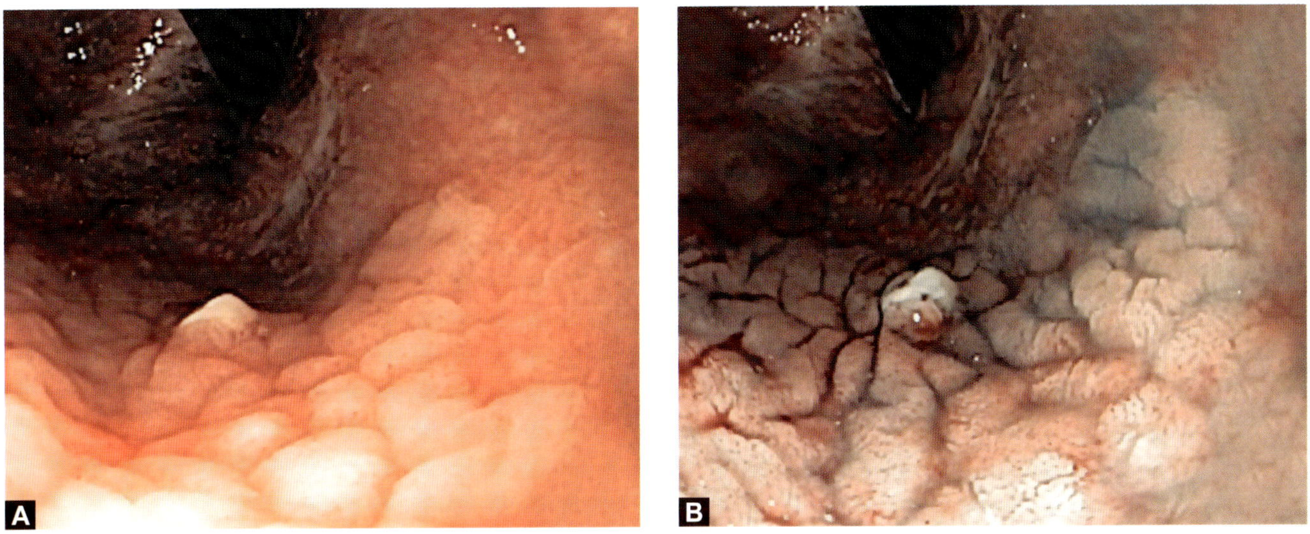

FIGURE 12-1 Dysplasia associated lesion mass in a patient with chronic inflammatory bowel disease. **A,** High-definition endoscopy imaging. **B,** Chromoendoscopy imaging.

conventional SD colonoscopy, and, of these, only one confirmed a significant increase in the detection of small adenomas but at the cost of longer withdrawal time and procedure.[40] In a tandem study,[42] chromocolonoscopy increased detection of additional adenomas in the second chromocolonoscopy examination, but the difference was not significant. A Cochrane review comparing chromoscopy vs. conventional endoscopy for the detection of colorectal polyps revealed that chromoscopy is likely to yield significantly more patients with at least one neoplastic lesion and significantly more with three or more neoplastic lesions.[43]

In these studies, all enrolled patients were considered to be at high risk for colorectal cancer. On the other hand, in a recent study of average cancer risk patients, HD panchromocolonoscopy marginally increased overall adenoma detection and yielded only a modest increase in flat and small adenoma detection as compared to HD white light colonoscopy.[31] Therefore, these findings do not support the routine use of HD chromocolonoscopy for colorectal cancer screening in average risk patients.[44]

On the other hand, targeted chromoendoscopy has been demonstrated to be beneficial in characterization of flat and depressed colorectal lesions.[8]

A more definite benefit for chromoendoscopy has been found in dysplasia surveillance in ulcerative colitis. Several trials[45-49] have found that chromoendoscopy with targeted biopsies increased the diagnostic yield for dysplastic lesions, including flat lesions in patients with long-term ulcerative colitis as opposed to using SC and required fewer biopsies per patient. A recent meta-analysis confirmed an overall benefit of using chromoendoscopy in ulcerative colitis.[50] Thus, chromoendoscopy has been suggested to be a part of new surveillance guidelines in patients with long-standing ulcerative colitis, but it has not been yet routinely implemented.[49]

The advantage of chromoendoscopy to improve detection of adenomas has also been demonstrated in patients with hereditary nonpolyposis colorectal cancer (HNPCC).[51]

However, chromoendoscopy has not been widely adopted into clinical practice in the US, because of difficulty in standardization of techniques, requirement for specialized disposable equipment, and increased procedure time.[52,53] This limited application of dye-based chromoendoscopy has led to efforts to develop so-called virtual chromendoscopy with no requirements for the use of topical stains.

VIRTUAL CHROMOENDOSCOPY

Narrow Band Imaging

NBI is an available method of virtual chromendoscopy that has a potential to improve detection of mucosal abnormalities without the application of chromic agents (Figure 12-2). While conventional white light endoscopy uses the full visible wavelength range (400–700 nm) to produce a red/green/blue image, NBI illuminates the tissue surface using special filters that narrow the red/

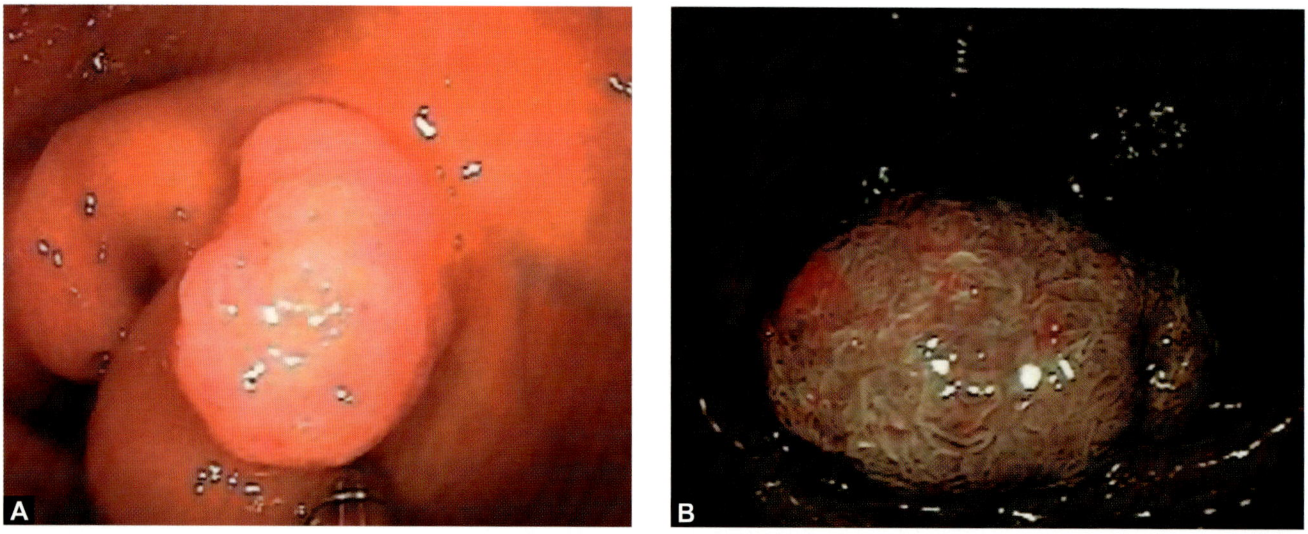

FIGURE 12-2 A large tubulovillous adenoma of the colon. **A,** High-definition white light imaging. **B,** High-definition narrow band imaging.

green/blue bands and simultaneously increase the relative intensity of the blue band. The resulting "narrow band" blue-green light improves imaging of mucosal patterns because of the limited optical scattering and shallow penetration depth, and thus it enhances the color contrast between the neoplastic lesions and adjacent normal mucosa. This blue light is also absorbed by hemoglobin for optimal detection of mucosal glandular, vascular patterns, and the presence of abnormal blood vessels that are associated with dysplasia.

NBI technique is a potentially useful tool in the detection of colorectal lesions, as well as their characterization.[54,55] For characterization, NBI has been used extensively with or without optical magnification.

However, recent randomized studies demonstrated no improvement of adenoma detection rates.[30,56,57] In a study by Adler et al.,[58] 401 patients were randomized to undergo either SD colonoscopy or NBI colonoscopy, a higher adenoma detection rate in the NBI group compared to the standard group (23 vs. 17%) was demonstrated only in the initial phase of the study, suggesting that exposure to NBI leads to both increased adenoma detection with both conventional and image enhanced methods (learning effect concept). In a study by Rex et al., 434 patients undergoing NBI or conventional examination with HD colonoscopies by a highly experienced endoscopist found no difference in detection between white light and NBI imaging. However, there was nearly doubling of the adenoma detection rate compared to their own well-documented historical controls,[30] suggesting a benefit primarily from HD.

Results of another prospective randomized back-to-back trial comparing NBI to conventional colonoscopy for adenoma detection demonstrated that the miss-rate for polyps and for adenomas was lower with HD-NBI than for SC.[59]

The use of NBI in long-standing ulcerative colitis has not led to improvement of dysplasia detection.[60] On the other hand, East et al.[61] demonstrated that NBI improved adenoma detection in high-risk group patients with HNPCC, in whom a second additional colonoscopic examination with NBI doubled the total number of detected adenomas. However, the study was not randomized and the increased detection could not be attributed with confidence to NBI.

A systematic review by van den Broek et al.[57] summarized the data on the performance and clinical utility of NBI during colonoscopy, and it did not demonstrate a significant improvement in adenoma detection using NBI but did confirm the value of NBI for differentiation of neoplastic from nonneoplastic colon polyps when used by experts.

The main advantage of NBI appears to be characterization, as NBI has a relatively high sensitivity of 90–95% and specificity of 80–85% for differentiation of neoplastic from nonneoplastic lesions rather than detection.[62] This level of accuracy is comparable to that of expert chromoendoscopist based on the available studies.[63,64] Several investigators examined the role of NBI for colorectal polyps' differentiation.[30,65-72] NBI was shown to be able to differentiate neoplastic and nonneoplastic polyps based on Kudo pit pattern and surface vascular patterns with a sensitivity and specificity of 91 and 89%, respectively, and it was comparable with dye-based chromoendoscopy.[65,68,71,72]

Recent trials confirmed very high accuracy of NBI for the diagnosis of small colorectal lesions, below 10 mm, in selected cases of high quality and high confidence stored images interpreted offline.[68,71] Rex et al. introduced a concept of confidence levels to the endoscopic interpretation of colorectal polyp histology.[68] This allowed sufficient accuracy (over 91%) for the use of NBI in the identification of distal hyperplastic polyps that do not need resection, as well as to plan post-polypectomy surveillance without pathologic evaluation of polyps 5 mm in size or smaller.[68]

Ignjatovic et al. demonstrated that for polyps less than 10 mm in size, *in vivo* optical diagnosis using NBI as virtual chromoendoscopy or in few cases dye-based chromoendoscopy can represent an acceptable approach for polyp characterization.[71] Wada et al. demonstrated that both NBI and chromoendoscopy can be useful in distinguishing between neoplastic and nonneoplastic colorectal lesions based on pit pattern and vascular patterns analysis.[73]

Rastogi et al. also showed that using a simple surface mucosal and vascular pattern classification, NBI without magnification was highly accurate and significantly superior to HD white light imaging for prediction of adenomas.[65] Thus, it is anticipated that with appropriate training, NBI can be used routinely for better lesion discrimination and characterization.

Fujinon Intelligent Color Enhancement and i-Scan

While NBI depends on optical filters within the light source, the "FICE" system, introduced by Fujinon, known as Fujinon intelligent color enhancement system, is based on a computed spectral estimation technology processing of the reflected photons to reconstruct virtual images with a choice of different wavelengths. A similar system, i-Scan has also been developed by Pentax. Both of these systems are based on similar physical principles as NBI, but they are not dependent on optical filters. These systems lead to enhancement of the tissue microvasculature as a result of differential optical absorption of light by hemoglobin in the mucosa.

The application of FICE system for detection and classification of colorectal lesions has also been investigated.[67,74,75] When FICE was compared with SD white light or with targeted chromoendoscopy, there was no improvement in adenoma detection rates.[76] A recent large randomized trial by Aminalai et al.[77] demonstrated no advantage of the FICE technique over conventional HD endoscopy. The overall adenoma detection rate (ADR) (0.28 in both groups), the total number of adenomas (184 vs. 183), or detection of subgroups of adenomas for both screening and diagnostic colonoscopy subgroups were similar.[77]

In another prospective randomized trial of tandem colonoscopy trial by Chung et al.,[78] there was also no objective advantage of FICE technique over conventional high-resolution endoscopy in terms of improved ADR. The adenoma miss rate with FICE showed no significant difference compared to that of white light endoscopy (6.6 vs. 8.3%, $p = 0.59$).

In a prospective randomized trial by Pohl et al.,[67] computed virtual chromoendoscopy system was compared with other modalities, such as SC and conventional chromoendoscopy with indigo carmine in low- and high-magnification modes for determination of colonic lesion histology. Based on this study, FICE system was able to identify morphological details that efficiently predicted adenomatous histology, and was superior to SC and equivalent to conventional chromoendoscopy.

Hoffman et al.[79,80] demonstrated that HD endoscopy combined with i-Scan system was significantly superior in detecting colorectal neoplasia as compared to standard videocolonoscopy, and it allowed prediction of histology of the identified lesions and surface enhancement. In their study, HD+ colonoscopy with i-Scan identified significantly more patients with at least one neoplasm compared with standard resolution endoscopy (38 vs. 13%; $p < 0.001$). However, given the poor results for improved adenoma detection using NBI and FICE, and the very low level of adenoma detection in the control arm of the i-Scan study (13%), additional study will be needed before understanding whether i-Scan improves adenoma detection. The histology of polyps was predicted accurately with i-Scan with a sensitivity of 98% and a specificity of 100% (95% confidence interval: sensitivity 90.6–99.6; specificity 92.8–100).

While these techniques of NBI, FICE, and i-Scan are very promising, further studies are needed to evaluate their final application in routine endoscopy practice, including efficiency and cost-effectiveness for both detection and characterization of malignant gastrointestinal lesions.

AUTOFLUORESCENCE IMAGING

Autofluorescence endoscopy is based on techniques that distinguish tissue types based on their differences in fluorescence emission. When the tissue is exposed to short-wavelength light, endogenous flurophores are excited leading to emission of fluorescent light of a longer wavelength AFI. Because of changes of endogenous fluorophores in normal, dysplastic, and neoplastic mucosa, the altered autofluorescence is reflected by a pseudocolored image of normal mucosa (green color) and dysplasia/neoplasia with varying tones of red/purple color. AFI has been incorporated into trimodel imaging endoscopes that combine high-resolution white light endoscopy and virtual chromoendoscopy with NBI.

In a prospective randomized study, autofluorescence endoscopy significantly increased the diagnostic yield of surveillance endoscopy to detect intraepithelial neoplasia in a high-risk patient group with ulcerative colitis.[81] However, AFI has not been demonstrated to enhance the diagnostic yield of screening colonoscopy in average-risk patients in a tandem colonoscopy trial by the same group.[72] Matsuda et al. showed that AFI detected more polyps in the right-sided colon compared to white light colonoscopy.[82] van den Broek et al.[83] evaluated interobserver agreement and accuracy for polyps' differentiation among experienced and nonexperienced gastroenterologists and confirmed that AFI had higher interobserver agreement and accuracy for diagnosing polyps than NBI. A recent randomized prospective trial by Takauchi et al. demonstrated that AFI colonoscopy with a transparent hood detected significantly more colorectal neoplasm than conventional colonoscopy without a hood.[84] Overall, studies on autofluorescence have demonstrated mixed results and the future application is still to be determined.

REALTIME *IN VIVO* HISTOLOGIC ASSESSMENT USING POINT FIELD TECHNOLOGIES

As noted above, chromoendoscopy and virtual or electronic chromoendoscopy methods, such as NBI, FICE, and i-Scan can identify surface patterns on lesions that correspond with lesion histology. However, more detailed realtime *in vivo* histologic assessment can be achieved with ultra-high magnifications systems (1,000 times magnification), such as CLE and ECS. These methods differ from NBI, FICE, and i-Scan, in that they are not standard equipment on commercial colonoscopes (they require investment in special equipment), and they require specific point interrogation of colorectal lesions. Therefore, their primary use in the colorectum is in diagnosing the lesions that have been already detected by other means.

Confocal Laser Endomicroscopy

CLE is a novel tool that allows *in vivo* imaging of gastrointestinal mucosa at cellular and subcellular levels during endoscopy and thus yields *in vivo* histopathology (Figure 12-3). It has the potential to replace traditional biopsies with *in vivo* histology.

CLE can be performed using one of the two FDA approved devices: endoscope-based CLE (eCLE) and a stand-alone through-the-scope probe CLE system (pCLE). CLE systems can be used in combination with virtual chromoendoscopy (NBI, i-Scan, and FICE) for initial detection and characterization of subtle mucosal abnormalities and circumscribed lesions. Once the

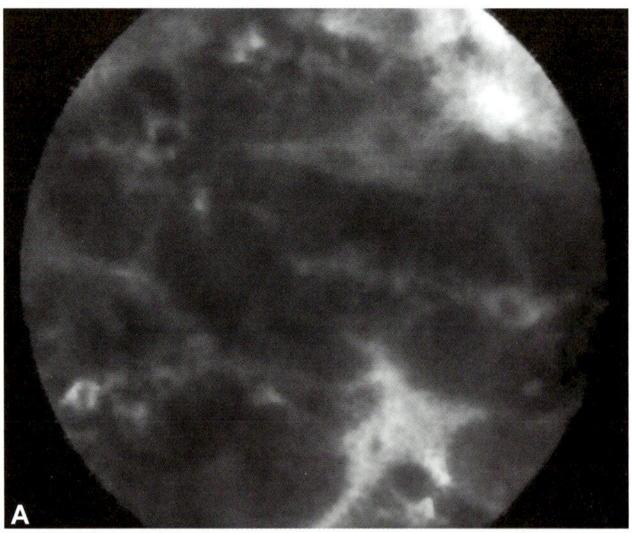

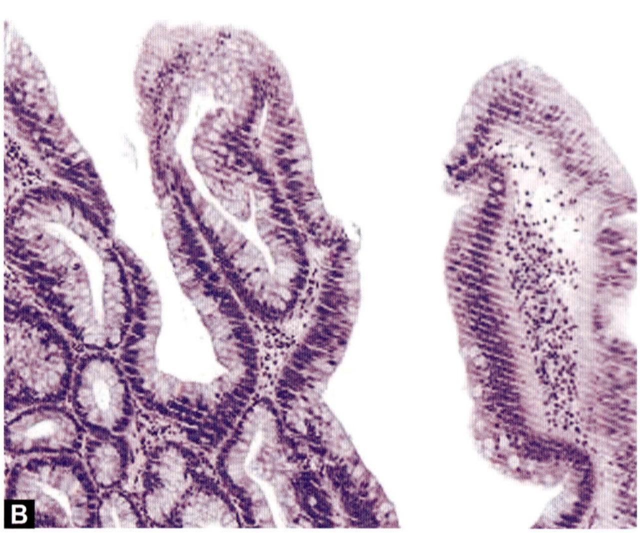

FIGURE 12-3 Tubulovillous adenoma. **A,** Confocal endomicroscopy imaging. **B,** Corresponding histopathology.

targeted lesion or mucosal abnormality is detected, it can be then interrogated further by the confocal system for *in vivo* histology.

The principle of CLE is based on tissue illumination with a low power laser allowing a better spatial resolution with 1,000 times magnification. Since both illumination and detection systems are on the same plane, images are not contaminated by light scattering from other planes. To obtain images, exogenous fluorescence contrast is required with agents, such as fluorescein (10% solution, intravenous application), acriflavine hydrochloride, or cresyl violet (topical applications). Intravenous fluorescein (1.0–5.0 mL of 10% solution) distributes throughout the capillary network and connective matrix, whereas acriflavine accumulates in superficial epithelial cells and nuclei, which raised a concern for potential mutagenic risk and limited its broader use. In a recent cross-sectional survey of 16 international medical centers with active research protocols involving 2,272 patients, no serious adverse events were reported with the use of intravenous fluorescein.[85]

Recent studies have supported the application of both CLE systems, eCLE and pCLE systems, as novel tools for *in vivo* histopathology of colorectal polyps and ulcerative colitis.[86-89] Both systems have been also shown to improve accuracy in distinguishing colorectal neoplasia.[87,89]

Kiesslich et al.[87] published the first report of the use of eCLE in 42 patients during ongoing colonoscopy in diagnosing intraepithelial neoplasia and colorectal cancer. A total of 134 small lesions (mean size 4 mm) were identified during colonoscopy after staining with methylene blue. With the help of the confocal endoscope, intraepithelial neoplasia could be predicted with a sensitivity of 97% and a specificity of 99% (accuracy 99%). Buchner et al.[89] compared virtual chromoendoscopy systems with pCLE for colorectal polyps classification and confirmed higher sensitivity of pCLE with similar specificity in accurate differentiation between neoplastic and nonneoplastic lesions. Furthermore, Sanduleanu et al.[90] demonstrated that the eCLE system can reliably distinguish low-grade from high-grade dysplasia in colorectal lesions with very good inter- and intraobserver agreement.

The chromoscopy-guided endomicroscopy technique has also been recently evaluated in patients with long-term ulcerative colitis.[88] The results confirmed that the presence of dysplastic changes could be predicted by endomicroscopy with high accuracy (sensitivity 94.7%; specificity 98.3%; and accuracy 97.8%). Thus, endomicroscopy has a potential to determine if ulcerative colitis lesions identified by chromoscopy should undergo biopsy examination and, thereby, increase the diagnostic yield and reduce the need for biopsy examinations. Therefore, chromoscopy-guided endomicroscopy may lead to significant improvement in the long-term, clinical management of ulcerative colitis.

In spite of these promising results, CLE is used mainly as a research tool in academic centers.

Endocytoscopy

Endocytoscopy (ECS) is based on the technology of light-contact microscopy. The current ECS system consists of two prototypes; Prototype I (XEC300) has a maximal 450× magnification and field of view of 300 × 300 μm, whereas Prototype II (XEC120) provides a maximal 1,100× magnification and a field of view of 120 × 120 μm. In contrast to confocal endomicroscopy, the endocytoscopes can be easily passed through an accessory channel of the conventional therapeutic endoscope. This method does not require the use of intravenous contrast agents; instead, it uses topical stains, such as methylene blue or crestyl violet, which are applied routinely in chromoendoscopy techniques in standard endoscopy.

A prospective study from Japan used ECS in 113 patients to obtain realtime histological images *in vivo* during colonoscopy.[91] With ECS system, it was possible to observe lesions at the cellular level, evaluate cellular atypia, and distinguish between neoplastic and non-neoplastic lesions when compared to histology. The correlation between the endocytoscopic and histological diagnosis was statistically significant.

These point field enhancement technologies, CLE and ECS with ultra-magnification, require specialized training, and expensive equipment and are overall time consuming; therefore, they have not been utilized in general practice yet. However, they can play an important role in prediction of neoplasia, especially in small colorectal lesions as compared to traditional histopathology analysis and, thus, prevent unnecessary biopsies or resection of small nonneoplastic colorectal lesions.

CONCLUSION

Recent quality recommendations for colonoscopy emphasize the effective application of white light examination using standard instruments. However, some lesions may be difficult to detect even with careful technique, because of their location behind folds or their subtle endoscopic appearance. Cap-assisted colonoscopy and the TER device have both shown a promise for detection of lesions in hidden areas in the colon. A practical method of enhancing detection of flat and depressed, and serrated lesions has proven difficult to identify, though HD optics appears to be promising. Chromoendoscopy is impractical for routine use for screening and surveillance, because of limited benefit and time consuming application. Chromoendoscopy is both effective and practical when used for dysplasia surveillance in ulcerative colitis, since it enhances detection and reduces the number of biopsies required. NBI and FICE have not yet proven effective for polyp detection, and additional data are needed to assess i-Scan for this purpose. The use of image enhancement technologies to determine the histology of detected lesions is much better developed. NBI, FICE, and i-Scan have all proven effective in differentiating adenomas from hyperplastic lesions by analysis of surface structures. CLE provides images that are equivalent to histology in their detail. ECS is a very high-magnification system that allows detailed histologic assessment. Although techniques for realtime assessment have not yet entered clinical practice, they may be eventually used to correctly identify distal hyperplastic polyps that do not require resection, thereby, reducing costs and risks,[92] or for application of the resect and discard policy for small or diminutive colorectal lesions.

REFERENCES

1. Hawk ET, Levin B. Colorectal cancer prevention. *J Clin Oncol.* 2005;23:378-91.
2. Rex DK, Cutler CS, Lemmel GT, Rahmani EY, Clark DW, Helper DJ, et al. Colonoscopic miss rates of adenomas determined by back-to-back colonoscopies. *Gastroenterology.* 1997;112:24-8.
3. Postic G, Lewin D, Bickerstaff C, Wallace MB. Colonoscopic miss rates determined by direct comparison of colonoscopy with colon resection specimens. *Am J Gastroenterol.* 2002;97:3182-5.
4. van Rijn JC, Reitsma JB, Stoker J, Bossuyt PM, van Deventer SJ, Dekker E. Polyp miss rate determined by tandem colonoscopy: a systematic review. *Am J Gastroenterol.* 2006;101:343-50.
5. Baxter NN, Goldwasser MA, Paszat LF, Saskin R, Urbach DR, Rabeneck L. Association of colonoscopy and death from colorectal cancer. *Ann Intern Med.* 2009;150:1-8.
6. Lakoff J, Paszat LF, Saskin R, Rabeneck L. Risk of developing proximal versus distal colorectal cancer after a negative colonoscopy: a population-based study. *Clin Gastroenterol Hepatol.* 2008;6:1117-21.
7. Winawer SJ. Colorectal cancer screening comes of age. *N Engl J Med.* 1993;328:1416-7.
8. Soetikno RM, Kaltenbach T, Rouse RV, Park W, Maheshwari A, Sato T, et al. Prevalence of nonpolypoid (flat and depressed) colorectal neoplasms in asymptomatic and symptomatic adults. *JAMA.* 2008;299:1027-35.
9. Hetzel JT, Huang CS, Coukos JA, Omstead K, Cerda SR, Yang S, et al. Variation in the detection of serrated polyps in an average risk colorectal cancer screening cohort. *Am J Gastroenterol.* 2010;105:2656-64.
10. Kahi CJ, Hewett DG, Norton DL, Eckert GJ, Rex DK. Prevalence and variable detection of proximal colon serrated polyps during screening colonoscopy. *Clin Gastroenterol Hepatol.* 2011;9:42-6.
11. Rex DK, Chadalawada V, Helper DJ. Wide angle colonoscopy with a prototype instrument: impact on miss rates and efficiency as determined by back-to-back colonoscopies. *Am J Gastroenterol.* 2003;98:2000-5.
12. Fatima H, Rex DK, Rothstein R, Rahmani E, Nehme O, Dewitt J, et al. Cecal insertion and withdrawal times with wide-angle versus standard colonoscopes: a randomized controlled trial. *Clin Gastroenterol Hepatol.* 2008;6:109-14.
13. Deenadayalu VP, Chadalawada V, Rex DK. 170 degrees wide-angle colonoscope: effect on efficiency and miss rates. *Am J Gastroenterol.* 2004;99:2138-42.
14. Tribonias G, Theodoropoulou A, Konstantinidis K, Vardas E, Karmiris K, Chroniaris N, et al. Comparison of standard versus high-definition, wide-angle colonoscopy for polyp detection: a randomized controlled trial. *Colorectal Dis.* 2010;12:e260-6.
15. Horiuchi A, Nakayama Y. Improved colorectal adenoma detection with a transparent retractable extension device. *Am J Gastroenterol.* 2008;103:341-5.
16. Horiuchi A, Nakayama Y, Kato N, Ichise Y, Kajiyama M, Tanaka N. Hood-assisted colonoscopy is more effective in detection of colorectal adenomas than narrow-band imaging. *Clin Gastroenterol Hepatol.* 2010;8:379-83.
17. Matsushita M, Hajiro K, Okazaki K, Takakuwa H, Tominaga M. Efficacy of total colonoscopy with a transparent cap in comparison with colonoscopy without the cap. *Endoscopy.* 1998;30:444-7.
18. Lee YT, Hui AJ, Wong VW, Hung LC, Sung JJ. Improved colonoscopy success rate with a distally attached mucosectomy cap. *Endoscopy.* 2006;38:739-42.
19. Conio M, Blanchi S, Repici A, Ruggeri C, Fisher DA, Filiberti R. Cap-assisted endoscopic mucosal resection for colorectal polyps. *Dis Colon Rectum.* 2010;53:919-27.
20. Harada Y, Hirasawa D, Fujita N, Noda Y, Kobayashi G, Ishida K, et al. Impact of a transparent hood on the performance of total colonoscopy: a randomized controlled trial. *Gastrointest Endosc.* 2009;69:637-44.
21. Hewett DG, Rex DK. Cap-fitted colonoscopy: a randomized, tandem colonoscopy study of adenoma miss rates. *Gastrointest Endosc.* 2010;72:775-81.
22. Tada M, Inoue H, Yabata E, Okabe S, Endo M. Colonic mucosal resection using a transparent cap-fitted endoscope. *Gastrointest Endosc.* 1996;44:63-5.

23. Pickhardt PJ, Nugent PA, Mysliwiec PA, Choi JR, Schindler WR. Location of adenomas missed by optical colonoscopy. *Ann Intern Med.* 2004;141:352-9.
24. Triadafilopoulos G, Watts HD, Higgins J, Van Dam J. A novel retrograde-viewing auxiliary imaging device (Third Eye Retroscope) improves the detection of simulated polyps in anatomic models of the colon. *Gastrointest Endosc.* 2007;65:139-44.
25. DeMarco DC, Odstrcil E, Lara LF, Bass D, Herdman C, Kinney T, et al. Impact of experience with a retrograde-viewing device on adenoma detection rates and withdrawal times during colonoscopy: the Third Eye Retroscope study group. *Gastrointest Endosc.* 2010;71:542-50.
26. Waye JD, Heigh RI, Fleischer DE, Leighton JA, Gurudu S, Aldrich LB, et al. A retrograde-viewing device improves detection of adenomas in the colon: a prospective efficacy evaluation (with videos). *Gastrointest Endosc.* 2010;71: 551-6.
27. Leufkens AM, DeMarco DC, Rastogi A, Akerman PA, Azzouzi K, Rothstein RI, et al. Effect of a retrograde-viewing device on adenoma detection rate during colonoscopy: the TERRACE study. *Gastrointest Endosc.* 2011;73: 480-9.
28. Kaltenbach T, Sano Y, Friedland S, Soetikno R; American Gastroenterological Association. American Gastroenterological Association (AGA) Institute technology assessment on image-enhanced endoscopy. *Gastroenterology.* 2008; 134:327-40.
29. Paggi S, Radaelli F, Amato A, Meucci G, Mandelli G, Imperiali G, et al. The impact of narrow band imaging in screening colonoscopy: a randomized controlled trial. *Clin Gastroenterol Hepatol.* 2009;7:1049-54.
30. Rex DK, Helbig CC. High yields of small and flat adenomas with high-definition colonoscopes using either white light or narrow band imaging. *Gastroenterology.* 2007;133:42-7.
31. Kahi CJ, Anderson JC, Waxman I, Kessler WR, Imperiale TF, Li X, et al. High-definition chromocolonoscopy vs. high-definition white light colonoscopy for average-risk colorectal cancer screening. *Am J Gastroenterol.* 2010;105: 1301-7.
32. East JE, Stavrindis M, Thomas-Gibson S, Guenther T, Tekkis PP, Saunders BP. A comparative study of standard vs. high definition colonoscopy for adenoma and hyperplastic polyp detection with optimized withdrawal technique. *Aliment Pharmacol Ther.* 2008;28:768-76.
33. Buchner AM, Shahid MW, Heckman MG, McNeil RB, Cleveland P, Gill KR, et al. High-definition colonoscopy detects colorectal polyps at a higher rate than standard white-light colonoscopy. *Clin Gastroenterol Hepatol.* 2010;8:364-70.
34. Pellise M, Fernández-Esparrach G, Cárdenas A, Sendino O, Ricart E, Vaquero E, et al. Impact of wide-angle, high-definition endoscopy in the diagnosis of colorectal neoplasia: a randomized controlled trial. *Gastroenterology.* 2008;135:1062-8.
35. Burke CA, Choure AG, Sanaka MR, Lopez R. A comparison of high-definition versus conventional colonoscopes for polyp detection. *Dig Dis Sci.* 2010;55:1716-20.
36. Kudo S, Tamura S, Nakajima T, Yamano H, Kusaka H, Watanabe H. Diagnosis of colorectal tumorous lesions by magnifying endoscopy. *Gastrointest Endosc.* 1996;44:8-14.
37. Rembacken BJ, Fujii T, Cairns A, Dixon MF, Yoshida S, Chalmers DM, et al. Flat and depressed colonic neoplasms: a prospective study of 1000 colonoscopies in the UK. *Lancet.* 2000;355:1211-4.
38. Kiesslich R, von Bergh M, Hahn M, Hermann G, Jung M. Chromoendoscopy with indigocarmine improves the detection of adenomatous and nonadenomatous lesions in the colon. *Endoscopy.* 2001;33:1001-6.
39. Brooker JC, Saunders BP, Shah SG, Thapar CJ, Thomas HJ, Atkin WS, et al. Total colonic dye-spray increases the detection of diminutive adenomas during routine colonoscopy: a randomized controlled trial. *Gastrointest Endosc.* 2002;56:333-8.
40. Hurlstone DP, Cross SS, Slater R, Sanders DS, Brown S. Detecting diminutive colorectal lesions at colonoscopy: a randomised controlled trial of pan-colonic versus targeted chromoscopy. *Gut.* 2004;53:376-80.
41. Lapalus MG, Helbert T, Napoleon B, Rey JF, Houcke P, Ponchon T, et al. Does chromoendoscopy with structure enhancement improve the colonoscopic adenoma detection rate? *Endoscopy.* 2006;38:444-8.
42. Le Rhun M, Coron E, Parlier D, Nguyen JM, Canard JM, Alamdari A, et al. High resolution colonoscopy with chromoscopy versus standard colonoscopy for the detection of colonic neoplasia: a randomized study. *Clin Gastroenterol Hepatol.* 2006;4:349-54.
43. Brown SR, Baraza W. Chromoscopy versus conventional endoscopy for the detection of polyps in the colon and rectum. *Cochrane Database Syst Rev.* 2010;10:CD006439.
44. Kahi CJ, Imperiale TF, Juliar BE, Rex DK. Effect of screening colonoscopy on colorectal cancer incidence and mortality. *Clin Gastroenterol Hepatol.* 2009;7:770-5.
45. Kiesslich R, Fritsch J, Holtmann M, Koehler HH, Stolte M, Kanzler S. Methylene blue-aided chromoendoscopy for the detection of intraepithelial neoplasia and colon cancer in ulcerative colitis. *Gastroenterology.* 2003;124:880-8.
46. Hurlstone DP, McAlindon ME, Sanders DS, Koegh R, Lobo AJ, Cross SS. Further validation of high-magnification chromoscopic-colonoscopy for the detection of intraepithelial neoplasia and colon cancer in ulcerative colitis. *Gastroenterology.* 2004;126:376-8.
47. Rutter M, Caspi A, Fergusson D, Horwood LJ, Goodman R, Maughan B, et al. Sex differences in developmental reading disability: new findings from 4 epidemiological studies. *JAMA.* 2004;291:2007-12.
48. Perret-Vivancos C, Marion K, Renaud FN, Freney J. Efficient removal of attached biofilm in a naturally contaminated colonoscope using detachment-promoting agents. *J Hosp Infect.* 2008;68:277-8.
49. Hurlstone DP, Sanders DS, Lobo AJ, McAlindon ME, Cross SS. Indigo carmine-assisted high-magnification chromoscopic colonoscopy for the detection and characterisation of intraepithelial neoplasia in ulcerative colitis: a prospective evaluation. *Endoscopy.* 2005;37:1186-92.

50. Buchner AM. Does the dye-based chromoendoscopy improve dysplasia detection in patients undergoing serveillance colonoscopy for long term ulcerative colitis (UC)? Meta-analysis [2010 ACG Abstract]. *Am J Gastroenterol.* 2010;105:S1-571.
51. Lecomte T, Cellier C, Meatchi T, Barbier JP, Cugnenc PH, Jian R, et al. Chromoendoscopic colonoscopy for detecting preneoplastic lesions in hereditary nonpolyposis colorectal cancer syndrome. *Clin Gastroenterol Hepatol.* 2005;3:897-902.
52. Chiu HM, Chang CY, Chen CC, Lee YC, Wu MS, Lin JT, et al. A prospective comparative study of narrow-band imaging, chromoendoscopy, and conventional colonoscopy in the diagnosis of colorectal neoplasia. *Gut.* 2007; 56:373-9.
53. Helbig C. Chromoendoscopy and its alternatives for colonoscopy: useful in the United States? *Rev Gastroenterol Disord.* 2006;6:209-20.
54. Su MY, Hsu CM, Ho YP, Chen PC, Lin CJ, Chiu CT. Comparative study of conventional colonoscopy, chromoendoscopy, and narrow-band imaging systems in differential diagnosis of neoplastic and nonneoplastic colonic polyps. *Am J Gastroenterol.* 2006;101:2711-6.
55. Hirata M, Tanaka S, Oka S, Kaneko I, Yoshida S, Yoshihara M, et al. Magnifying endoscopy with narrow band imaging for diagnosis of colorectal tumors. *Gastrointest Endosc.* 2007;65:988-95.
56. Kaltenbach T, Friedland S, Soetikno S. A randomised tandem colonoscopy trial of narrow band imaging versus white light examination to compare neoplasia miss rates. *Gut.* 2008;57:1406-12.
57. van den Broek FJ, Reitsma JB, Curvers WL, Fockens P, Dekker E. Systematic review of narrow-band imaging for the detection and differentiation of neoplastic and nonneoplastic lesions in the colon (with videos). *Gastrointest Endosc.* 2009;69:124-35.
58. Adler A, Pohl H, Papanikolaou IS, Abou-Rebyeh H, Schachschal G, Veltzke-Schlieker W, et al. A prospective randomised study on narrow-band imaging versus conventional colonoscopy for adenoma detection: does narrow-band imaging induce a learning effect? *Gut.* 2008; 57:59-64.
59. Gross SA, Buchner AM, Cangemi JR, Wolfsen HC, DeVault KR, Crook J. A prospective randomized back-to-back trial comparing narrow band imaging to conventional colonoscopy for adenoma detection. *Gastroenterology.* 2008;134:A47-8.
60. Dekker E, van den Broek FJ, Reitsma JB, Hardwick JC, Offerhaus GJ, van Deventer SJ, et al. Narrow-band imaging compared with conventional colonoscopy for the detection of dysplasia in patients with longstanding ulcerative colitis. *Endoscopy.* 2007;39:216-21.
61. East JE, Suzuki N, Stavrinidis M, Guenther T, Thomas HJ, Saunders BP. Narrow band imaging for colonoscopic surveillance in hereditary non-polyposis colorectal cancer. *Gut.* 2008;57:65-70.
62. East JE, Saunders BP. Narrow band imaging at colonoscopy: seeing through a glass darkly or the light of a new dawn? *Expert Rev Gastroenterol Hepatol.* 2008;2:1-4.
63. East JE, Suzuki N, Saunders BP. Comparison of magnified pit pattern interpretation with narrow band imaging versus chromoendoscopy for diminutive colonic polyps: a pilot study. *Gastrointest Endosc.* 2007;66:310-6.
64. Machida H, Sano Y, Hamamoto Y, Muto M, Kozu T, Tajiri H, et al. Narrow-band imaging in the diagnosis of colorectal mucosal lesions: a pilot study. *Endoscopy.* 2004; 36:1094-8.
65. Rastogi A, Keighley J, Singh V, Callahan P, Bansal A, Wani S, et al. High accuracy of narrow band imaging without magnification for the real-time characterization of polyp histology and its comparison with high-definition white light colonoscopy: a prospective study. *Am J Gastroenterol.* 2009;104:2422-30.
66. Sikka S, Ringold DA, Jonnalagadda S, Banerjee B. Comparison of white light and narrow band high definition images in predicting colon polyp histology, using standard colonoscopes without optical magnification. *Endoscopy.* 2008;40:818-22.
67. Pohl J, Nguyen-Tat M, Pech O, May A, Rabenstein T, Ell C. Computed virtual chromoendoscopy for classification of small colorectal lesions: a prospective comparative study. *Am J Gastroenterol.* 2008;103:562-9.
68. Rex DK. Narrow-band imaging without optical magnification for histologic analysis of colorectal polyps. *Gastroenterology.* 2009;136:1174-81.
69. Togashi K, Konishi F, Ishizuka T, Sato T, Senba S, Kanazawa K. Efficacy of magnifying endoscopy in the differential diagnosis of neoplastic and non-neoplastic polyps of the large bowel. *Dis Colon Rectum.* 1999;42:1602-8.
70. Tung SY, Wu CS, Su MY. Magnifying colonoscopy in differentiating neoplastic from nonneoplastic colorectal lesions. *Am J Gastroenterol.* 2001;96:2628-32.
71. Ignjatovic A, East JE, Suzuki N, Vance M, Guenther T, Saunders BP. Optical diagnosis of small colorectal polyps at routine colonoscopy (Detect InSpect ChAracterise Resect and Discard; DISCARD trial): a prospective cohort study. *Lancet Oncol.* 2009;10:1171-8.
72. van den Broek FJ, Fockens P, Van Eeden S, Kara MA, Hardwick JC, Reitsma JB, et al. Clinical evaluation of endoscopic trimodal imaging for the detection and differentiation of colonic polyps. *Clin Gastroenterol Hepatol.* 2009;7:288-95.
73. Wada Y, Kashida H, Kudo SE, Misawa M, Ikehara N, Hamatani S. Diagnostic accuracy of pit pattern and vascular pattern analyses in colorectal lesions. *Dig Endosc.* 2010;22:192-9.
74. Pohl J, May A, Rabenstein T, Pech O, Ell C. Computed virtual chromoendoscopy: a new tool for enhancing tissue surface structures. *Endoscopy.* 2007;39:80-3.
75. Liu YX, Huang LY, Bian XP, Cui J, Xu N, Wu CR. Fuji Intelligent Chromo Endoscopy and staining technique for the diagnosis of colon tumor. *Chin Med J (Engl).* 2008;121: 977-82.

76. Pohl J, Lotterer E, Balzer C, Sackmann M, Schmidt KD, Gossner L, et al. Computed virtual chromoendoscopy versus standard colonoscopy with targeted indigocarmine chromoscopy: a randomised multicentre trial. *Gut.* 2009; 58:73-8.
77. Aminalai A, Rösch T, Aschenbeck J, Mayr M, Drossel R, Schröder A, et al. Live image processing does not increase adenoma detection rate during colonoscopy: a randomized comparison between FICE and conventional imaging (Berlin Colonoscopy Project 5, BECOP-5). *Am J Gastroenterol.* 2010;105:2383-8.
78. Chung SJ, Kim D, Song JH, Park MJ, Kim YS, Kim JS, et al. Efficacy of computed virtual chromoendoscopy on colorectal cancer screening: a prospective, randomized, back-to-back trial of Fuji Intelligent Color Enhancement versus conventional colonoscopy to compare adenoma miss rates. *Gastrointest Endosc.* 2010;72:136-42.
79. Hoffman A, Kagel C, Goetz M, Tresch A, Mudter J, Biesterfeld S, et al. Recognition and characterization of small colonic neoplasia with high-definition colonoscopy using i-Scan is as precise as chromoendoscopy. *Dig Liver Dis.* 2010;42:45-50.
80. Hoffman A, Sar F, Goetz M, Tresch A, Mudter J, Biesterfeld S, et al. High definition colonoscopy combined with i-Scan is superior in the detection of colorectal neoplasias compared with standard video colonoscopy: a prospective randomized controlled trial. *Endoscopy.* 2010;42:827-33.
81. van den Broek FJ, Fockens P, van Eeden S, Reitsma JB, Hardwick JC, Stokkers PC, et al. Endoscopic tri-modal imaging for surveillance in ulcerative colitis: randomised comparison of high-resolution endoscopy and autofluorescence imaging for neoplasia detection; and evaluation of narrow-band imaging for classification of lesions. *Gut.* 2008;57:1083-9.
82. Matsuda T, Saito Y, Fu KI, Uraoka T, Kobayashi N, Nakajima T, et al. Does autofluorescence imaging videoendoscopy system improve the colonoscopic polyp detection rate?—a pilot study. *Am J Gastroenterol.* 2008;103:1926-32.
83. van den Broek FJ, van Soest EJ, Naber AH, van Oijen AH, Mallant-Hent RCh, Böhmer CJ, et al. Combining autofluorescence imaging and narrow-band imaging for the differentiation of adenomas from non-neoplastic colonic polyps among experienced and non-experienced endoscopists. *Am J Gastroenterol.* 2009;104:1498-507.
84. Takeuchi Y. Autofluorescence imaging with a transparent hood for detection of colorectal neoplasms: a prospective, randomized trial. *Gastrointestinal Endoscopy.* 2010;72: 1006-13.
85. Wallace MB, Meining A, Canto MI, Fockens P, Miehlke S, Roesch T, et al. The safety of intravenous fluorescein for confocal laser endomicroscopy in the gastrointestinal tract. *Aliment Pharmacol Ther.* 2010;31:548-52.
86. Kiesslich R, Gossner L, Goetz M, Dahlmann A, Vieth M, Stolte M, et al. In vivo histology of Barrett's esophagus and associated neoplasia by confocal laser endomicroscopy. *Clin Gastroenterol Hepatol.* 2006;4:979-87.
87. Kiesslich R, Burg J, Vieth M, Gnaendiger J, Enders M, Delaney P, et al. Confocal laser endoscopy for diagnosing intraepithelial neoplasias and colorectal cancer in vivo. *Gastroenterology.* 2004;127:706-13.
88. Kiesslich R, Goetz M, Lammersdorf K, Schneider C, Burg J, Stolte M, et al. Chromoscopy-guided endomicroscopy increases the diagnostic yield of intraepithelial neoplasia in ulcerative colitis. *Gastroenterology.* 2007;132:874-82.
89. Buchner AM, Shahid MW, Heckman MG, Krishna M, Ghabril M, Hasan M, et al. Comparison of probe-based confocal laser endomicroscopy with virtual chromoendoscopy for classification of colon polyps. *Gastroenterology.* 2010;138:834-42.
90. Sanduleanu S, Driessen A, Gomez-Garcia E, Hameeteman W, de Bruïne A, Masclee A. In vivo diagnosis and classification of colorectal neoplasia by chromoendoscopy-guided confocal laser endomicroscopy. *Clin Gastroenterol Hepatol.* 2010;8:371-8.
91. Sasajima K, Kudo SE, Inoue H, Takeuchi T, Kashida H, Hidaka E, et al. Real-time in vivo virtual histology of colorectal lesions when using the endocytoscopy system. *Gastrointest Endosc.* 2006;63:1010-7.
92. Rabeneck L, Paszat LF, Hilsden RJ, Saskin R, Leddin D, Grunfeld E, et al. Bleeding and perforation after outpatient colonoscopy and their risk factors in usual clinical practice. *Gastroenterology.* 2008;135:1899-906.

13 Endoscopic Resection of Advanced Mucosal Neoplasia and Early Cancer in the Colon

Michael Bourke

ABSTRACT

Colon cancer is the third most common cause of cancer and cancer deaths. Colon cancer screening and surveillance has reduced the incidence of colorectal cancer and has led to the detection of more early stage neoplasia. Early stage colon cancer can be managed safely by endoscopic methods. These methods involve assessment of the colonic lesion, excision by endoscopic resection, or submucosal dissection, followed by continued surveillance. There is a wide variation in the use of these methods worldwide. The Western world has favored endoscopic resection, while endoscopic submucosal dissection has been limited to Japan and parts of Asia. This chapter deals with the pros and cons of both the techniques.

INTRODUCTION

Colonoscopy and colonoscopic polypectomy are critical therapies in the prevention and treatment of colorectal cancer. Mathematical modeling suggests that colonoscopic polypectomy reduces the anticipated incidence of colorectal malignancy in patients with significant adenomas by approximately 80% in long-term follow-up.[1-3] With the advent of worldwide colorectal cancer screening and the rapid increase in colonoscopy utilization, many more adenomas and early stage colorectal cancers are being detected. Between 80 and 90% of polyps are ≤10 mm in size, and endoscopic treatment has been the accepted standard for more than three decades. They do not pose a significant challenge to an appropriately trained and skilled colonoscopist.[4] However, the assessment and treatment of larger lesions greater than 20 mm in maximum dimension is an evolving field of knowledge.

Recent data confirm that most patients with large refractory or difficult polyps enrolled on an intention-to-treat (ITT) basis can be safely and effectively treated endoscopically. A small percentage subsequently found to have invasive cancer or technically unresectable lesions and required surgical review, but ultimately more than 90% of patients avoid surgery with substantial clinical gains and major cost savings of approximately 6 hospital days and US$ 7000 per patient treated.[5] In the past, these patients were simply referred for surgery, and anecdotally in 2010, this probably was the most commonly utilized treatment, particularly in the West.[6,7] However, colonic surgery may be associated with significant morbidity and potential mortality, especially amongst those of advanced age or significant comorbidity.[8-10] Thirty days mortality is in the order of 4%, and in contrast to other major surgical procedures, this is largely independent of hospital or individual surgeon case volume, primarily reflecting the physiological impact of the surgery and the clinical status of the patients rather than any technical challenge related to the surgery.

LESION ASSESSMENT

Large sessile or flat lesions of the colon are best described according to the Paris system of endoscopic classification of superficial neoplastic lesions (Figure 13-1).[11,12] This classification system is now widely used in Japan. Application of a widely accepted reproducible classification system has numerous potential advantages, including standardization of polyp morphology descriptions and improved lesion categorization. By improving lesion categorization, a better understanding of the variations in lesion characteristics and biology is achieved, and lesion-specific treatment and surveillance algorithms

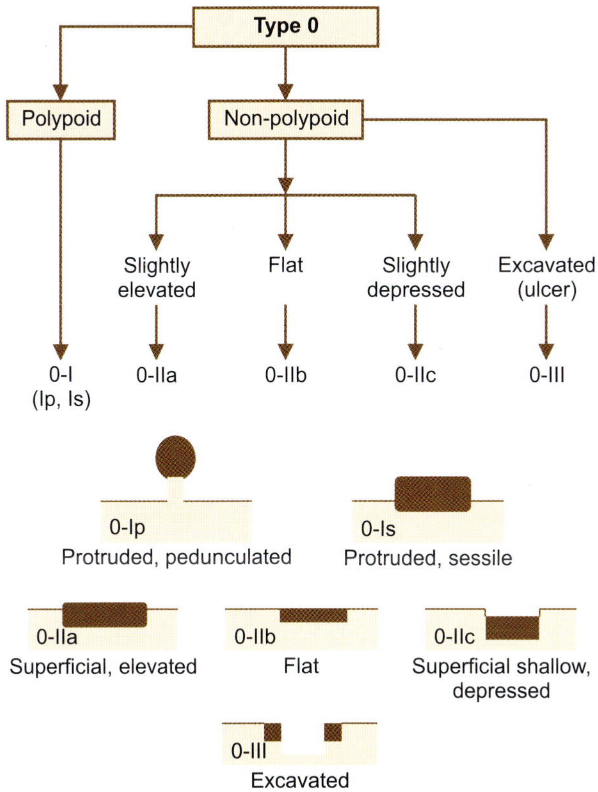

FIGURE 13-1 Paris classification. Schematic representation of the major variants of type 0 neoplastic lesions of the digestive tract: polypoid (Ip and Is), non-polypoid (IIa, IIb, and IIc), non-polypoid and excavated (III). Terminology as proposed in a consensus macroscopic description of superficial neoplastic lesions (Reproduced from the Paris classification of superficial neoplastic lesions).

can be developed.[13] Within the Paris system, polypoid lesions may be pedunculated (0-Ip), sessile (0-Is), or with a mixed pattern (0-Isp). Nonpolypoid lesions are either slightly elevated, termed 0-IIa (elevation <2.5 mm above the level of the mucosa), completely flat (0-IIb), or uncommonly slightly depressed (0-IIc). In addition, 0-IIa and 0-IIb lesions are ≥10 mm in diameter with a low vertical axis, but they are extending laterally along the interior luminal wall and are termed laterally spreading tumors (LSTs). LSTs may be either adenomas or serrated lesions. Adenomatous LSTs are further subclassified according to their surface morphology as either granular (G) or smooth nongranular (NG) (Figures 13-2 and 13-3). The application of this classification system has important implications for the risk of submucosal invasion (SMI).[14,15] Currently, Western endoscopists tend to group 0-Is, 0-Isp and 0-IIa lesions together, which are then simply described as 'sessile.' 0-IIb lesions may also be included in this group or described as being flat, although they are not frequently detected. Little attention is paid to the surface morphology, although large granular LSTs may be described as 'carpet lesions.' Such a simplification and unified grouping of all these different types of lesions with their differing tumor biology has retarded progress in understanding.[13] In addition, failure to detect these various flat lesions, which have a predilection for the right colon may explain the lack of protection conferred by screening colonoscopy in preventing right sided cancer in contrast to the clear benefits in the left colon, where there is a significant reduction with a relative risk of 0.33, when compared to non-screened aged matched controls.[16,17]

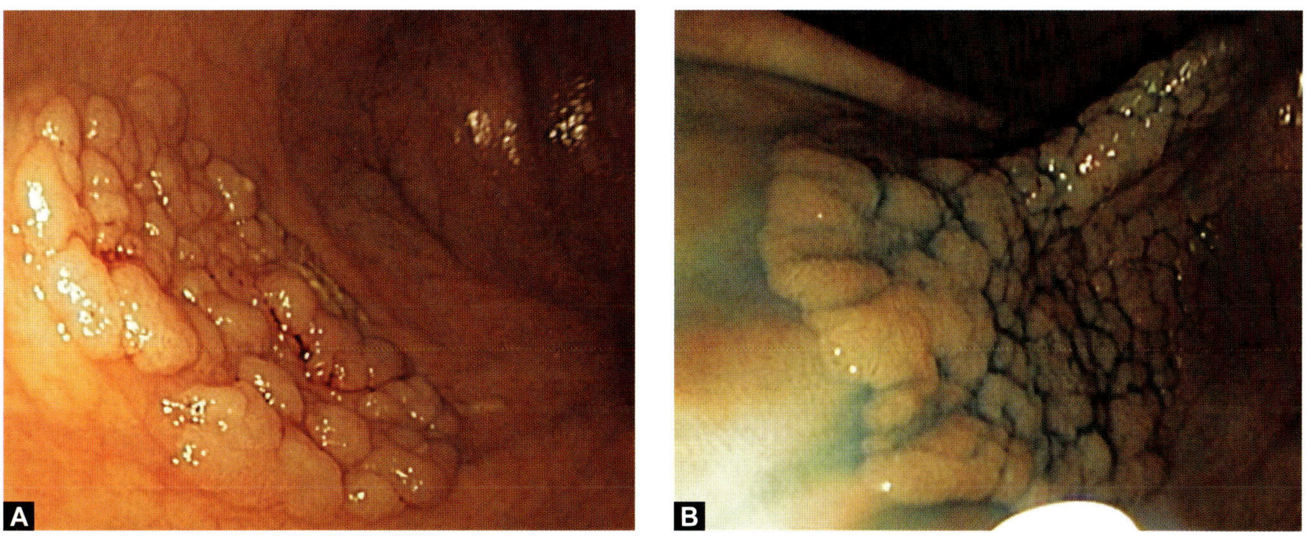

FIGURE 13-2 Paris 0-IIa granular laterally spreading tumors. **A,** Under white light endoscopy. **B,** After indigo carmine spray.

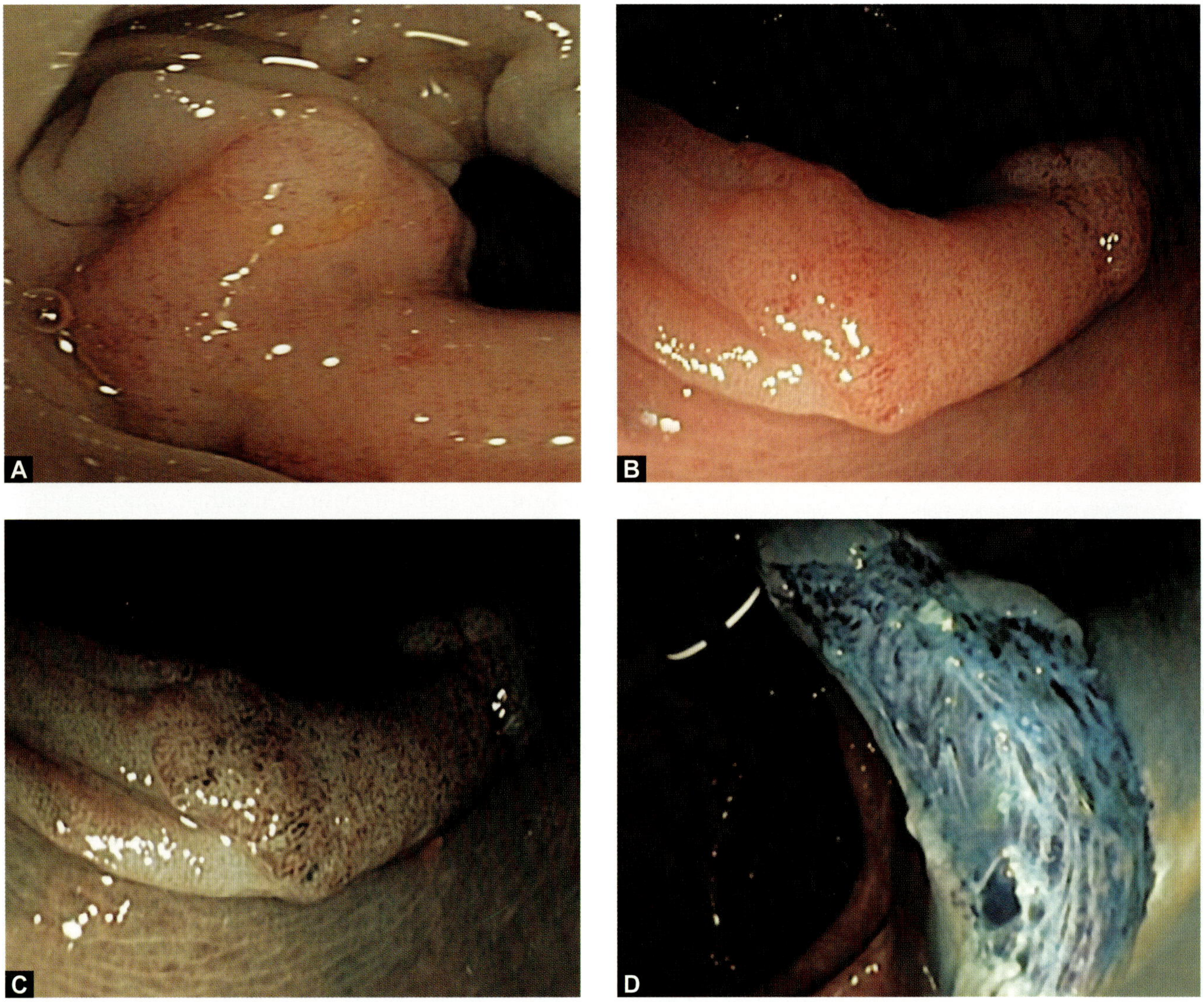

FIGURE 13-3 Paris 0-IIa nongranular laterally spreading tumor. **A,** Under white light endoscopy. **B,** Under magnification endoscopy. **C,** Under narrow band imaging. **D,** After endoscopic resection.

Amongst lesions greater than 20 mm (excluding obvious invasive cancer), a large prospective multicenter study, the Australian Colonic Endoscopic Resection Study (ACE) (n > 600) has recorded lesion morphology as follows: 0-IIa: 45%, 0-Is: 33%, and 0-IIa + Is: 15%. 0-IIa + Ic (flat lesions with central depression) and 0-IIb (completely flat lesions) each account for between 3 and 5% of the total. Approximately 90% of 0-IIa and 0-IIa + Is lesions are G in morphology.[15] Combining lesion granularity and morphology is very useful in predicting the risk of SMI. A homogeneous 0-IIa G lesion has a risk of SMI of approximately 1% in both Japanese and Western cohorts.[14,15] In contrast, 0-IIa + c NG lesions have the greatest risk of SMI at approximately 67% (relative risk 54; $p < 0.001$). The risk of SMI in 0-IIa NG lesions without a depressed component is intermediate at 15–20%. Amongst 0-IIa + Is lesion, the risk of SMI is 10–15%, and if it occurs, it is most frequently beneath the Is component.[14] Thus, resection of this component first, and as large as possible, is advocated if piecemeal excision is planned for a 0-IIa + Is lesion. If at all feasible, this specimen should be retrieved separately for histopathological analysis.

Kudo pit pattern should also be employed to further characterize lesions. In the era of high-resolution endoscopes and narrow band imaging (NBI) and other "push button" enhanced imaging systems, there is an ongoing debate as to whether clinically relevant assessment of epithelial microarchitecture requires the addition of magnification.[18] This is not routinely used in the colon by most Western endoscopists.[19] This is discussed in detail in Chapter 12: Endoscopic Imaging of Colorectal Polyps and Cancer. Pit pattern type IV is the predominant finding in G LSTs. Type III is seen in NG lesions as is type V. Pit pattern type V reliably predicts SMI, whereas type III generally implies noninvasive disease.[20,21]

ENDOSCOPIC RESECTION

General Principles

Endoscopic mucosal resection (EMR), which is also known as endoscopic resection (ER), was first described by Deyhle et al.[22] in 1973 as an endoscopic technique for resecting sessile colonic polyps. The technique involves injecting a liquid solution (usually normal saline) into the submucosal layer of the colon wall. This expands the submucosal space and elevates the polyp, providing a safety cushion, heat sink, and an expanded plane of resection, allowing safe snare excision of the lesion. Since the technique involves deliberate excision of the superficial layer of the submucosa in addition to the mucosa, some believe that EMR is a misnomer, and the term ER should be used instead.

Endoscopic submucosal dissection (ESD) is an alternative technique developed for en bloc upper gastrointestinal (GI) lesion excision in Japan and is now being applied to special situations in the colon. It will be discussed in a later section.

The goal of ER is to remove the entire lesion in as few pieces as safely possible. For lesions of maximum dimension, 20–25 mm in the right colon and 25–30 mm in the left colon (particularly rectum), en bloc or Ro resection should be considered but may not always be technically possible. In the colon, Ro excision should be consistently achievable for lesions less than 20 mm in maximum dimension. En bloc resection has many proven and theoretical advantages, including more accurate histological assessment, negligible recurrence, and potential cure in low risk submucosal invasive disease.[13] In the colon, if the depth of SMI is less than 1000 microns (termed SM1), the tumor is histologically well differentiated, and there is no lymphovascular invasion, then Ro endoscopic excision is curative.[23-25] This is particularly advantageous in those patients of advanced age or significant comorbidity, where the risk of surgery is substantial. Modifications of standard EMR technique may enhance the limits of en bloc resection (see later sections).

During piecemeal ER, if each resection is considered as an opportunity for error at the interface between successive excisions due to incomplete excision leading to recurrence, or overlap between successive resections with potential transmural injury, then excising the lesion in as few pieces as safely possible is clearly logical. The greater the number of pieces for any given piecemeal ER, the greater the total perimeter of excision becomes, and hence the greater the opportunity for error. A convenient means of comparing ER efficacy for lesions of varying dimensions is to divide the lesion size by the number of pieces required to completely resect it. This is termed the Sydney resection quotient.[26] A lesion of a given size resected in a fewer pieces gives a larger value and by inference, a safer and more efficacious outcome.

Equipment

Snare selection is to some extent an individual choice, but stiff type snares have clear advantages for tissue capture. We prefer a snare with a serrated wire to facilitate entrapment of normal tissue at the margin of the lesion. A range of sizes and configurations is required including oval, round, and hexagonal from 10 to 20 mm for flat lesions. For large pedunculated and bulky exophytic lesions, large snares of 3 × 6 cm, oval or hexagonal, are necessary. The 20 mm spiral snare is our standard instrument for large en bloc (15–20 mm and above) and extensive piecemeal ER. The diameter of the wire is 0.48 mm. Small residuals at the margins are excised using a thin wire mini oval snare. The smaller wire diameter of 0.3 mm facilitates better tissue capture in this case.

Microprocessor-controlled electrosurgical generators capable of delivering alternating cycles of high frequency short pulse cutting with more prolonged coagulation current are required. These generators sense tissue impedance via signals from the return electrode and adjust power output accordingly. In the authors view, generators without these features do not provide an acceptable level of electrosurgical safety for extensive and complex ER.

Injection Solution

The ideal solution should be inexpensive, readily available, nontoxic, easy to prepare and inject, and provide a long-lasting submucosal cushion.[27] Ideally, it should also provide a well circumscribed rather than diffuse elevation and thus, a substantial difference in elevation between the target lesion and the uninvolved non-neoplastic surrounding tissue.[28] This greatly facilitates the technical ease of resection.

Although normal saline is most commonly used, there are a wide variety of alternatives, each with their own limitations, reflecting the absence of a clearly superior solution. Normal saline's advantages include ease of use, isotonicity, nonallergenicity, and lack of toxicity, if injected transmurally. However, the submucosal cushion is relatively short-lived and the mucosal elevation is not as marked as other products, nor as well circumscribed. It is also limited by its dispersion within the submucosal plane, and thus it is unable to achieve a well circumscribed tissue elevation. Numerous alternatives, including hyaluronic acid, hydroxypropylmethyl cellulose, glycerol, fibrinogen, hypertonic saline, dextrose, and/or autologous blood are limited by expense, complex prepatory requirements, localized tissue inflammation and damage, and administration difficulties.[27,29] Succinylated gelatin (SG) is a widely available inexpensive safe colloidal solution that is commonly used for intravenous fluid resuscitation. It exerts an oncotic pressure comparable to that of human albumin. In a blinded randomized *in vivo* porcine study, when compared to normal saline, SG resulted in a 42% increase in the surface area for en bloc EMR.[29] In a randomized double blind human trial of colonic ER in 80 patients with lesions ≥20 mm, when compared to normal saline, SG greatly improved technical outcomes, including significantly few injections, a lower injection volume, a 50% reduction in procedure time, and a more than doubling of the Sydney resection quotient. There was also a doubling of the en bloc resection rate from 15 to 30%, but this did not reach statistical significance most likely due to underpowering.[26]

A biologically inert blue dye, such as indigo carmine in a concentration of 0.04% (equating to 1 mL from the standard 4 mg/L solution) is used in the injection solution. The benefits are three-fold:[30]

- The dye defines the perimeter of the lesion. This is especially beneficial in subtle pathology where the neoplasm may merge imperceptibly with the surrounding mucosa, for example, 0-IIb NG lesions or sessile serrated adenomas. This eliminates the need for preresection thermal marking of the margins of the target, which is usually not necessary in the colon
- The blue coloration delineates the extent of the submucosal cushion, thus, defining the safe ER zone
- Dyes, such as indigo carmine and methylene blue are avid for the loose areolar connective tissue of the submucosa, staining this layer blue. This is very helpful to confirm that one is working in the correct tissue plane. The dye is not taken up by the muscularis propria and thus, if this plane is entered, a disruption to the almost uniformly blue appearance will be seen.

Dilute epinephrine in a concentration of 1:100,000 is also added to the injection solution. It has no role in preventing delayed bleeding but is useful for creating a bloodless field during ER, analogous to its use in cutaneous surgery. Small amounts of bleeding during the resection disrupt the endoscopic view. The epinephrine by its local vasoconstrictive action may also limit dispersion of the submucosal injection solution, and thus potentially enhance the magnitude and duration of tissue elevation.

Injection Technique

The first few submucosal injections set the stage for a successful procedure, and great care should be taken at this point. Poorly placed or excessive injections, particularly within relatively narrow lumens (e.g., stenosing sigmoid diverticular disease) may create major difficulties and potentially render the procedure impossible. A carefully placed submucosal injection should make the procedure easier by lifting the lesion out into the lumen and towards the colonoscope. This is particularly important for poorly accessible lesions located on the proximal sides of folds or within tight angulations. A transparent short cap can be used to deflect folds and facilitate access to the proximal aspect of lesions saddling folds. For extensive piecemeal ER, we prefer a sequential inject and resect technique and thus avoid elevating the entire lesion at the outset. We perform one or two resections each 1–2 sequential injections. Elevating the entirety of a large lesion (>40 mm) may create difficulty with access but also excessive tension within the cushion limiting purchase of the snare and decreasing the size of sequential piecemeal resections.

Where access is unrestricted and en bloc excision is being considered (<25–30 mm from distal colon and rectum and <20–25 mm from right colon), the injection is pressed to elevate the lesion towards the colonoscope.

Procedure

- Divide the lesion into three and make the initial injection at the junction of the middle and furthest third (from the scope tip)
- Position the needle tip tangentially to the mucosal surface and gently touch the surface
- Ask your assistant to commence the injection whilst simultaneously "stabbing" the mucosa with the

needle tip by a rapid 1–2 cm movement with the right hand holding the injection catheter. This technique accesses the submucosal plane swiftly and accurately

- The correct plane is confirmed by an immediate elevation of the mucosa. Ongoing injection without tissue elevation or intraluminal fluid escape indicates transmural placement of the needle tip with extramural injection. Slowly withdraw the needle and the tissue should elevate
- Pull back slightly on the injection catheter or colonoscope whilst maintaining the position of the needle tip in the submucosal plane. This will reduce the deformity on the mucosal surface and maximize fluid deposition immediately beneath the lesion, limiting dispersion of the fluid cushion beyond the perimeter of the lesion. You may even gently rotate the mucosa (which is impaled on the needle tip) out into the lumen by torque on the endoscope shaft
- After satisfactory tissue elevation (usually a 5–8 mL submucosal injection), resect this area first
- In cases of submucosal fibrosis where the needle tip is placed correctly, but the submucosal plane is obliterated by fibrosis, a “jet sign” (Figure 13-4) may be seen; a jet of fluid exits the lesion at high pressure
- Alternatively, a canyoning effect may occur where the lesion remains anchored in its original position but the tissue of the perimeter elevates. The injection should be terminated immediately. The peripheral elevation will make the lesion very difficult to access, ensnare, and resect

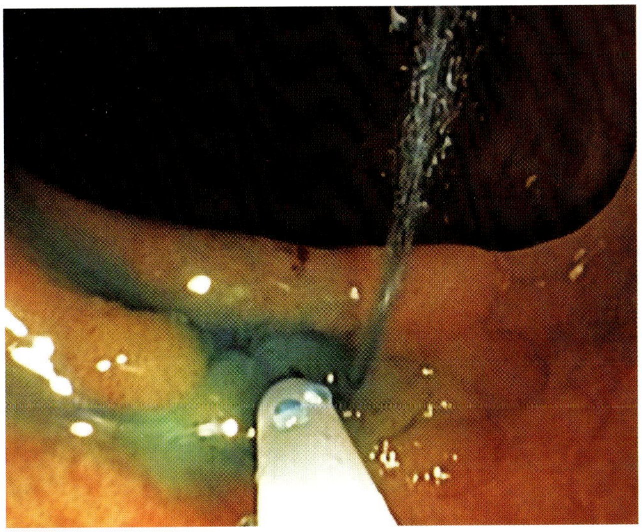

FIGURE 13-4 Jet sign. When the submucosal plane is obliterated by fibrosis, a jet of fluid exits the lesion at high pressure during injection.

- For more extensive lesions, beyond or straddling haustral folds or angulations, plan to resect the least accessible area first and use the first injection to facilitate access to this area.

Resection Technique

After careful lesion assessment, an endoscopic resection plan is loosely formulated, taking into account the orientation, size, and position of the lesion in relation to the endoscope and its location in the colon. Generally, a more aggressive approach can be adopted in the rectum, whereas great care needs to be taken in the cecum. Plan to remove the lesion in as few pieces, as safely as possible. En bloc and oligopiecemeal resections create fewer opportunities for error, more accurate histological assessment, and theoretically, a reduced risk of recurrence in comparison to when lesions are removed in numerous pieces (polypiecemeal excision). Figures 13-5 to 13-11 provide illustrative examples of ER of lesions of varying sizes, locations, and morphology.

Procedure

- Orientate the target so that it is in the 5–6 o’clock position
- Resect the most inaccessible and difficult aspect first
- Work sequentially from the point of first entry into the submucosal plane using the edge of the defect as the base for subsequent piecemeal resections
- Excise a 2–3 mm margin of normal tissue at the edge of the lesion. This eliminates the risk of small amounts of residual tissue at the edge of the defect. These can be difficult to treat
- Align the snare at the edge of the advancing mucosal defect to minimize occurrence of tissue islands within the defect. These are difficult to remove subsequently
- Open the snare completely above your target and push down firmly on the fluid cushion with the up/down control whilst aspirating air. Deflating the lumen reduces colonic wall tension and decreases the footprint of the neoplasm on that wall, maximizing tissue capture
- Close the snare tightly. If a spiral or serrated snare of more than 10 mm diameter is used, it is not possible to resect the tissue without the use of diathermy. Individual snares have different handling characteristics. Endoscopists who perform advanced ER should become familiar with the performance characteristics of their preferred snares. We use 20 mm spiral snare as the general work horse of

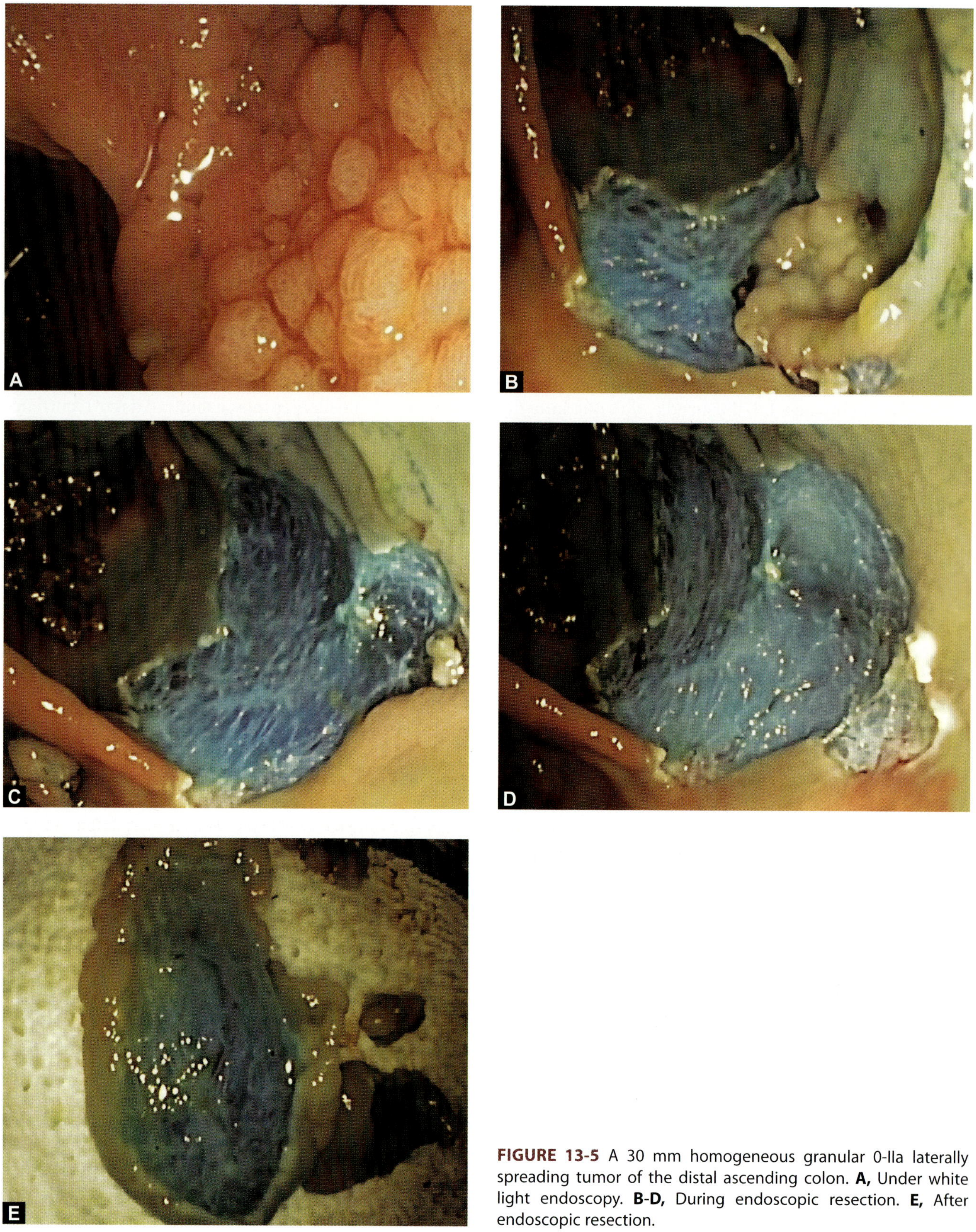

FIGURE 13-5 A 30 mm homogeneous granular 0-IIa laterally spreading tumor of the distal ascending colon. **A,** Under white light endoscopy. **B-D,** During endoscopic resection. **E,** After endoscopic resection.

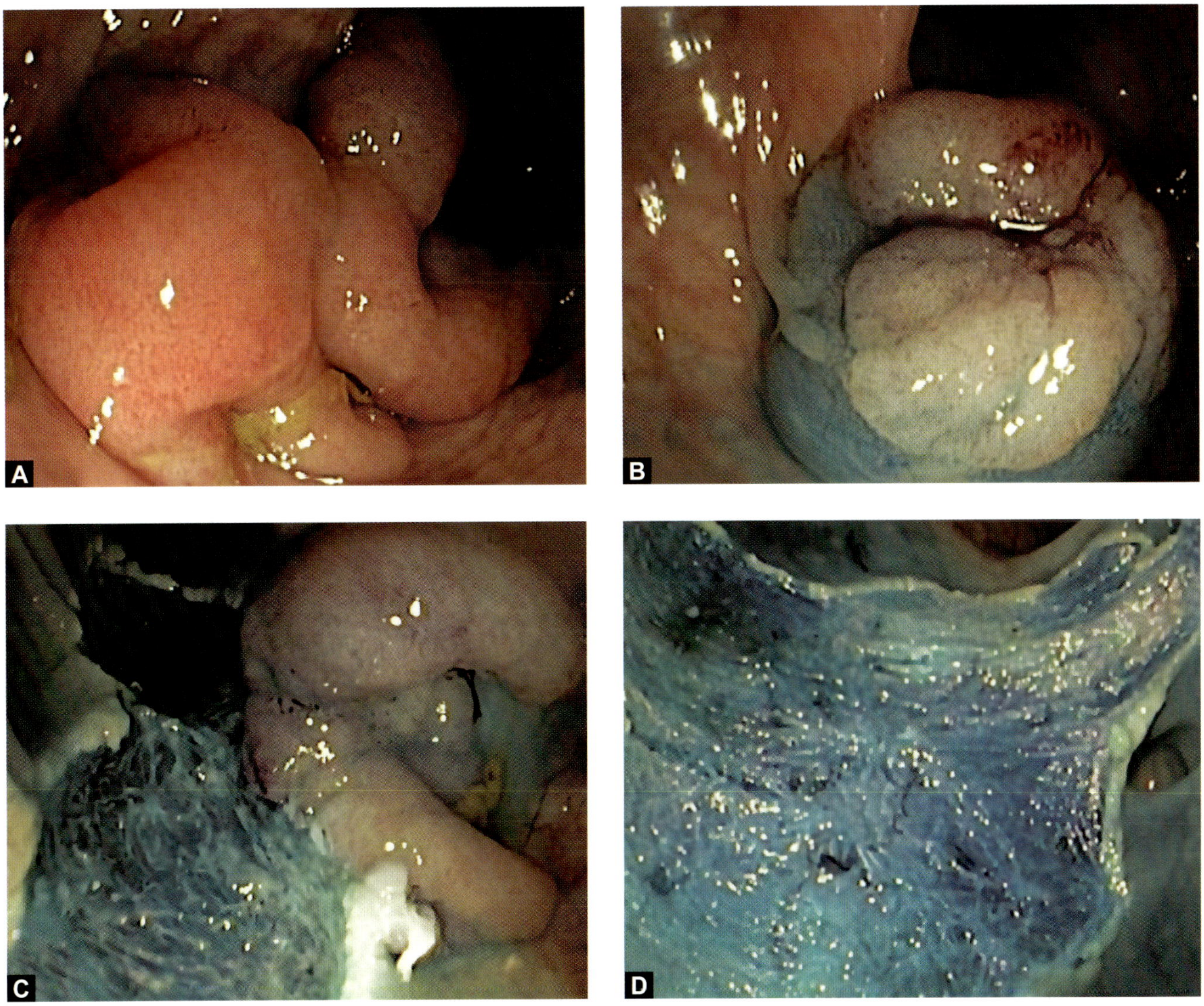

FIGURE 13-6 A 45 mm hemicircumference 0-IIa + Is nongranular laterally spreading tumor of descending colon. **A,** Before resection under white light endoscopy. **B,** After raising with saline. **C,D,** After endoscopic resection.

extended piecemeal and en bloc EMR. Closing the snare maximally excludes muscularis propria from the captured tissue, analogous to the use of rubber band ligation during multiband mucosectomy in the esophagus. As endoscopists, we prefer to close the snare handle ourselves during the final transection phase. The sensory feedback is invaluable to inform on the safety and efficacy of the excision. Safe tissue capture is confirmed by three maneuvers:[28,30]

1. Assessing mobility of the ensnared tissue relative to the adjacent colonic wall—the captured tissue should be able to move back and forth quickly and seemingly slide a short distance over the surface of the colon
2. The degree of closure of the snare handle—for a spiral snare, the snare handle should be such that the distance between the thumb and fingers is less than 1 cm
3. The speed of transection—this phase should be short lived. The snare is kept tightly closed whilst the foot pedal is depressed. With a microprocessor controlled generator, between 1 and 3 pulses transect the tissue. A more prolonged transection phase indicates either potential entrapment of the muscularis propria or deeper neoplastic invasion. In the right colon, we generally tap the pedal, essentially cutting the tissue from the colonic wall in a fashion similar to ESD.

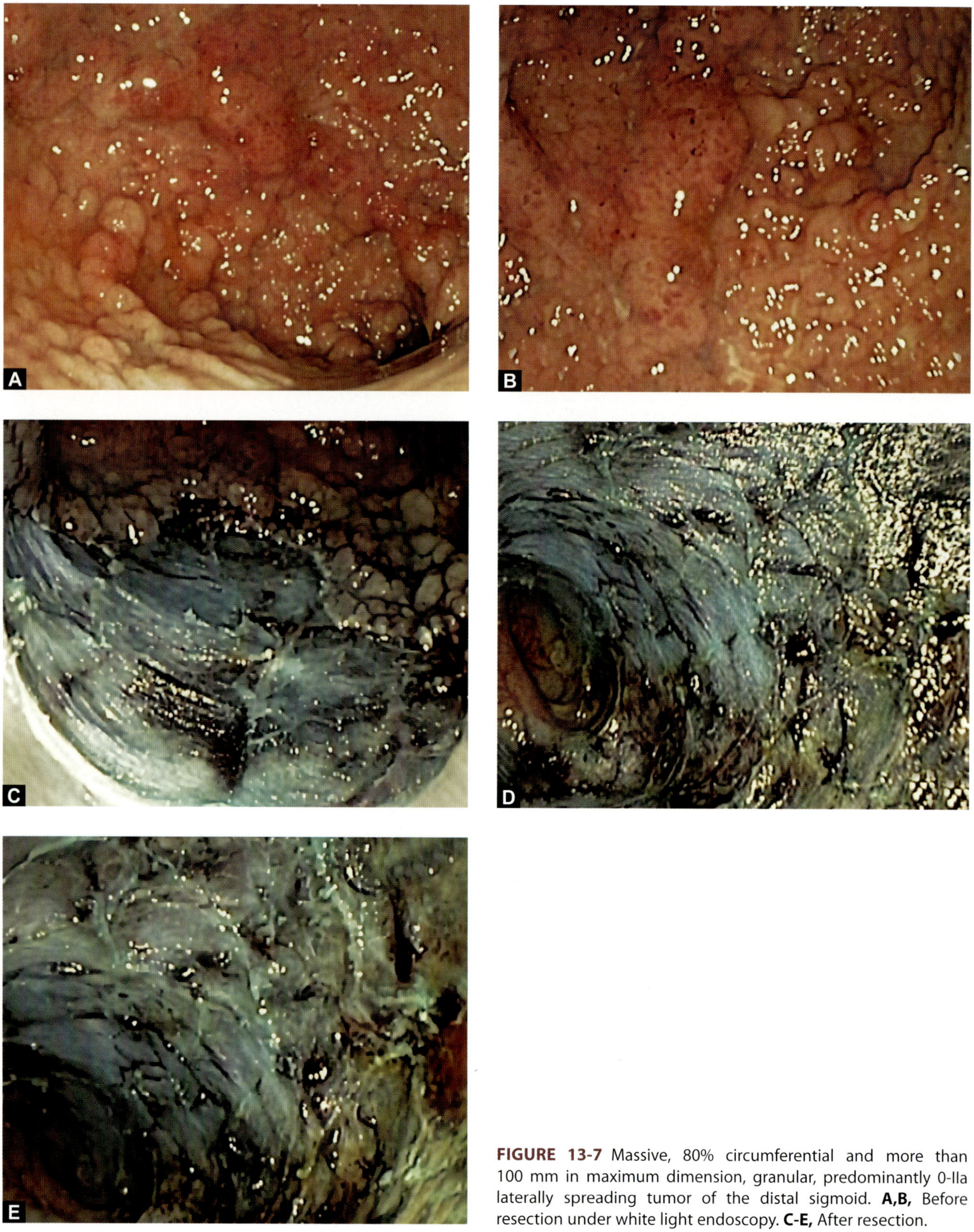

FIGURE 13-7 Massive, 80% circumferential and more than 100 mm in maximum dimension, granular, predominantly 0-IIa laterally spreading tumor of the distal sigmoid. **A,B,** Before resection under white light endoscopy. **C-E,** After resection.

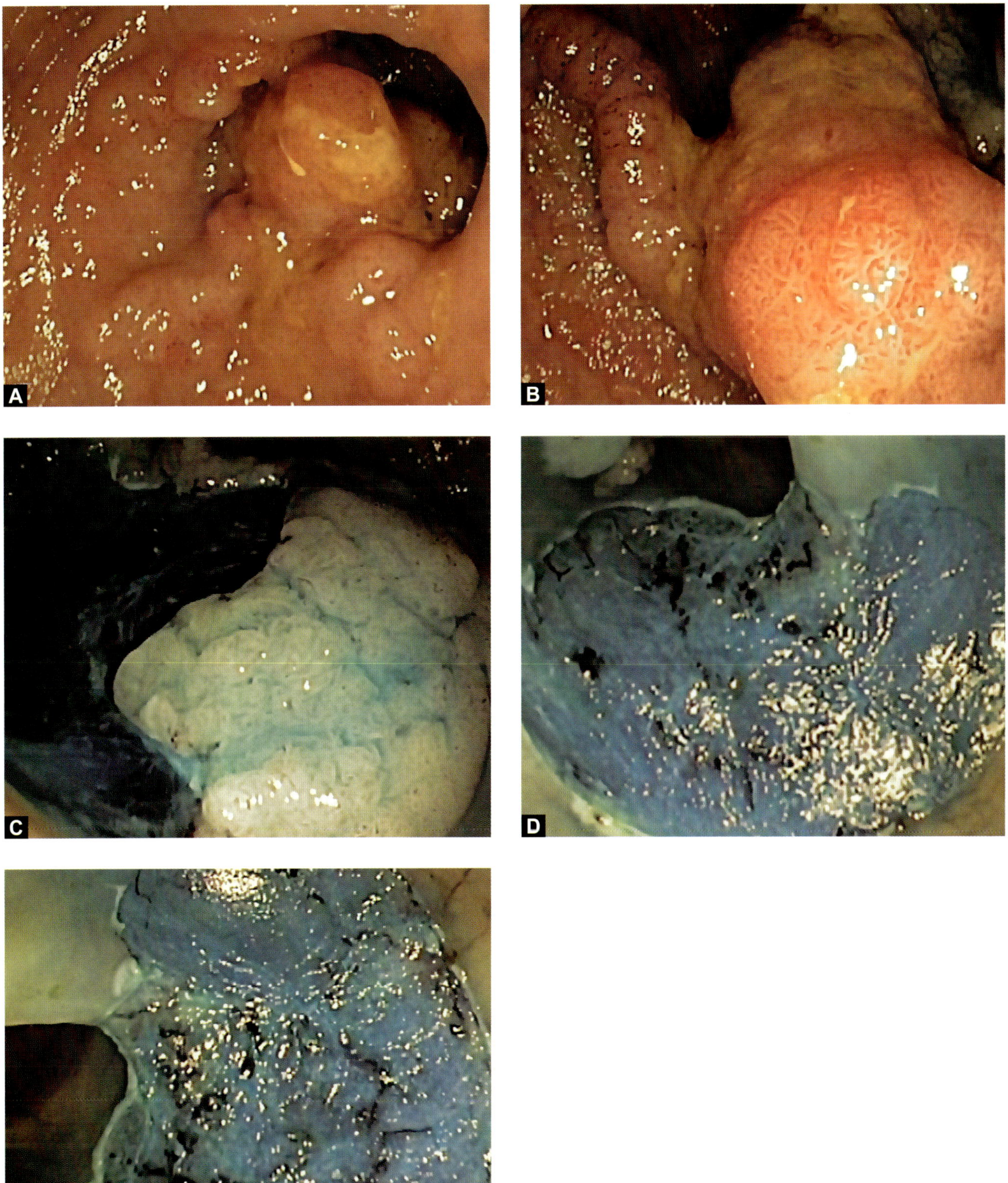

FIGURE 13-8 A 50 mm 0-IIa + Is granular lesion of the recto-sigmoid. **A,B,** Under white light endoscopy. **C,** During endoscopic resection. **D,E,** After endoscopic resection.

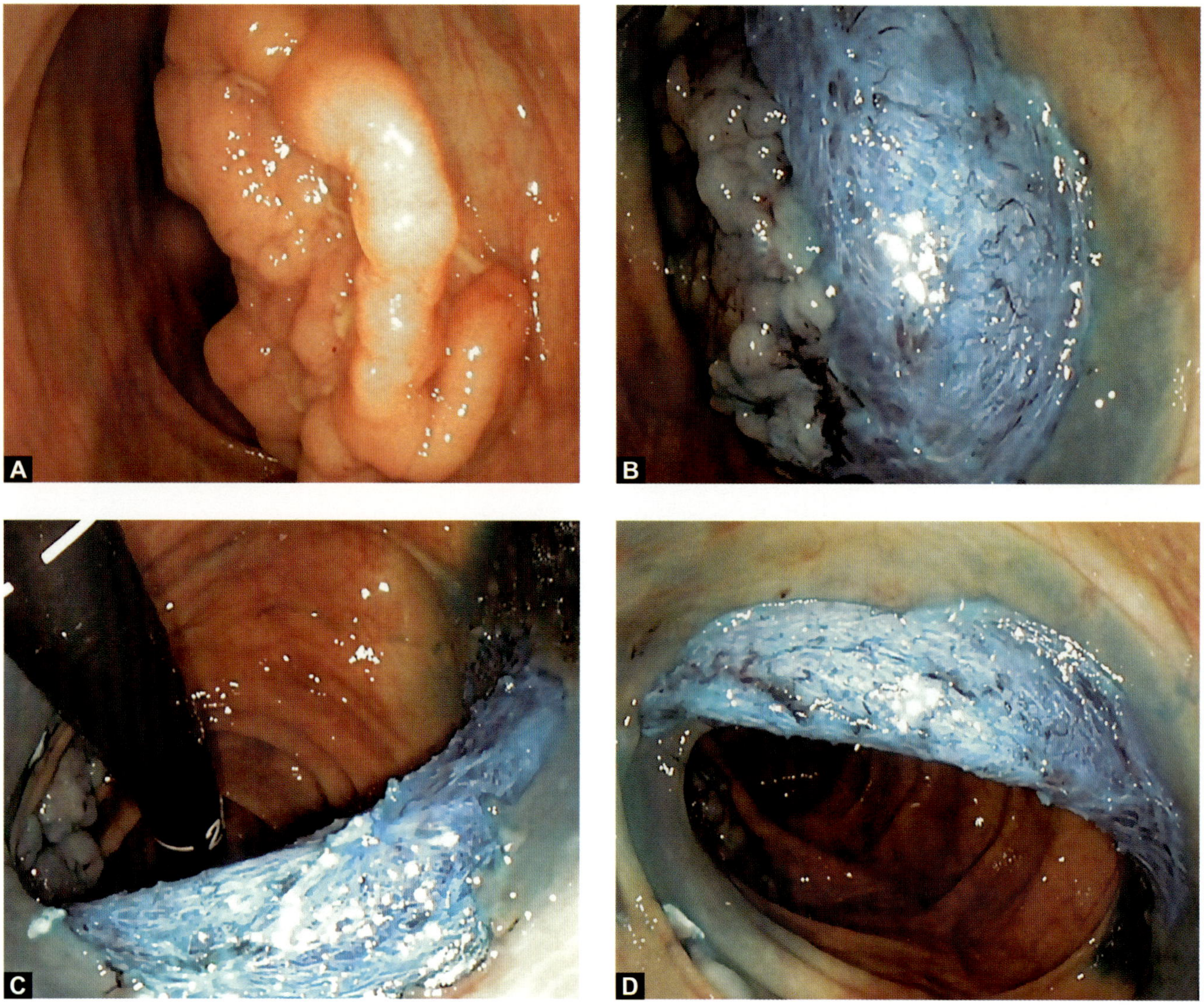

FIGURE 13-9 A 50 mm hemicircumferential saddle, granular laterally spreading tumor of the ascending colon. **A,** Under white light endoscopy. **B,** During endoscopic resection. **C,D,** After resection.

Specimen Processing, Postprocedural Care, and Endoscopic Follow-up

All specimens should be retrieved for histological assessment. Commercially available 2–3 cm nets are the best option for multiple specimen retrieval. With very extensive ER specimen, retrieval can be a challenge and may require several passages of the colonoscope. The larger 4 cm net is less maneuverable, and, whilst helpful with extensive polypiecemeal ER, it may be difficult to open completely in tight angulations, such as within the cecum. It almost completely occludes the 3.7 mm channel of the pediatric colonoscope, making aspiration of air and decompression of the distended colon during the final stages of the procedure difficult.

Those specimens larger than 15 mm should be flattened on a cork board and their margins pinned. Pinning of specimens (particularly after en bloc excision) prevents curling of the tissue within the formalin and facilitates more accurate histological assessment allowing the histopathologist to report on lateral and deep margins of excision.

Location of the lesion should be precisely noted to facilitate accurate endoscopic follow-up. In the left

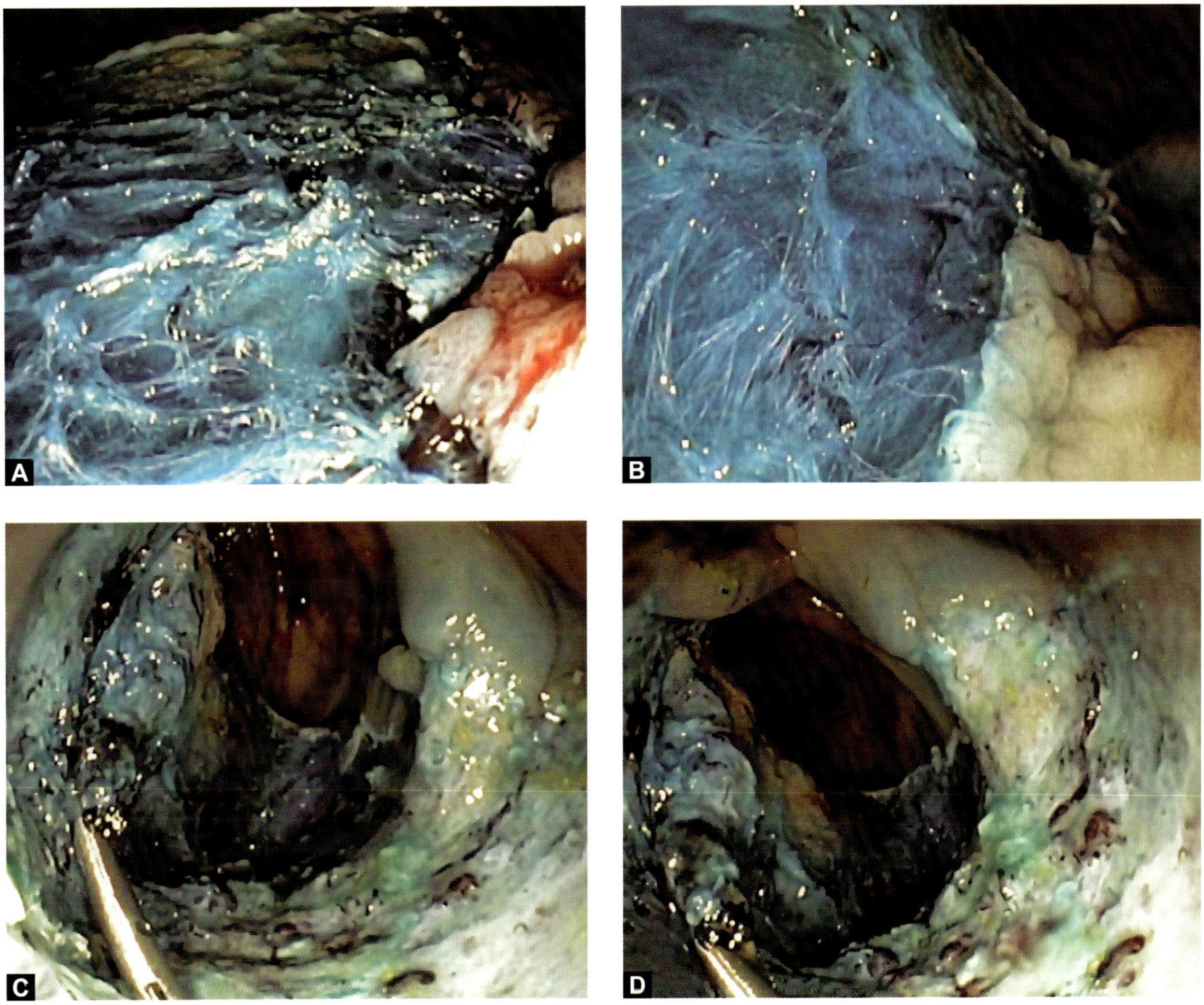

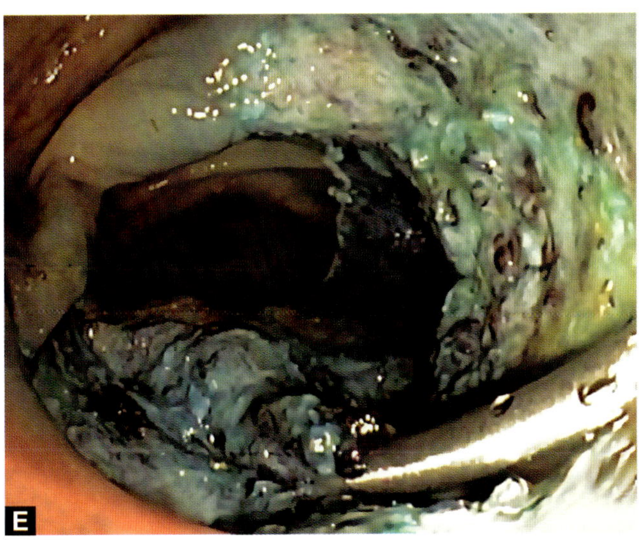

FIGURE 13-10 Massive (80 mm), more than 2/3rd circumferential, 0-IIa nongranular laterally spreading tumor, occupying most of the proximal ascending colon and involving the ileocecal valve. **A-E,** During and after endoscopic resection.

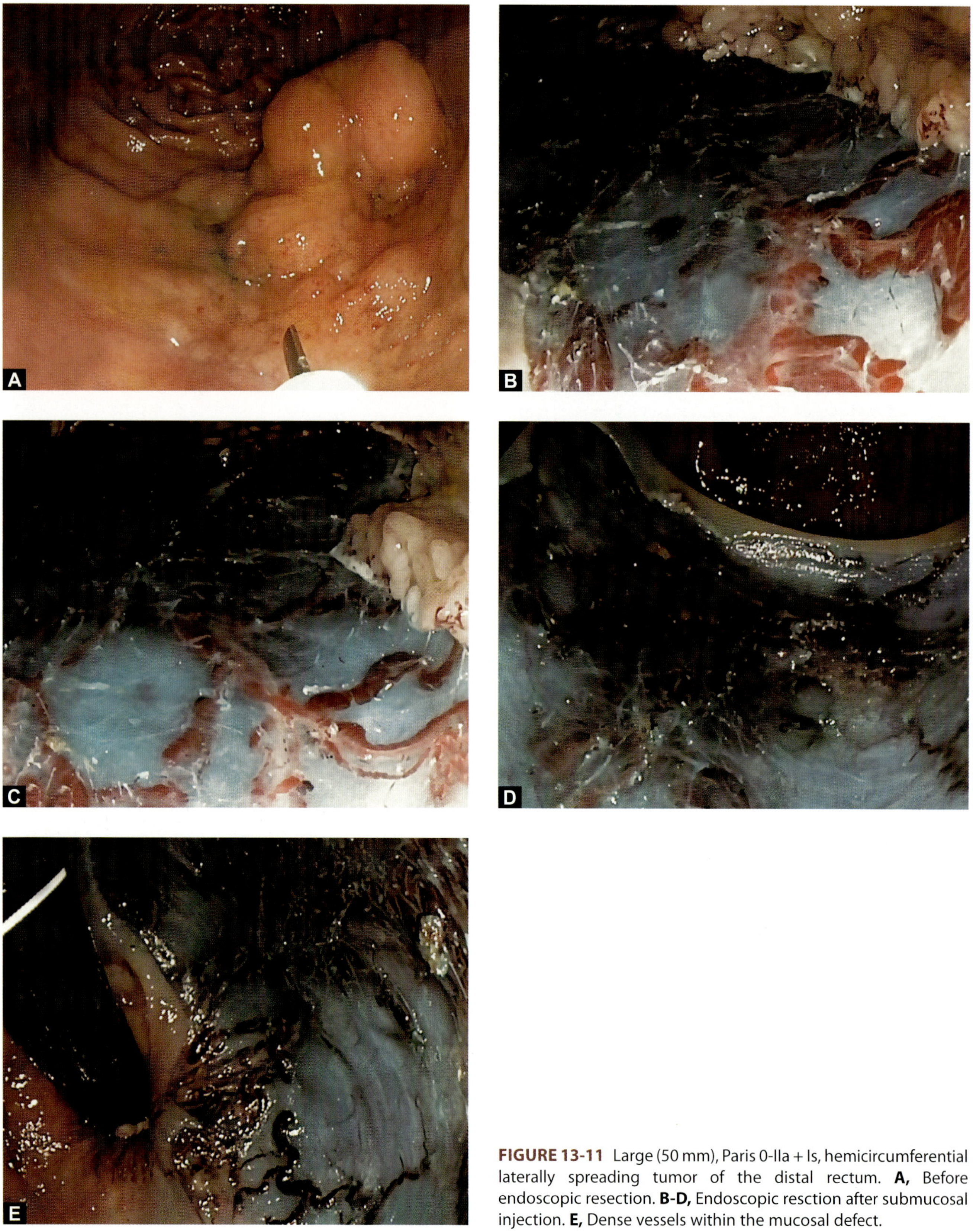

FIGURE 13-11 Large (50 mm), Paris 0-IIa + Is, hemicircumferential laterally spreading tumor of the distal rectum. **A,** Before endoscopic resection. **B-D,** Endoscopic resction after submucosal injection. **E,** Dense vessels within the mucosal defect.

colon, the anatomical location and the precise distance from the anus on withdrawal with a straight scope should be recorded. If the lesion is located beyond the fold in a difficult position to directly visualize, this must also be recorded. In the right colon (ascending colon and cecum), it is useful to note the number of folds above the fold of the ileocecal valve and the orientation with reference to the ileocecal valve, considering the valve as being on the medial wall in the 9 o'clock position. Thus, in reference to this, a 6 o'clock position would be the posterior wall of the ascending colon. For sites that will be difficult to localize subsequently, such as the transverse or sigmoid colon or medial wall of the distal ascending colon, marking the contralateral wall 2–3 cm distal to the ER site (to ensure that the submucosal carbon solution does not contaminate the ER site) with one or two injections of sterile carbon particle suspension is invaluable. It is important to avoid transmural injection, as carbon markers have been reported to cause fat necrosis, and a localized inflammatory reaction may cloud clinical interpretation after the procedure.[31] A 2-step injection technique is preferred. Saline is used to find the submucosal plane and create a small cushion, which can then be injected with the carbon suspension.[32]

After complex ER procedures, patients are kept nil by mouth for two hours and assessed in first stage recovery with abdominal examination before moving to second stage recovery. They remain for an additional 4 hours postprocedure on a clear liquid diet. If they are well at that point, they are discharged on a clear fluid diet overnight to commence a normal diet in the morning, provided they remain well. We perform all our complex ER procedures in the morning and retain the patients in the second stage recovery, where they can read or otherwise occupy themselves sitting in a comfortable chair for most of the day. This allows most of these patients to be managed as outpatients.[5,26] Where there is a clinical concern, patients are assessed and admitted to hospital as required.

After extensive ER, surveillance colonoscopy is undertaken at 4–6 months to directly assess the scar with both high resolution white light and NBI to look for any residual/recurrent disease, which can easily be treated at that time. If there is a residual, this is generally diminutive and unifocal and easily excised/ablated.[5] Subsequent to that, colonoscopy is repeated annually for the next three years, with direct visualization and biopsy of the scar, and with surveillance intervals gradually lengthening subsequent to that.

Summary of Colonic Endoscopic Resection, Outcomes, and Limitations

In the colon, the overwhelmingly predominant ER method is snare resection following submucosal injection, also termed EMR. Whilst colonic ER is known to be effective, a precise assessment of its efficacy in routine practice is lacking, as the majority of published studies are predominantly single center, often single operator, retrospective, and without an IIT case accrual methodology or comprehensive follow-up protocol.[33-36] Thus, the true denominator of lesions assessed to generate these study outcomes is not clear. A lesion-specific approach has not been defined, and limited data are available regarding the factors that are associated with successful ER.[13] For example, it seems logical that technical efficacy would vary between 0-IIa G and 0-IIb NG (completely flat) LSTs; however, this has not been prospectively studied.

The optimal technique of piecemeal ER for extensive lesions has not been defined. There is no expert consensus on whether the entire lesion should be elevated initially or whether a sequential inject and resect approach should be taken. Similarly, there is no agreement or evidence base on snare selection. Although normal saline solution is most commonly used, the optimal solution or the volume to be injected is not known, with wide variations in the amount used. The search for the ideal submucosal injection solution continues.[26,27,29,37] Complex lesion competencies, which would include extensive ER, have also not been determined. Large LSTs greater than 30 mm are uncommon and require special skills for safe removal.[5,38] They are best managed on a tertiary referral basis, but such pathways have not yet been developed or clearly defined.[39]

Most large studies from tertiary centers report technical success in the order of 100% with few major complications, no deaths, and perforation at a frequency of 0–2%.[33-36,40] Nearly all suffer from the limitations described above, particularly retrospective design and lack of comprehensive ITT enrolment. The ACE study[15,41] is a large national collaborative effort to address these deficiencies. Patients with colonic LSTs and large sessile polyps ≥20 mm were enrolled on an ITT basis with 60 demographic, endoscopic, and technical data points initially recorded and comprehensive clinical and/or endoscopic follow-up at 2 weeks, 4 months, and annually for 5 years. Till date, 600 patients have been enrolled and technical success for single session endoscopic resection is approximately 90%. Significant risk factors for failure include a previous attempt at ER and ileocecal valve involvement.

Despite these limitations, ER has been a very useful tool and clearly is the primary therapy in the management of large LSTs and sessile lesions in the colon. However, because there has been limited prospective study to refine the best practice approach, the optimal technique, including snare and solution selection, has not been defined and further substantial gains in technical efficacy for colonic ER might be reasonably anticipated.

Complications and Management

The most serious complications are nonspecific post-procedural pain, serositis, delayed bleeding, and perforation. Identification of high risk patients, early recognition of complications, and aggressive management ameliorate their frequency and severity.

Perforation and Serositis

Management of perforation commences before such a complication has occurred. It starts with a careful inspection of the resection defect.[42] The defect in the mucosa should appear as a relatively homogeneous blue expanse in which, on closer inspection, one can see a mat of white connective tissue fibers corresponding to the loose areolar tissue of the submucosa (Figure 13-12). This connective tissue is avid for the dyes used in the injection solution, hence, the characteristic blue staining.[5,30] Running across this blue expanse and sometimes herniating out (Figure 13-13), transversely oriented blood vessels can also be seen. They are predominantly small venules. After snare-based ER, usually the true muscle layer cannot be seen. Fibers that are well oriented and appear to run transversely across the lumen correspond to the inner circular muscle layer of the colon. Occasionally, these may be exposed during endoscopic resection.

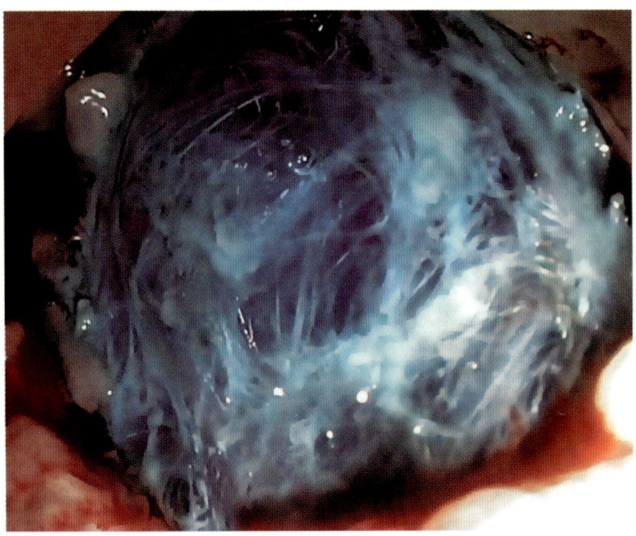

FIGURE 13-12 Exposed submucosa demonstrating a sponge-like mat of loose areolar connective tissue expanded by the injection solution.

If there is a concern for injury to the muscularis propria layer, this can be assessed in two ways:

1. Examining the undersurface of the resected specimens may reveal a small firm gray/white disk, which represents excised muscularis propria. This we term a "target sign" (Figure 13-14).[42] This finding should prompt careful inspection of the defect
2. A mirror target may also be evident within the mucosal defect and appreciated as a white cautery ring where the muscularis propria has been incised and excised (Figure 13-15). In cases of en bloc excision, this white cautery ring is of varying size and generally centrally placed. However, for extensive piecemeal resection, it may be located anywhere within the defect. The depth of injury may either be full or partial thickness, the latter may result in presentation after discharge with delayed perforation. The finding of a target or mirror target sign should prompt the endoscopist to completely close the mirror target defect with endoscopic clip application (Figure 13-16).

Postprocedural pain should prompt clinical examination for signs of peritonism. After extensive resection, nonspecific abdominal pain is not uncommon and may be due to:

- Excessive transmural fluid injection—generally no localizing signs are found. This usually resolves with simple analgesia
- Serositis—localized signs of peritonism may be present
- Gaseous distension of the colon and small bowel (in cases of incompetent ileocecal valve—endoscopic decompression of the colon will not improve pain). CO_2 insufflation has a clear clinical advantage in long ER procedures
- Perforation—signs are usually progressive, but presentation may be delayed.

Ongoing pain should prompt radiological assessment and surgical review. The finding of free intraperitoneal or subdiaphragmatic air on plain X-rays is uncommon.[43,44] Computed tomography is more sensitive and is required, if symptoms continue. Multidisciplinary management

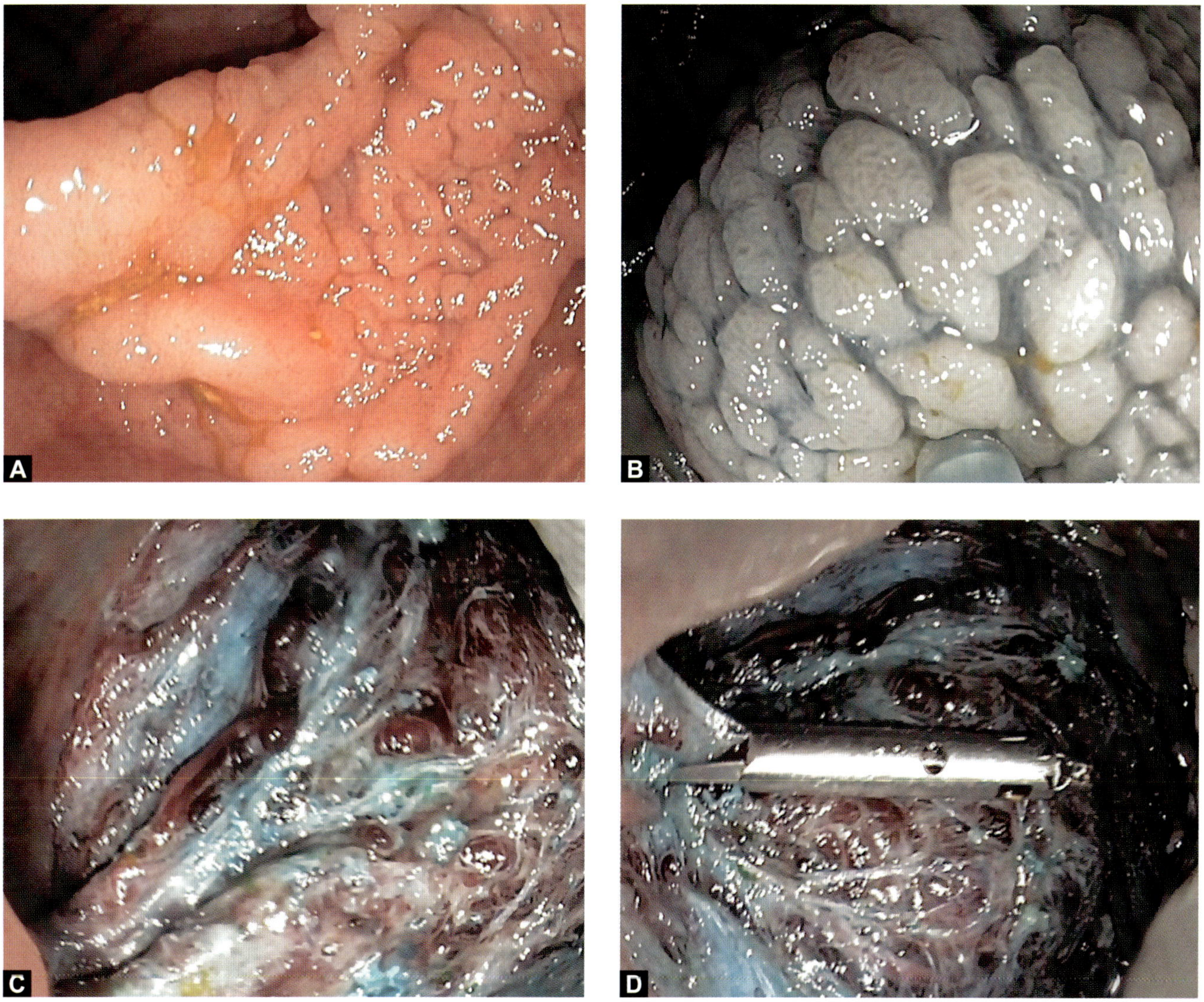

FIGURE 13-13 Laterally spreading granular tumor. **A,** Under WLE. **B,** Under NBI. **C,D,** Segments of the vessels may herniate out above the loose areolar connective tissue transversely oriented blood vessels within a large mucosal defect after endoscopic resection.

between medical and surgical teams is necessary to achieve the best possible clinical outcome.

Bleeding

Clinically significant delayed bleeding remains the most common complication. Risk factors for bleeding after conventional polypectomy have been well studied in small polyps less than 10-15 mm.[45,46] In general, there remains a lack of consensus and standardization on how postpolypectomy bleeding should be defined and treated, and this is particularly so for post-EMR bleeding. Clinically insignificant bleeding detected as blood in the stool but without other symptoms is not uncommonly described after ER, particularly in the distal colon, and this should not be seen as a complication. Anticoagulant use is clearly a risk factor for postconventional polypectomy bleeding, and this holds true for colonic ER; however, aspirin and nonsteroidals are not believed to increase conventional postpolypectomy bleeding, and their cessation is not advised, particularly amongst those who are taking aspirin as secondary prophylaxis.[47] We have recently shown that aspirin increases the risk of postcolonic EMR bleeding to an odds ratio of approximately 6, and we routinely cease it for 7 days prior to colonic EMR.[48] In this analysis of comprehensive prospective data in 290

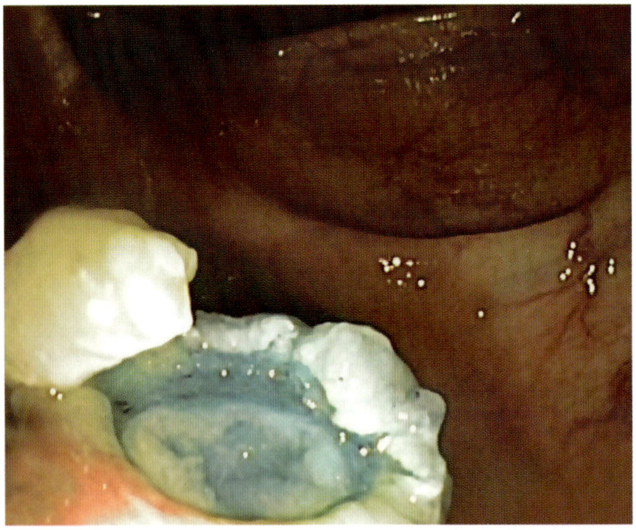

FIGURE 13-14 A target sign visible on the under surface of the resected tissue.

patients with LSTs ≥20 mm treated by EMR, proximal location in the colon, specifically cecum and proximal ascending, increased the risk of clinically significant post-ER bleeding (odds ratio 4.5; p = 0.01) in comparison to the remainder of the colon.[48] Bleeding rates were 12.3, 10.7, and 10% for cecum, ascending colon, and ileocecal valve, respectively. The bleeding risk for the hepatic flexure was intermediate at 7%. The entire distal colon exhibited a low bleeding rate at around 2–3%. Ninety percent bleeding occur in the first 48 hours and two-thirds of this within 24 hours. This finding may reflect a relative difference in the anatomical structure or physiology of the proximal colon or a difference in the number, caliber, and relative fragility of the submucosal vessels (Figure 13-17).[48]

The bleeding is generally venous in nature and will often settle spontaneously with conservative management alone. Patients who have continued hemodynamic instability following initial resuscitation require repeat colonoscopy with endoscopic hemostasis. This is best accomplished by mechanical means with clip hemostasis. At this stage in the treatment cycle, application of thermal modalities within a post-EMR defect will potentially lead to transmural injury or perforation.

ENDOSCOPIC SUBMUCOSAL DISSECTION

An insulated tip electrosurgical knife was developed in Japan to completely remove large superficial gastric lesions en bloc by the technique of ESD. ESD has produced excellent results in the stomach, rapidly becoming the standard of care for these lesions.[49,50] A variety of other knives are also now in use. Recently, there has been a substantial interest in applying ESD to large LSTs and sessile lesions in the colorectum.[23,25] The application of ESD to these lesions enables en bloc excision, which brings with it a number of potential advantages, including complete and accurate histological assessment, negligible recurrence, and potentially

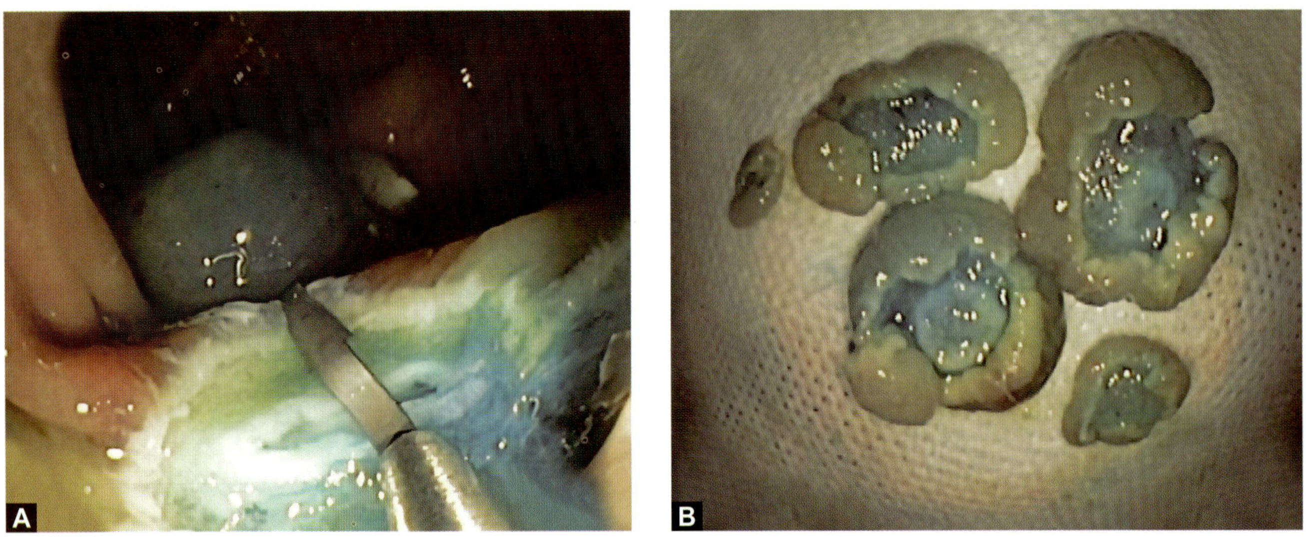

FIGURE 13-15 Complication of endoscopic resection. **A,** Mirror target sign is seen within the mucosal defect. There is an outer white rim where the mucosa has been intentionally resected corresponding to the effect of the diathermy. **B,** Excised white oval disk of muscularis propria.

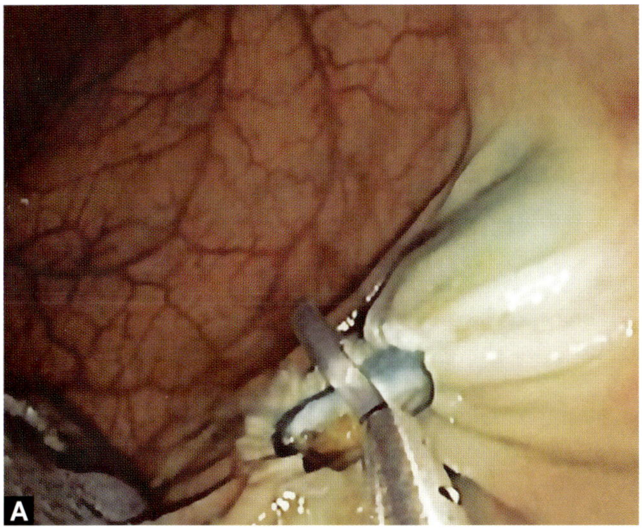

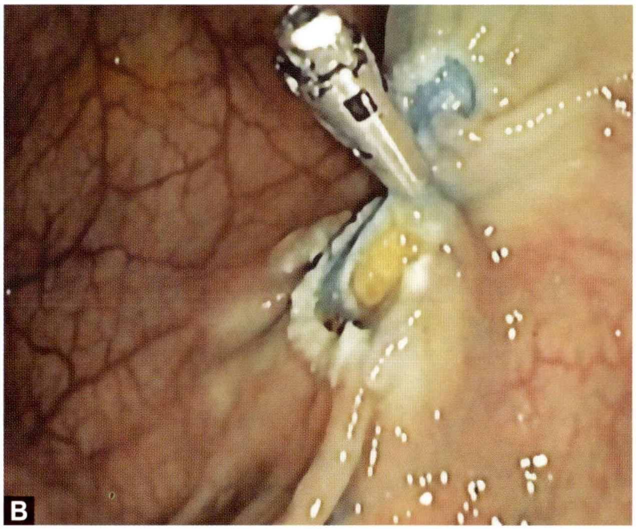

FIGURE 13-16 Complication of endoscopic resection. **A,** Postendoscopic resection full thickness defect with exposed pericolonic fat evident in the base. **B,** Closure of the defect using clips.

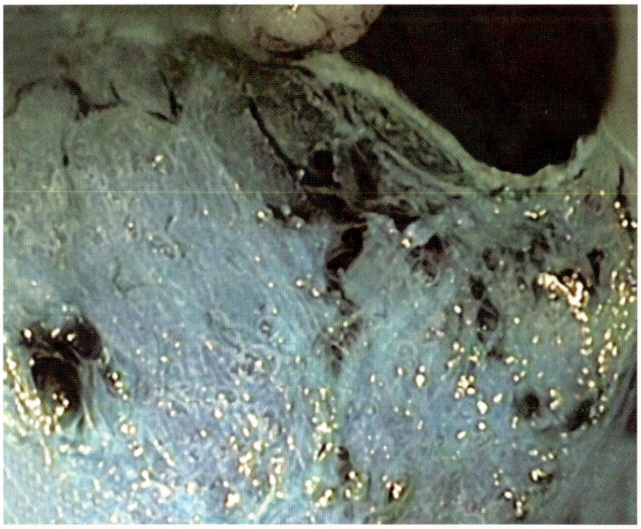

FIGURE 13-17 Nonbleeding visible vessels within a large mucosal defect.

curative endoscopic treatment for superficial submucosal invasive cancers with favorable histology (moderate or well differentiated with no lymphovascular invasion), particularly in poor operative risk candidates. Results are promising with two large series, each of 200 patients describing en bloc excision rates of 80–90% for lesions of mean size of 30–38 mm.[27,28] However, operative time was in the order of 90 minutes and perforation occurred in 5–6% of cases and has been reported in up to 10% of cases.[23] Mean hospital length of stay was 5 days.

In contrast, colonic EMR is mostly an outpatient procedure, relatively fast and efficient, being completed in less than 30–40 minutes (mean 20 minutes) and has an incidence of perforation of less than 1%.[34,41] It is a snare-based technique with which all colonoscopists are comfortable, additional training requirements are limited, and there are no additional devices or solutions. Although recurrence in expert centers occurs with a frequency of up to 20% (in the absence of en bloc excision), this is usually small and easily treated.[35,41,51]

Barriers to Colonic Endoscopic Submucosal Dissection in the West

Whilst conceptually appealing to Western endoscopists, there are a number of technical and theoretical obstacles to the widespread use of colonic ESD in the West. Currently, colonic ESD technology is immature, limited to experts even in Japan, and not standardized. The procedure is technically difficult with a steep learning curve.[23] Western endoscopists have limited exposure to upper GI ESD as early gastric or esophageal lesions are uncommon outside Japan and Korea.[52] This scarcity of suitable lesions in low-risk locations means that an incremental technique acquisition pathway does not exist for Western endoscopists. Those who wish to perform colonic ESD can either commence directly in this high-risk location or undergo extensive training in animal models. Data on the learning curve for ESD are lacking; however, it has been shown that for an experienced endoscopist, approximately

40 cases of gastric circumferential submucosal injection (CSI) EMR are necessary to establish satisfactory safety and efficacy in this comparatively low risk location.[53] As currently practiced, colonic ESD, requiring a mean of 5 days inpatient admission, is time consuming, and has an incidence of perforation of approximately 5%.[24,25] The necessity for inpatient postprocedural care diminishes the superiority of ESD over laparoscopic colectomy, which, it could be argued, has a similar postoperative care plan but includes full thickness and regional lymph node excision.[54]

In a Western population, most advanced mucosal neoplasms referred for endoscopic resection are G 0-IIa LSTs, or 0-Is lesions, or a combination of these and SMI is uncommon. Residual/recurrent adenoma at 4 months surveillance occurs with a frequency of 10–20% and is usually unifocal and diminutive and easily excised and/or ablated. Thus, comparative outcomes for ESD/en bloc excision against 12 and 24 months colonic ER results are unlikely to be different. NG lesions are uncommon but clearly represent a case for en bloc excision.[14] However, if SMI is found in a sessile lesion (in contrast to pedunculated lesions), then in the West, this generally mandates surgical treatment if the patient is medically fit. Thus, en bloc excision in this group may not confer significant clinical gain. In Japan, data are being accumulated on the role of nonoperative management in low risk submucosal disease, and this appears to be a viable therapeutic strategy.[21,23] Another important consideration is the varying operative risks in the lower and upper digestive tract. In the case of superficial low-risk submucosal invasive malignancy in the esophagus or stomach, an argument can be made for endoscopic treatment alone, as esophagectomy or gastrectomy carries significant risks of long-term morbidity and perioperative mortality in excess of the risk of regional lymph node metastasis.[8,55] Thus, the small risk if the patient has not been cured endoscopically may be exceeded by the risk of perioperative death. In contrast, with colonic surgery, permanent morbidity is unlikely, and the risk of perioperative mortality is acceptable in the majority of patients in a setting of SMI.

Hybrid Endoscopic Mucosal Resection-Endoscopic Submucosal Dissection Techniques and Other Innovations

Modification of conventional EMR/ER technique is an option for enhancing en bloc outcomes. CSI-EMR is a hybrid of EMR and ESD technique that releases the lateral margins of the lesion, thereby, enhancing vertical elevation after submucosal injection and enabling a greater area of mucosa to fall within the snare for ER.[56] CSI also provides a "trench" or "groove" in which the snare can anchor and accurately demarcates the edges of the lesion, which can be difficult to perceive during conventional snare-based ER. CSI-EMR is technically more attainable for Western endoscopists, as it avoids the need for dissection beneath the lesion, which is the most challenging, hazardous, and time consuming component of ESD. In a randomized *in vivo* porcine trial, CSI-EMR was superior to conventional EMR for en bloc resection of 40 mm diameter artificial flat lesions. The en bloc rate was 70% with CSI-EMR and nil with conventional EMR ($p = 0.016$). The depth of submucosal resection obtained with CSI-EMR (mean 1,107 μm) was deeper than with EMR.

Limited human data have been accumulated. Twenty-nine heterogeneous lesions sized ≥3 cm with en bloc resection at 55% has been published.[57] Experience with gastric CSI-EMR is more extensive.[58,59] For lesions sized ≤20 mm, en bloc resection rates are approximately 90%, but ESD is superior for larger lesions. There are no randomized trials comparing CSI-EMR and ESD. Such studies for intermediate sized lesions of 20–30 mm would be of clinical relevance. These should also take account of procedural time, complication rate, and duration of hospital stay. In the colon "saddle" lesions and those overlying sharp angulations will not be suitable for CSI-EMR.

Modifications to traditional ESD devices or the submucosal injection solution may make ESD more accessible to Western endoscopists. The Hybrid-Knife (HK) is a novel device that combines endoscopic dissection with the ability to inject fluid submucosally.[60] This device may enhance procedural efficiency and safety, as device exchange is not necessary. The HK with dual function allows easy switching between injection and dissection, which facilitates erring on the side of extra-submucosal injection. Ready access to repeated injection keeps the cutting plane maximally expanded throughout the ESD, making dissection easier and safer.[61] This is especially important for ESD novices, who are likely to be less capable of readily identifying the respective tissue planes at the dissection interface and less precise with their cuts. The ease with which the endoscopist can reinject and expand the cutting zone enhances safety. Prospective data are still limited, but promising results in the upper GI have been reported by Western endoscopists.[62,63] Yahagi et al. compared HK ESD with conventional ESD for 30 mm

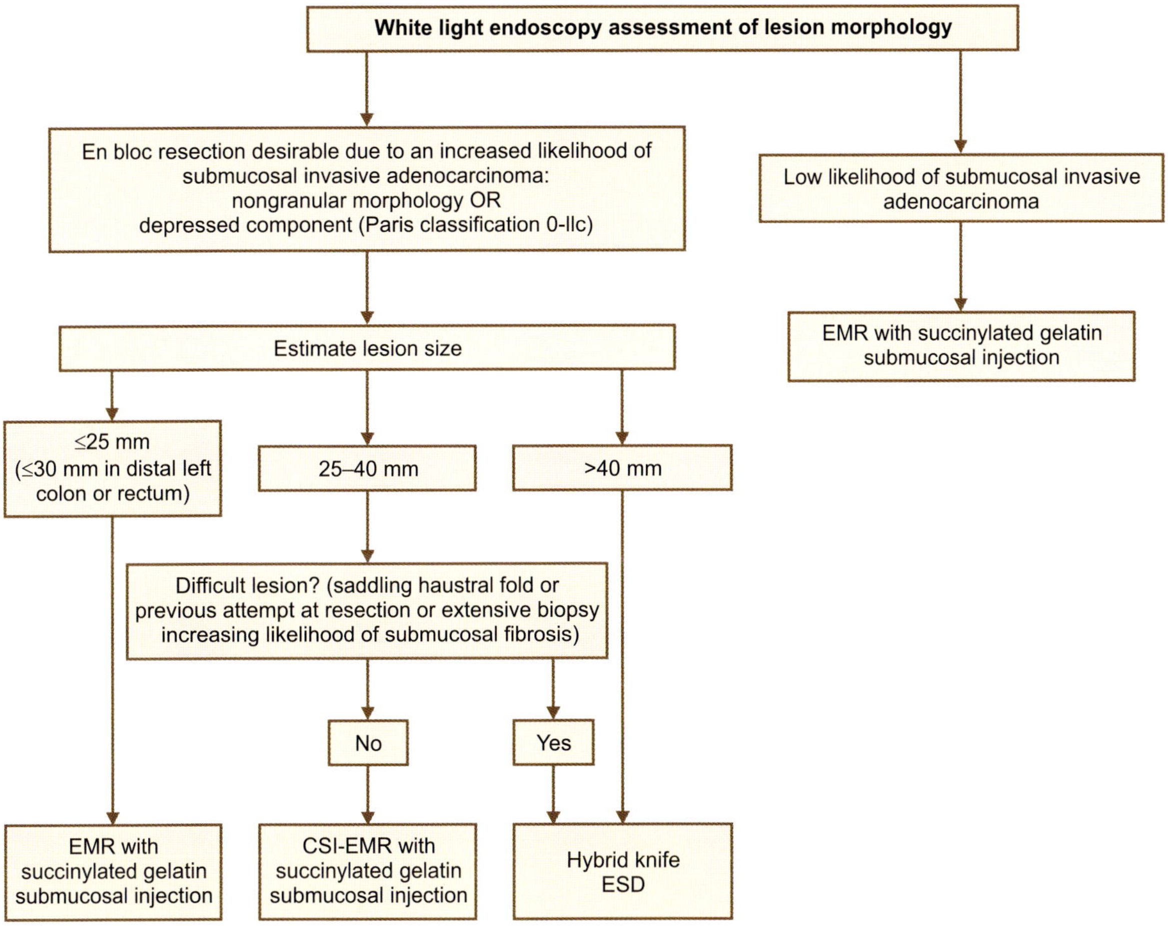

FIGURE 13-18 An algorithm for lesion-specific endoscopic treatment.

artificial lesions in a porcine colon using normal saline for submucosal injection.[64] All procedures were performed by a single Japanese expert with more than 1,000 human ESD case experience, and the HK was associated with a significantly lower perforation rate in this high-risk animal model (12.5%) than with standard equipment ESD (25%). Human studies of colonic ESD with the HK device performed by multiple operators are required for confirmation.

CONCLUSION

There still remains significant philosophical differences in the endoscopic approach to LSTs and large sessile colonic lesions between the West and East. Evidence-based lesion-specific endoscopic treatment algorithms are required. A potential approach is summarized in figure 13-18. Postprocedural care, procedure duration, and endoscopic complications are major considerations in the West, which influence the approach. Further prospective studies will hopefully clarify the optimal treatment strategy in both environments. Amongst typical referral cases seen at tertiary centers in the West, NG lesions are uncommon, and thus absolute indications for en bloc resection, for example, by ESD are infrequent.[5,35,41] Japanese experts now also increasingly accept that en bloc resection is not necessary for most LSTs.[65]

The last decade has seen major advances in ER through the entire GI tract and particularly the colon. Even more aggressive endoscopic interventions are now possible with minimal disruption to the underlying anatomy or physiology of the patient, shortened recovery, and limited interference with usual activities. The future of ER for the management of early colorectal neoplasm looks promising.

REFERENCES

1. Winawer SJ, Zauber AG, Ho MN, O'Brien MJ, Gottlieb LS, Sternberg SS, et al. Prevention of colorectal cancer by colonoscopic polypectomy. The National Polyp Study Workgroup. *N Engl J Med.* 1993;329:1977-81.
2. Dove-Edwin I, Sasieni P, Adams J, Thomas HJ. Prevention of colorectal cancer by colonoscopic surveillance in individuals with a family history of colorectal cancer: 16 year, prospective, follow-up study. *BMJ.* 2005;331:1047.
3. Zauber A, Winawer SJ, Lansdorp-Vogelaar I, van Ballegooijen M, O'Brien MJ. Effect of initial polypectomy versus surveillance polypectomy on colorectal cancer mortality reduction: microsimulation modeling of the national polyp study. *Am J Gastroenterol.* 2007;102:S558.
4. Waye JE. Polypectomy: basic principles. In: Waye JD, Rex D, Williams CB, editors. Colonoscopy: principles and practice. Oxford, UK: Blackwell Publishing; 2003. p. 410-9.
5. Swan MP, Bourke MJ, Alexander S, Moss A, Williams SJ. Large refractory colonic polyps: is it time to change our practice? A prospective study of the clinical and economic impact of a tertiary referral colonoscopic polypectomy service. *Gastrointest Endosc.* 2009;70:1128-36.
6. Voloyiannis T, Snyder MJ, Bailey, Pidala M. Management of the difficult colon polyp referred for resection: resect or rescope? *Dis Colon Rectum.* 2008;51:292-5.
7. Onken JE, Friedman JY, Subramanian S, Weinfurt KP, Reed SD, Malenbaum JH, et al. Treatment patterns and costs associated with sessile colorectal polyps. *Am J Gastroenterol.* 2002;97:2896-901.
8. Birkmeyer JD, Siewers AE, Finlayson EV, Stukel TA, Lucas FL, Batista I, et al. Hospital volume and surgical mortality in the United States. *N Engl J Med.* 2002;346:1128-37.
9. Birkmeyer JD, Stukel TA, Siewers AE, Goodney PP, Wennberg DE, Lucas FL. Surgeon volume and operative mortality in the United States. *N Engl J Med.* 2003;349: 2117-27.
10. McNicol L, Story DA, Leslie K, Myles PS, Fink M, Shelton AC, et al. Postoperative complications and mortality in older patients having non-cardiac surgery at three Melbourne teaching hospitals. *Med J Aust.* 2007;186:447-52.
11. The Paris endoscopic classification of superficial neoplastic lesions: esophagus, stomach, and colon: November 30 to December 1, 2002. *Gastrointest Endosc.* 2003;58:S3-43.
12. Endoscopic Classification Review Group. Update on the Paris classification of superficial neoplastic lesions in the digestive tract. *Endoscopy.* 2005;37:570-8.
13. Bourke MJ. Current status of colonic endoscopic mucosal resection in the West and the interface with endoscopic submucosal dissection. *Dig Endosc.* 2009;21:S22-7.
14. Uraoka T, Saito Y, Matsuda T, Ikehara H, Gotoda T, Saito D, et al. Endoscopic indications for endoscopic mucosal resection of laterally spreading tumours in the colorectum. *Gut.* 2006;55:1592-7.
15. Moss A, Bourke MJ, Williams SJ, Hourigan LF, Brown GJ, Singh R, et al. Lesion morphology, Paris classification and pit pattern but not size predict and stratify risk of submucosal invasive adenocarcinoma within laterally spreading tumours (LSTs) and large sessile colonic polyps in a multicenter setting: Results of the Australian Colonic Endoscopic mucosal resection (ACE) study. *Gastrointest Endosc.* 2010;71:AB185-6.
16. Baxter NN, Goldwasser MA, Paszat LF, Saskin R, Urbach DR, Rabeneck L. Association of colonoscopy and death from colorectal cancer. *Ann Intern Med.* 2009;150:1-8.
17. Brenner H, Hoffmeister M, Arndt V, Arndt V, Stegmaier C, Altenhofen L, et al. Protection from right- and left-sided colorectal neoplasms after colonoscopy: population-based study. *J Natl Cancer Inst.* 2010;102:89-95.
18. Rex DK. Narrow-band imaging without optical magnification for histologic analysis of colorectal polyps. *Gastroenterology.* 2009;136:1174-81.
19. Uraoka T, Sano Y, Saito Y, Saito H, Matsuda T, Yamamoto K. Narrow-band imaging for improving colorectal adenoma detection: appropriate system function settings are required. *Gut.* 2009;58:604-5.
20. Kanao H, Tanaka S, Oka S, Hirata M, Yoshida S, Chayama K. Narrow-band imaging magnification predicts the histology and invasion depth of colorectal tumors. *Gastrointest Endosc.* 2009;69:631-6.
21. Matsuda T, Fujii T, Saito Y, Nakajima T, Uraoka T, Kobayashi N, et al. Efficacy of the invasive/non-invasive pattern by magnifying chromoendoscopy to estimate the depth of invasion of early colorectal neoplasms. *Am J Gastroenterol.* 2008;103:2700-6.
22. Deyhle P, Largiader F, Jenny S, Fumagali I. A method for endoscopic electroresection of sessile colonic polyps. *Endoscopy.* 1973;5:38-40.
23. Tanaka S, Oka S, Kaneko I, Hirata M, Mouri R, Kanao H, et al. Endoscopic submucosal dissection for colorectal neoplasia: possibility of standardization. *Gastrointest Endosc.* 2007;66:100-7.
24. Fujishiro M, Yahagi N, Kakushima N, Kodashima S, Muraki Y, Ono S. Outcomes of endoscopic submucosal dissection for colorectal epithelial neoplasms in 200 consecutive cases. *Clin Gastroenterol Hepatol.* 2007;5:678-83.
25. Saito Y, Uraoka T, Matsuda T, Emura F, Ikehara H, Mashimo Y, et al. Endoscopic treatment of large superficial colorectal tumors: a case series of 200 endoscopic submucosal dissections (with video). *Gastrointest Endosc.* 2007;66:966-73.
26. Moss A, Bourke MJ, Metz A. A randomized, double-blind trial of succinylated gelatin submucosal injection for endoscopic resection of large sessile polyps of the colon. *Am J Gastroenterol.* 2010;105:2375-82.
27. ASGE Technology Committee, Kantsevoy SV, Adler DG, Conway JD, Diehl DL, Farraye FA, et al. Technology status evaluation report: endoscopic mucosal resection and endoscopic submucosal dissection. *Gastrointest Endosc.* 2008;68:11-8.
28. Bourke MJ. Mucosal resection in the upper GI tract. *Gastrointest Endosc.* 2010;12:18-25.

29. Moss A, Bourke MJ, Kwan V, Tran K, Godfrey C, McKay G, et al. Succinylated gelatin substantially increases en bloc resection size in colonic EMR: a randomised blinded trial in a porcine model. *Gastrointest Endosc.* 2010;71:589-95.
30. Alexander S, Bourke MJ, Williams SJ, Bailey A, Co J. EMR of large sporadic nonampullary duodenal adenomas: technical aspects and long term outcome. *Gastrointest Endosc.* 2009;69:66-73.
31. Coman E, Brandt LJ, Brenner S, Frank M, Sablay B, Bennett B. Fat necrosis and inflammatory pseudotumor due to endoscopic tattooing of the colon with India ink. *Gastrointest Endosc.* 1991;37:65-8.
32. Sawaki A, Nakamura T, Suzuki T, Hara K, Kato T, Kato T. A two-step method for marking polypectomy sites in the colon and rectum. *Gastrointest Endosc.* 2003;57:735-7.
33. Doniec JM, Lohnert MS, Schniewind B, Bokelmann F, Kremer B, Grimm H. Endoscopic removal of large colorectal polyps: prevention of unnecessary surgery? *Dis Colon Rectum.* 2003;46:340-8.
34. Conio M, Repici A, Demarquay JF, Blanchi S, Dumas R, Filiberti R. EMR of large sessile colorectal polyps. *Gastrointest Endosc.* 2004;60:234-41.
35. Arebi N, Swain D, Suzuki N, Fraser C, Price A, Saunders BP. Endoscopic mucosal resection of 161 cases of large sessile or flat colorectal polyps. *Scand J Gastroenterol.* 2007;42:859-66.
36. Bergmann U, Beger HG. Endoscopic mucosal resection for advanced non-polypoid colorectal adenoma and early stage carcinoma. *Surg Endosc.* 2003:17:475-9.
37. Giday SA, Magno P, Buscaglia JM, Canto MI, Ko CW, Shin EJ, et al. Is blood the ideal submucosal cushioning agent? A comparative study in a porcine model. *Endoscopy.* 2006; 38:1230-4.
38. Rex DK. Have we defined best colonoscopic polypectomy practice in the United States? *Clin Gastroenterol Hepatol.* 2007;5:674-7.
39. Bourke MJ. Making every colonoscopy count: ensuring quality in endoscopy. *J Gastroenterol Hepatol.* 2009;24: S43-50.
40. Puli SR, Kakugawa Y, Gotoda T, Antillon D, Saito Y, Antillon MR. Meta-analysis and systematic review of colorectal endoscopic mucosal resection. *World J Gastroenterol.* 2009;15:4273-7.
41. Moss A, Bourke MJ, Williams SJ, Hourigan LF, Brown GJ, Singh R, et al. Predictors of therapeutic success for endoscopic mucosal resection (EMR) of laterally spreading tumours (LSTs) and large sessile colonic polyps: Results of the prospective multicenter Australian Colonic EMR (ACE) study. *Gastrointest Endosc.* 2010;71:AB111.
42. Swan MP, Bourke MJ, Moss A, Williams SJ, Hopper AD, Metz A. The target sign: an endoscopic marker for the resection of the muscularis propria during colonic endoscopic mucosal resection. *Gastrointest Endosc.* 2011; 73:79-85.
43. Hainaux B, Agneessens E, Bertinotti R, De Maertelaer V, Rubesova E, Capelluto E, et al. Accuracy of MDCT in predicting site of gastrointestinal tract perforation. *AJR Am J Roentgenol.* 2006;187:1179-83.
44. Kim SH, Shin SS, Jeong YY, Heo SH, Kim JW, Kang HK. Gastrointestinal tract perforation: MDCT findings according to the perforation sites. *Korean J Radiol.* 2009;10:63-70.
45. Kim HS, Kim TI, Kim WH, Kim YH, Kim HJ, Yang SK. Risk factors for immediate postpolypectomy bleeding of the colon: a multicenter study. *Am J Gastroenterol.* 2006; 101:1333-41.
46. Hui AJ, Wong RM, Ching JY, Hung LC, Chung SC, Sung JJ. Risk of colonoscopic polypectomy bleeding with anticoagulants and antiplatelet agents: analysis of 1657 cases. *Gastrointest Endosc.* 2004;59:44-8.
47. Eisen G, Baron TH, Dominitz JA, Faigel DO, Goldstein JL, Johanson JF, et al. Guideline on the management of anticoagulation and antiplatelet therapy for endoscopic procedures. *Gastrointest Endosc.* 2002;55:775-9.
48. Metz A, Bourke MJ, Moss A, Williams SJ, Swan MP, Byth K. Factors that predict bleeding following endoscopic mucosal resection of large colonic lesions. *Endoscopy.* 2011;43:506-11.
49. Ohkuwa M, Hosokawa N, Boku N, Ohtu A, Tajiri H, Yoshida S. New endoscopic treatment for intramucosal gastric tumors using an insulated-tip diathermic knife. *Endoscopy.* 2001;33:221-6.
50. Ono H, Kondo H, Gotoda T, Shirao K, Yamaguchi H, Saito D, et al. Endoscopic mucosal resection for treatment of early gastric cancer. *Gut.* 2001;48:225-9.
51. Kaltenbach T, Friedland S, Maheshwari A, Ouyang D, Rouse RV, Wren S, et al. Short- and long-term outcomes of standardized EMR of nonpolypoid (flat and depressed) colorectal lesions > or = 1 cm (with video). *Gastrointest Endosc.* 2007;65:857-65.
52. Kojma T, Parra-Blanco A, Takahashi H, Fujita R. Outcome of endoscopic mucosal resection for early gastric cancer: review of Japanese literature. *Gastrointest Endosc.* 1998;48: 550-4; discussion 554-5.
53. Choi IJ, Kim CG, Chang HJ, Kim SG, Kook MC, Bae JM. The learning curve for EMR with circumferential mucosal incision in treating intramucosal gastric neoplasm. *Gastrointest Endosc.* 2005;62:860-5.
54. Clinical Outcomes of Surgical Therapy Study Group. A comparison of laparoscopically assisted and open colectomy for colorectal cancer. *N Engl J Med.* 2004;350: 2050-9.
55. Birkmeyer JD, Sun Y,Wong SL, Stukel TA. Hospital volume and late survival after cancer surgery. *Ann Surg.* 2007;245: 277-83.
56. Moss A, Bourke MJ, Tran KL, Godfrey C, McKay G, Chandra AP, et al. Lesion isolation by circumferential submucosal incision prior to endoscopic mucosal resection (CSI-EMR) substantially improves en bloc resection rates for 40-mm colonic lesions. *Endoscopy.* 2010;42: 400-4.
57. Repici A, Conio M, De Angelis C, Sapino A, Malesci A, Arezzo A, et al. Insulated-tip knife endoscopic mucosal

resection of large colorectal polyps unsuitable for standard polypectomy. *Am J Gastroenterol.* 2007;102: 1617-23.

58. Miyamoto S, Muto M, Hamamoto Y, Boku N, Ohtsu A, Baba S, et al. A new technique for endoscopic mucosal resection with an insulated-tip electrosurgical knife improves the completeness of resection of intramucosal gastric neoplasms. *Gastrointest Endosc.* 2002;55:576-81.
59. Yamamoto H, Kawata H, Sunada K, Satoh K, Kaneko Y, Ido K, et al. Success rate of curative endoscopic mucosal resection with circumferential mucosal incision assisted by submucosal injection of sodium hyaluronate. *Gastrointest Endosc.* 2002;56:507-12.
60. Lingenfelder T, Fischer K, Sold MG, Post S, Enderle MD, Kaehler GF. Combination of water-jet dissection and needle-knife as a hybrid knife simplifies endoscopic submucosal dissection. *Surg Endosc.* 2009;23:1531-5.
61. Neuhaus H, Wirths K, Schenk M, Enderle MD, Schumacher B. Randomized controlled study of EMR versus endoscopic submucosal dissection with a water-jet hybrid-knife of esophageal lesions in a porcine model. *Gastrointest Endosc.* 2009;70:112-20.
62. Neuhaus H, Mayershofer R, Charton JP, Seelhoff A, Vieth M, Schumacher B. Endoscopic submucosal resection (ESD) of early Barrett's neoplasia (EBN) with a water-jet hybrid knife (ESDH): first prospective clinical trial. *Gastrointest Endosc.* 2010;71:AB125.
63. Schumacher B, Mayershofer R, Charton JP, Seelhoff A, Vieth M, Neuhaus H. Endoscopic submucosal resection of early gastric neoplasia with a water-jet hybrid knife (ESDH): a prospective Western study in 31 patients. *Gastrointest Endosc.* 2010;71:AB124.
64. Yahagi N, Neuhaus H, Schumacher B, Neugebauer A, Kaehler GF, Schenk M, et al. Comparison of standard endoscopic submucosal dissection (ESD) versus an optimized ESD technique for the colon: an animal study. *Endoscopy.* 2009;41:340-5.
65. Fujiya M, Moriichi K, Saitoh Y, Watari J, Kohgo Y. Endoscopic piecemeal resection is a practical option to cure colorectal tumors. *Dig Endosc.* 2009;21:S28-30.

Index

Page numbers with *t* and *f* indicate table and figure, respectively.

D

E